Date Due

Lessons from the First Twenty Years of Medicare

Research Implications for Public and Private Sector Policy

Lessons from the First Twenty Years of Medicare □ ᵃ □

Research Implications for Public and Private Sector Policy

Mark V. Pauly · William L. Kissick
EDITORS

L A U R A E. R O P E R, *Associate Editor*

upp

UNIVERSITY OF PENNSYLVANIA PRESS
Philadelphia

Series in Health Economics, Health Management, and Health Policy

Mark V. Pauly, Editor

Based on the proceedings of a conference October 8–10, 1986, sponsored by the Leonard Davis Institute of Health Economics, University of Pennsylvania.

Support for this conference was provided by the CIGNA Foundation, Smith Kline & French, Inc., and the Metropolitan Life Foundation.

Publication of this project was supported by grant number HS05680 from the National Center for Health Services Research and Health Care Technology Assessment

Library of Congress Cataloging-in-Publication Data

Lessons from the first twenty years of medicare : research implications for public and private sector
    policy/Mark V. Pauly, William L. Kissick, editors; Laura E. Roper, associate editor.
        p.   cm.—(Series in health economics, health management, and health policy)
    Includes bibliographies and index.
    ISBN 0-8122-8118-7
    1. Medicare—History—Congresses.   I. Pauly, Mark V., 1941–
II. Kissick, William L.   III. Roper, Laura E.   IV. Series.
HD7102.U4L47 1988
368.4'26'00973—dc19   88-17368
                                                                                         CIP

Contents

III   Medicare Payment and Provider Behavior

IV   Medicare Benefits and Private Burdens

V   Medicare and Appropriate Medical Care

Preface

The Leonard Davis Institute of Health Economics of the University of Pennsylvania elected to convene a conference in 1986 on the subject, "Lessons from the First Twenty Years of Medicare: Research Implications for Public and Private Sector Policy," on the twentieth anniversary of the implementation of Medicare. The purpose of the conference was to assess what research has to tell us about the effects of Medicare policy over the last twenty years, to analyze the impact of changing economic and demographic conditions on Medicare policy, and to consider future policy directions and their potential impact. We were particularly interested in identifying areas of consensus and disagreement. In the latter case we were also interested in exploring whether disagreement resulted from matters of fact or from matters of value (e.g., the appropriate role of government).

On October 8, 1986, sixty health policy researchers gathered in Philadelphia for two-and-one-half days to consider Medicare policy. The size of the conference was limited in order to provide ample opportunity for full discussion of research strategies, findings, and their implications. Invited researchers came from the private sector, academe, and government, and represented many disciplines, including economics, sociology, gerontology, medicine, law, and political science.

The keynote address of the conference was given by the Honorable Wilbur Cohen, who discussed the social, political, and philosophical objectives of the Medicare legislation enacted in 1965. As Assistant Secretary for Legislation in the Department of Health, Education, and Welfare during the Kennedy and Johnson administrations, Cohen was responsible for drafting and articulating the administration's position during the development and passage of the Medicare bill. Subsequently, as Undersecretary and then Secretary of HEW, he guided the program's implementation. According to Cohen, Medicare was born more of social conviction than of research findings. From this beginning, the conference participants sought to identify what research could tell us about the legislation's shortcomings and accomplishments. Ultimately, our objective was to identify principles that could contribute to a future that incorporates lessons from the past.

The plenary and concurrent sessions focused on four broad themes:

I   Medicare: Issues, Accomplishments and Changing Needs
II   Effects of the New Payment System
III   Payors and Beneficiaries
IV   The Future of Medicare

In each session formal papers, both submitted and invited, were presented and followed by comments from recruited discussants. These contributions were followed by general participation of all those present. In addition to these sessions, Judy Miller Jones of the Health Policy Forum, Stanley J. Brody of the University of Pennsylvania, and Cecil Sheps of the University of North Carolina addressed the conference. (See the next section for a list of conference participants.)

This volume consists of the research papers presented at the four sessions, although in a different order from that in which they were presented. We begin with papers that offer a broad discussion of Medicare history and policy options, and then turn, in subsequent sections, to more specific research issues.

Introduction: Research on Twenty Years of Medicare— The Questions Posed

LAURA E. ROPER

MARK V. PAULY

WILLIAM L. KISSICK

Introduction

On July 30, 1965, at the Truman Library in Independence, Missouri, President Lyndon Baines Johnson signed the Social Security Amendments of 1965 (PL 89-97), which authorized payment of hospital and physician services for virtually all U.S. citizens aged sixty-five and over. For millions of Americans this represented a new dimension of Social Security and the rights of citizenship. For some, it was the culmination of a three-decade political struggle that had followed upon President Franklin Delano Roosevelt's signing of the Social Security Act in 1935 as a landmark initiative of the New Deal. As historically and politically significant as Medicare was, it was still a legislative compromise. Initial proposals had been much broader and included provision of national health insurance, a novel concept about which political consensus could not be achieved.

Nor was political support unanimous for the Medicare law of 1965. Organized medicine and organized labor had polarized the opposition, while the Golden Age lobbies, the American Hospital Association, and Blue Cross/Blue Shield provided the swing votes that insured the bill's passage. Even among supporters of the King–Anderson legislation, as it had been known in Congress, a major debate had raged regarding the potential costliness of the program. At the time, physicians controlled the use and, to a large extent, the pricing of health services. In their solo practices, the predominant form of medical practice at the time, physicians were compensated for their services on the basis of fees they themselves had established. They controlled hospital admissions and utilization as voluntary staff members. Hospitals, in turn, were for the most part compensated retrospectively by third-party insurers on a cost basis. In both instances, for physicians and hospitals alike, higher utilization resulted in increased revenues without any regulatory checks.

Many articulate champions of public-sector coverage for hospital and physician services for the elderly (then perceived as a vulnerable segment of the population) nevertheless cautioned vigorously about the risks of open-ended funding of a medical care enterprise that was undisciplined by either the marketplace or government regulation. At the time, our society had some thirty-five years of experience with traditional hospital and physician financing, which began with the birth of Blue Cross/Blue Shield in the 1930s. Beyond that, little was known about the behavior of medical services under a particular payment scheme. The exceptions were the prepaid group practice, as exemplified by the Kaiser Foundation Health Plan and a few others, and the more widely disseminated multispecialty group practice patterned after the Mayo Clinic. These were not, however, models that achieved wide support. Arguments for organization, restructuring, cost control, and quality assurance were unpersuasive, and the old political adage, "You can't fight something with nothing" carried the day. The result was passage of legislation that guaranteed funding for services controlled by individual physicians and hospitals.

On July 1, 1966, nineteen million Americans aged sixty-five years and older became eligible for physician and hospital services covered by Medicare. Less than one year later, in June 1967, Health, Education, and Welfare (HEW) Secretary John Gardner convened a national conference on the crisis in medical costs. Considering that the planning for this conference commenced in the fall of 1966, it took only a few months for the grave concerns of the proponents of organization, restructuring, and cost containment to see their prophecies acknowledged. This national acknowledgment and discussion of the cost crisis would be repeated with increasing momentum over the ensuing two decades.

During this time questions about the quality and efficacy of the Medicare program would also arise. Contrasts in the rates of utilization of services by the elderly before and after Medicare coverage provoked a number of questions concerning need and demand, appropriate utilization, cost effectiveness, equity, and outcomes, questions that are being debated up to the present day. While these are important issues, the impact of Medicare on health status, disability, and quality of life is difficult to measure; costs are less so and consequently have been the focus of debate. The cost of the program increased from $1 billion in 1966 to $70.5 billion in 1985, which represents an annual growth rate of 23.7 percent. The Consumer Price Index had an average annual growth rate of 5.3 percent during the same period, while the covered elderly population increased from 19.1 million in 1966 to 27.3 million in 1985, reflecting an annual growth rate of slightly under 1.9 percent.

Through the 1970s the government and private sector made only modest attempts to contain costs. The tentativeness of those attempts stemmed from a reluctance to limit the autonomy, authority, and prerogative of physicians, including their control of hospital utilization. By the late 1970s President Jimmy Carter viewed the problem to be serious enough to call for national hospital cost-containment legislation. Although the proposal, by Health and Human Services Secretary Joseph Califano, was defeated, it did draw important segments of the electorate into debate over national health care cost containment.

It was not until early in Ronald Reagan's administration that the U.S. Congress took the initiative and addressed hospital costs under Medicare, enacting the landmark Prospective Payment System (PPS), which established diagnosis-related groups (DRGs) under the Tax Equity and Fiscal Responsibility Act of 1982. This health policy ended what might be called Phase I of the Medicare financing reform, which had been tentative and partial, and launched Phase II.

The impact of this legislation on the health sector has been tremendous, yet one could argue that the impact of DRGs, which were originally designed for internal hospital management as mechanisms for fiscal allocation, will be found more in long-term development, demonstration, and innovation in the health sector and in the opening of an arena for research. In other words, long-term developments are likely to be far more important than the short-term financial dislocations and reallocations that PPS has generated. Albeit in ways perhaps unimagined, proponents of organization, restructuring, monitoring, and control of health care in the debates of 1965 are seeing endorsement of both their concerns and the options and strategies they proposed. Nonetheless, the imposition of DRGs not only has failed to contain costs to the degree proponents had hoped, but did not (nor was ever intended to) address other important issues, such as the predicament of the small number of Medicare beneficiaries who are left destitute by the costs of care for catastrophic illness not covered by Medicare. Much remains to be done in the continuing effort to improve health care service delivery and access to health care. As part of this effort, it is imperative to conduct research to understand policy outcomes and research that will help policy makers anticipate both the short- and long-term effects of new policy initiatives.

What Research Has to Tell Us

Medicare policy generates debate on a wide range of issues, both normative and behavioral. Discussions about Medicare can embrace topics as divergent as physician practice patterns, the behavior of insurance markets, and who should bear the burden of the elderly's medical costs. Research can help form and inform those discussions. While a great deal of research has been undertaken on Medicare issues, analysts only now are beginning to address a number of important research questions. This volume presents both broad policy papers that target research areas and specific research results that are relevant to various Medicare policy questions.

The book is divided into five parts. The first part, Medicare Policy: Past, Present, and Future, lays out the major policy options under consideration, their justifications, research findings, and the factors that led or might lead to their enactment. Judith Lave presents an overview of the development of the Medicare payment system, discusses the gaps in current coverage, and analyzes the implications of various reform proposals. Her own recommendations include simplification of the benefit package, mandatory assignment, and taxation of the elderly to fund Part B benefits. In effect, Medicare is to be expanded to include the types of benefits now provided to most but not all elderly by Medigap policies, with mandatory taxation of the elderly to replace voluntary premiums.

Randall Bovbjerg discusses the possibilities for converting Medicare into a voucher system redeemable for private insurance. While acknowledging problems of implementation, he is optimistic that such an arrangement could permit the elderly to choose plans that are both more efficient and more equitable than the current patchwork system.

Mark Pauly's contribution examines the likely political future of Medicare at a time in which the elderly will be more numerous, better educated, better off financially, longer lived, and more heterogeneous than was the case at the passage of Medicare. He concludes that support by the non-elderly for the current form of Medicare is likely to decline, at least after the turn of the century.

Ronald Vogel provides an analysis of the intergenerational transfer embodied in Medicare and shows that much of that transfer is currently being received by the relatively well-to-do elderly. He concludes that Medicare remains the only program for the elderly that "is not progressively financed, and whose expenditures on the acute care of the relatively well-to-do elderly could conceivably be used to . . . expand long-term care and other chronic care services for the poor and near-poor elderly."

The next part, Medicare as Insurance in Insurance Markets, discusses both the problems with current Medicare and private insurance coverage and possible reforms. Charles Phelps and Anne Reisinger show that Medicare fails to cover those expenses for which insurance coverage is most valuable—the costly but relatively rare serious illness. In part this gap arises from the limitation in coverage for long hospital stays, but a larger part comes from the copayments on physician services and excess physician fee payments. Private supplemental insurance reduces this risk, but also increases Medicare's cost burden.

Appropriate public policy will depend on an understanding of why people purchase front end supplemental coverage and sometimes eschew coverage of catastrophic costs. Richard Scheffler examines the behavior of individuals sixty-five years old and over who purchased nongroup coverage in sixty-three Blue Cross Medigap plans. His analysis, like that of Phelps and Reisinger, suggests that Medicare utilization increases with policies that provide first dollar coverage. He considers a number of policy scenarios that other analysts have proposed and their possible effects on utilization. He concludes that, because demand for supplemental insurance will grow, and because the form insurance policies take affects utilization, there is a basic need to coordinate public insurance with private supplemental coverage.

Bernard Friedman and Larry Manheim furnish convincing simulation evidence that, with the kind of administrative cost loadings that characterize private individual long-term care insurance, the market demand for such insurance is sure to remain small. They argue, however, that Medicare can best function in a kind of brokerage role, intended to make voluntary long-term care coverage available to nonpoor elderly at loading charges that reflect the cost advantages of group coverage.

Medicare Payment and Provider Behavior, the third part of this volume, presents research results regarding the impact on providers of changes from cost-based reimbursement to two new payment methods, prospective payment based on DRGs for hospital services and capitated payment for physicians. Gerald Kominski and his coauthors discuss one of the most critical aspects of the DRG system, the determination of the annual "update" factor that permits payments per admission to grow. They note that the Department of Health and Human Services has taken a more restrained view of the appropriate rate of growth in this factor than have others, especially the Prospective Payment Assessment Commission (ProPAC). Views about the form of technological change, about the appropriate sharing of productivity gains between Medicare and hospitals, and about the true change in case mix have been different, largely because of the absence of definitive research. Kominski and his colleagues also provide some important findings on the changes in length of stay that have followed PPS, arguing that the next research challenge is to discover how the out-of-hospital care being provided to these patients is being furnished and financed.

Custer and his coauthors look at some messages from theory and from preliminary empirical work on the impact of DRGs on physician-hospital relationships. They develop a theory in which a hospital administration, independent of direct physician control, must nevertheless account for the fact that hospital decisions affect the inputs physicians have available to use when they provide care to inpatients, and the inputs (primarily time) that physicians themselves furnish. They note that, in many ways, the best reaction of a medical staff is to cooperate (or collude), in order to deal with both the profits and the potential cost pressures that the DRG system furnishes. They also note the probable decline in some services of benefit to patients when the DRG system constrains hospital resources, though whether the lost benefit is more than offset by cost savings is not yet known.

The two final chapters in this section consider the efficacy of a payment mechanism just emerging from the demonstration-testing phase, capitation payment to providers. The most general form of capitation for Medicare patients would be to pay a health maintenance organization (HMO) for their coverage, a policy now available to many Medicare beneficiaries. Judith Kasper, Gerald Riley, and Jeffrey McCombs examine the past history and future prospects for Medicare HMOs. They conclude that, despite theoretical concerns about the impact of capitation on quality and access, Medicare use of capitation is certain to grow. They advocate the need for more research to identify which characteristics of HMOs perform best, and caution against complete reliance on capitation as a solution to all of the problems that arise in organizing care for Medicare beneficiaries.

Kathryn Langwell and her colleagues at Mathematica review the evidence and prospects for physician capitation. They note the beneficial incentives for cost control that would flow from physician capitation, incentives that could control the cost of services physicians order without the need to include the cost of those services under full capitation. They note, however, that the same dangers of underprovision and skimping of services exist under this arrangement as any other capitated arrangements. They call for the development of a delivery system in which receiving physician services from a capitated physician is one of the options available to Medicare beneficiaries.

The fourth part, Medicare Benefits and Private Burdens, presents two chapters that discuss the financial burdens borne by two nongovernmental payers for the elderly—beneficiaries and employers. There is concern regarding who might pick up any increased burden if the government is to reduce its own costs for financing health care. Private employers currently provide important levels of support through the provision of health coverage for employees after retirement, and there is interest in whether these levels should be increased or reduced. In their chapter, Pamela Farley Short and Alan Monheit examine current coverage practices of employers and observe that under existing conditions they will be financing an increasing percentage of the elderly's health care costs. They conclude that it is unlikely employers will accept even greater responsibility because liability is potentially high, given slow growth in the economy, increased longevity in a progressively larger retired community, and continued rapidly increasing costs in the health sector.

Marilyn Moon examines the direct and indirect changes in costs for beneficiaries since the imposition of PPS. She argues that, while the system has reduced costs for the government, there has been significant cost shifting to beneficiaries, especially when indirect costs are considered. In analyzing the efficacy of current policies, two questions must be directly addressed. First, has PPS led to overall savings, or just to savings for the government by shifting costs to other payers? Second, are the burdens on the elderly acceptable or are they too high?

The last part, Medicare and Appropriate Medical Care, addresses the question of what the government can and should do to promote better medical care for the elderly. The authors of the three concluding chapters suggest that their recommendations will increase the quality of care and might reduce costs. Fowles and her coauthors monitor mortality, complications, and charges for Medicare beneficiaries undergoing hip replacement surgery in north California. They found inverse relationships between surgical volume and mortality and between surgical volume and charges. On the basis of this and other studies they make an argument for the usefulness of Medicare claims data for evaluating hospitals' surgical performance and pricing. They observe that this trend is already under way, but caution that claims data must be used with care because of its limitations.

Sheldon Rovin and Zoe Boniface consider the issue of preventive care in the context of the Medicare population. They discuss the concept of prevention and review research evaluating the efficacy of investing in preventive care. While research has been limited and results have been inconclusive, especially regarding prevention for the elderly, they advocate that Medicare at least provide preventive services on a pilot basis as a low-cost way of improving the elderly's welfare. Moreover, they argue that the government is uniquely situated to take a leading role in evaluating the efficacy of prevention and should expand current efforts in that direction.

Robert Kane suggests that Medicare should be extended to cover post-acute care, noting the problems that arise in the current Medicare system, which covers acute care fairly generously but which provides much less coverage for post-acute care, including, but by no means limited to, nursing home care. He considers three options: PPS for post-acute care only, one that bundles post-acute care with acute (e.g., inpatient) care, and a capitation system that covers post-acute care. He notes that such coverage may increase cost in the short term but may eventually lead to lower costs in the long run.

Conclusion

One purpose of the conference was to determine areas of consensus about Medicare policy. Two such areas emerge from these chapters. One is that the current system does not provide appropriate coverage. Despite its accomplishments, there are serious gaps in Medicare coverage that need to be addressed, and there are other areas where coverage may be excessive or inefficiency may be increasing. The other area of consensus was that policymakers need to move with some caution in implementing payment changes or expansions in coverage, because not enough is known about consumer and provider responses to payment changes, insurance markets, or the efficacy of existing cost containment measures.

Another purpose was to delineate areas of disagreement and determine whether disagreement is based on questions of fact or questions of value. The conference papers and discussion clearly illustrate that there is fundamental disagreement over the role government should play, who should pay the costs of Medicare, and whether benefits should be expanded or contracted. Regardless, the research results contained in this volume, and similar work currently being conducted, will clearly contribute to the quality of future policy decisions.

Conference Participants

Ronald Andersen**, Ph.D., Director, Center for Health Administration Studies, Graduate School of Business, University of Chicago

Bernard S. Bloom, Ph.D., Research Associate Professor, Departments of Dentistry/Psychiatry/Health Care Systems, University of Pennsylvania

Zoe Boniface*, Ph.D. Candidate, Leonard Davis Institute, University of Pennsylvania

Randall R. Bovbjerg*, J.D., Senior Research Associate, The Urban Institute

Elaine Brody, M.S.W. Director, Department of Human Services, Philadelphia Geriatric Center

Stanley J. Brody°, J.D., Professor of Physical Medicine and Rehabilitation in Psychiatry, School of Medicine, University of Pennsylvania

The Honorable Wilbur Cohen°, Professor Emeritus, Lyndon Baines Johnson School of Public Affairs

William Custer*, Ph.D., Research Economist, Department of Health Systems Analysis, AMA

Patricia Danzon, Ph.D., Professor, Department of Health Care Systems, University of Pennsylvania

Haim Erder, Ph.D., Research Associate, Leonard Davis Institute, University of Pennsylvania

Claire M. Fagin, Ph.D., Dean, School of Nursing, University of Pennsylvania

Leonard Feldman, Director of Health Affairs, Smith Kline & French Laboratories

Jinnet Fowles*, Ph.D., Vice President, Research and Development, Health Services Research Center, Park Nicollet Medical Foundation

Bernard Friedman, Ph.D., Associate Director, Center for Health Services and Policy Research, Northwestern University

Lois Ginsberg, Program Manager, Advanced Education, Leonard Davis Institute, University of Pennsylvania

Willis B. Goldbeck**, President, Washington Business Group on Health

Merwyn Greenlick**, Ph.D., Vice President for Research, Kaiser Permanente Medical Group

John C. Hershey, Ph.D., Director of Research, Leonard Davis Institute, University of Pennsylvania

Barbara Holland**, J.D., Hangley, Connolly, Epstein, Chico, Foxmen, and Ewing

Edward F. X. Hughes, M.D., Director, Center for Health Services and Policy Research, Northwestern University

Robert P. Inman**, Ph.D., Professor, Departments of Finance and Economics, University of Pennsylvania

Judith Miller Jones°, Executive Director, National Health Policy Forum

Robert Kane*, M.D., Dean, School of Public Health, University of Minnesota

Judy Kasper*, Ph.D., Research Analyst, Office of Research, Health Care Financing Administration.

William L. Kissick, M.D., Professor, Research Medicine and Health Care Systems, University of Pennsylvania

Gerald F. Kominski*, Ph.D., Health Policy Analyst, Prospective Payment Assessment Commission

Kathryn Langwell*, Ph.D., Senior Economist, Mathematica Policy Research, Inc.

Judith Lave*, Ph.D., Professor of Health Economics, Graduate School of Public Health, University of Pittsburgh

Risa Lavizzo-Mourey**, M.D., M.B.A., Assistant Professor, School of Medicine, University of Pennsylvania

Joanne H. Levy, Assistant Director Research and Administration, Leonard Davis Institute, University of Pennsylvania

James Lubitz*, Ph.D., Branch Chief, Analytic Studies Branch, Office of Research, Health Care Financing Administration

Larry Manheim*, Senior Economist, Center for Health Services and Policy Research, Northwestern University

Ted Marmor°, Ph.D., Professor of Public Management and Political Science, School of Organization and Management and Department of Political Science, Yale University

Samuel P. Martin, M.D., Director, Clinical Scholars Program, Professor, Health Care Systems, University of Pennsylvania

Jeff McCombs*, Ph.D., Social Science Research Analyst, Division of Hospital Experimentation, Office of Research and Demonstration, Health Care Financing Administration

Dan M. McGill, Ph.D., Chair and Executive Director, Huebner Foundation, University of Pennsylvania

Diane McGivern, Ph.D., Associate Professor, School of Nursing, University of Pennsylvania

Alan Monheit*, Ph.D., Senior Economist, National Center for Health Services Research and Office of Technology Assessment

Marilyn Moon*, Ph.D., Director, Public Policy Institute, American Association of Retired Persons

Robert Musacchio*, Ph.D., Director, Department of Health Systems Analysis, American Medical Association

Lyle Nelson*, Ph.D., Economist, Mathematica Policy Research, Inc.

Patricia Patrizi, Research Associate, Leonard Davis Institute, University of Pennsylvania

Mark V. Pauly*, Ph.D., Executive Director, Leonard Davis Institute, Robert D. Eilers Professor of Health Care Management and Economics, University of Pennsylvania

Charles E. Phelps*, Ph.D., Director, Public Policy Analysis Program, Professor, Departments of Economics and Political Science, University of Rochester

Thomas Rice**, Ph.D., Assistant Professor, Department of Health Policy and Administration, School of Public Policy, University of North Carolina

Gerald Riley*, Ph.D., Research Analyst, Office of Research, Health Care Financing Administration

Laura E. Roper, Ph.D., Project Manager, Research, Leonard Davis Institute, University of Pennsylvania

Gerald Rosenthal**, Ph.D., Professor of Health Policy and Economics, Department of Humanities & Social Science, Hahnemann University

J. Arnold Rosoff**, L.D., Associate Professor, Departments of Legal Studies and Health Care Systems, University of Pennsylvania

Sheldon Rovin*, D.D.S., Chairman and Professor of Dental Care Systems, School of Dental Medicine, University of Pennsylvania

Robert J. Rubin**, M.D., Executive Vice President, ICF, Inc.

Mark Sager, M.D., Internist, Department of Medicine, University of Wisconsin

Richard M. Scheffler*, Ph.D., Director, Research Program in Health Economics, Professor of Economics and Public Policy, School of Public Health, University of California, Berkeley

Mark Schlesinger**, Ph.D., Research Coordinator, Center for Health Policy and Management, Kennedy School of Government, Harvard University

Cecil G. Sheps°, M.D., Taylor Grandy Distinguished Professor of Social Medicine, Health Services Research Center, University of North Carolina

Pamela Farley Short*, Ph.D., Senior Economist, National Center for Health Services Research and Health Care Technology Assessment

Linda Siegenthaler, Economist, Division of Extra-Mural Research, National Center for Health Services Research and Health Care Technology Assessment

Anne Ramsay Somers, Adjunct Professor, Department of Environmental and Community Medicine, Robert Wood Johnson Medical School

Rosemary A. Stevens, Ph.D., Professor of History and Sociology of Science, University of Pennsylvania

Ronald Stewart, Manager, Government Affairs, Smith Kline & French Laboratories

William Stewart°, M.D., Professor Emeritus, Department of Pediatrics, School of Medicine, Louisiana State University

Ira Strumwasser*, Ph.D., Director of Research, Michigan Health Care Education and Research Foundation

Anita A. Summers, Chair, Department of Public Policy and Management, University of Pennsylvania

Ronald Vogel*, Ph.D., Associate Professor of Management and Policy, College of Business and Public Administration, University of Arizona

Sankey V. Williams**, M.D., Associate Professor of Medicine, Hospital of the University of Pennsylvania

*Author; **discussant; °invited speaker

Additional Contributors
to This Volume

Meryl Bloomrosen, MBA, Manager, Health Information Management Services, Aspen Systems Corporation

John P. Bunker, M.D., Director, division of Health Services Research, Stanford University School of Medicine

Jolene A. Hall, M.B.A., Health Policy Analyst, Prospective Payment Assessment Commission

Margaret C. Loftus, Senior Medical Analyst, Blue Shield of California

James W. Moser, Ph.D., Economist, Center for Health Policy Research, American Medical Association

Shelly L. Nelson, M.H.A., Research Analyst, Mathematica Policy Research

Marjorie Oda, M.D., Robert Wood Johnson Clinical Scholar 1983–1985, Stanford University School of Medicine

Dena S. Puskin, Sc.D., Senior Health Policy Analyst, Prospective Payments Assessment Commission

Anne Lenhard Reisinger, Ph.D., Assistant Professor, Columbia University

David J. Schurman, M.D., Professor of Orthopedics Surgery, Stanford University Medical Center

Richard D. Willke, Ph.D., Economist, Center for Health Policy Research, American Medical Association

I

Medicare Policy: Past, Present, and Future

1. The Structure of the Medicare Benefit Package: Evolution and Options for Change

❑ ❑ ❑

JUDITH R. LAVE

Introduction

The Medicare program, established through the Social Security Amendments of 1965, became effective on July 1, 1966. The main goals of the program were to decrease the financial burdens that the elderly incur in obtaining health care services and to increase access to care. In the twenty years of its existence, the program has experienced some dramatic changes, although the basic structure of the program has been stable. The major changes have been the extension of eligibility to the recipients of Social Security disability payments and to people with end-stage renal disease (ESRD), as well as changes in the methods of paying providers as highlighted by the implementation of the Medicare Prospective Payment System (PPS). The basic financing mechanism (the methods of raising funds to pay for the program), the set of covered services, and the cost-sharing requirements have changed little since the initiation of the program.

In this chapter, I focus on the structure of the Medicare benefit package and examine options for change. The structure includes both the services covered by the program and the cost-sharing obligations (required deductibles, coinsurance, and premium payments) of the Medicare population. I begin with a brief overview of the Medicare benefit package and how it has evolved over time. How research and demonstration activity have influenced the changes that have occurred, as well as their possible role in influencing future changes, are then discussed. I go on to examine many of the current problems with the program. Then I discuss some of the recommendations that have been made for changing the benefit structure, with special emphasis on the acute care benefits. The proposals to turn Medicare into a voucher program will be discussed in the chapter by Bovbjerg, although it should be noted that the *level* of the voucher will depend upon the benefits it is supposed to purchase.

The nature of the benefit package, which affects the demand for services, is only one of the factors influencing the quantity and quality of services obtained by Medicare beneficiaries. The services obtained will depend as well on the method used by Medicare to pay providers for services rendered to program beneficiaries.

The Medicare Benefit Package

The Medicare program consists of two separate but complementary insurance programs: Hospital Insurance (HI or Part A) covers services furnished by hospitals, skilled nursing facilities (SNFs), and home health agencies; and Supplementary Medical Insurance (SMI or Part B) covers services provided by physicians and a few other health care providers, durable medical equipment, medical prostheses and supplies, and home health agencies (for people not enrolled under HI). Services covered under both parts are subject to substantial cost sharing. Enrollment in HI is almost automatic for the *entitled* population (people turning 65 who are eligible for Social Security, the Social Security disabled population after two years of benefits, and most people with ESRD). Enrollment in SMI is contingent upon paying a small monthly premium.

Table 1.1 provides a general description of the Medicare benefit structure on both July 1, 1966, and on July 1, 1986. There are a number of general observations to be made about the benefit structure.

1. *Many health services used by Medicare beneficiaries are not covered by the program.* These services include most preventive services, general long-term care services, hearing and eye exams, routine foot care, most dental care, and outpatient prescription drugs. Some of these services, such as routine foot care, were not covered because they are routine (and therefore should be budgetable); while other services (in particular, general long-term care services) were not covered because they were considered to be custodial services rather than medical care services. Medicare was designed to be, and continues to be, a program that pays for the costs of *acute illness* or the acute manifestations of chronic illness.

As is noted below, the Medicare program has not expanded in the depth of services covered, such as prescription drugs or long-term care services; however, it should be remembered that it has had a major expansion in breadth of coverage, with the inclusion of the disabled and the ESRD populations. The underlying reason why benefits have not expanded in depth has been the continuing concern about the escalation in costs since the program began and the continuing rise in the Social Security payroll tax to cover current commitments in benefits to people entitled to Medicare.

2. *Few services have been added to the Medicare benefit package as a result of legislative change.* The definition of physician has been broadened and hospice care, outpatient physical therapy, and speech pathology have been made covered services. In contrast, the nature of covered services has changed dramatically through the regulatory process. As new medical devices, types of durable medical equipment, and new treatments become available, the Health Care Financing Administration (HCFA) must decide whether the items meet criteria for coverage. The coverage decisions are critically important, and some of HCFA's decisions can even create a new industry (Ruby, Banta, and Burns 1985). For example, outpatient enteral and parenteral nutrition were defined to be prosthetic devices in 1981. A consulting firm has estimated that there will be a $16 billion market for this type of home care by 1990 (Somers 1983).

3. *A simple listing of covered services is deceptive.* To qualify for some benefits, the Medicare beneficiary must satisfy certain requirements. For example, to qualify for the Medicare SNF benefit, admission to the SNF must follow (within a specified time period) a three-day (or longer) hospital stay; the person must be admitted for a condition for which he or she was treated in the hospital and must need skilled nursing care. To qualify for home health, a person must be confined to the home and must need either skilled nursing care on an intermittent basis or speech and physical therapy. Very strict regulations have been written establishing the criteria needed to satisfy these conditions.

4. *The structure of the cost-sharing requirements has remained essentially unchanged.* Part A cost-sharing requirements depend on the size of the inpatient deductible (IPD), which in turn is directly related to the average cost of a day in a short-term general hospital. The beneficiary pays the deductible for the first day of hospitalization in a benefit period.[1] The copay for days 60 to 90 of the benefit period is one-quarter of the IPD; for the 61 lifetime reserve days, it is one-half the IPD; and for days 21 through 100 in an SNF, it is one-eighth of the IPD. Because Part A cost sharing is linked to the IPD, the proportion of total costs covered by beneficiary copayments has increased. Since the length of stay has fallen from 13.8 days to 9.1 days, the proportion of the total inpatient costs of the initial stay met by the deductible has increased from about 7.2 percent to 11 percent. In addition, since the cost of an inpatient day has increased much more than the cost of an SNF day, the proportion of the cost of SNF care covered by Medicare for days 21 through 100 has decreased. On average, the beneficiary pays about 70 percent of the cost of an SNF day for each of these days.[2]

In comparison with Part A, the Part B deductible has risen only slightly. With

TABLE 1.1
Medicare-Covered Services and Cost-Sharing Requirements

Benefit	July 1, 1966		July 1, 1986	
	Limits	Cost sharing	Limits	Cost sharing
Part A—HI				
Hospitalization	1–60 days of BP 61–90 days of BP	Initial deductible $40 Daily copay $10	1–60 days of BP 61–90 days of BP	Initial deductible $492 Daily copay $123
(Lifetime reserve days)	NC (limit of 190 days in specialty psychiatric hospitals)	NA	91–150 days (limit of 190 days in specialty psychiatric hospitals)	Daily copay $246
Skilled nursing facility (effective January 1967)	1–20 days 21–100 days	None Daily copay $5	1–20 days 21–100 days	None Daily copay $61.50
Home health	100 visits	None	Unlimited visits	None
Hospice	NC	NA	Beneficiary may elect hospice care in lieu of other service for two periods of 90 days and one period of 30 days	5% of cost to program for drugs and respite care
Outpatient hospital diagnostic testing		$20 deductible 20% coinsurance	Covered under Part B	
Part B—SMI				
Physician and other medical services including diagnostic testing	None	Monthly premium of $3 Annual deductible $50 20% of approved charges; excess of physician charges if physician does not take assignment	None	Monthly premium of $15.50 Annual deductible $75 20% of approved charges; excess of physician charges if physician does not take assignment

Service				
Durable medical equipment	Some limits	20% coinsurance depending on supplier	Some limits	20% coinsurance depending on provider
Home health	100 visits	20% coinsurance	Unlimited visits	None
Outpatient mental health	Limited	50% of reasonable charges up to $500 and 100% of charges thereafter	Limits	50% of reasonable charges up to $500 and 100% thereafter
Outpatient hospital expense	NC	NA	Unlimited	20% coinsurance
Outpatient physical therapy	NC	NA	Limited provided by private physical therapist	20% coinsurance (100% after $500 charges from private physical therapist)
Comprehensive outpatient rehabilitation services	NC	NA	None	20% coinsurance
Rural health	NC	NA	None	20% coinsurance
Immunization	NC	NA	Pneumococcal vaccine, hepatitis B for selected populations	None

Note: BP is the benefit period. It begins with an initial hospitalization and ends when the beneficiary has not been an inpatient in a hospital or skilled nursing facility for 60 days.

NC = not covered; NA = not applicable.

[a]Originally, professional inpatient services of pathologists and radiologists were not subject to deductibles.

the exception of home health, other cost-sharing requirements under Part B have remained essentially unchanged. One result of this stability is that real coverage for outpatient psychiatric care has decreased substantially. The cost-sharing requirements of Medicare are larger than those in most employer-sponsored health insurance plans. On average, Medicare covers about 69 percent of hospital and physician costs of the beneficiary population, while employer-based programs cover about 80 percent (Harvard Medicare Project 1986).

5. *The cost-sharing requirements under Part B are more confusing and have become more complicated over time than is indicated by Table 1.1.* The amount of cost sharing sometimes depends on the nature of the provider or the site of care. For example, if surgery is undertaken in an approved outpatient setting, and if the physician takes assignment, there is no cost sharing on physician services.

6. *Part A and Part B continue as two distinct programs despite the fact that 98 percent of HI beneficiaries were also enrolled in SMI* (either because they elected to pay the premium or because the states bought into Part B for Medicaid eligibles HCFA 1986A).

Furthermore, the distinctive characteristics of inpatient and outpatient care, which were quite clear at the time Medicare was enacted and which in part justified the creation of separate HI and SMI programs, have become blurred over time. This is because many procedures, such as cataract surgery, have been shifted from an inpatient to outpatient setting.

The Role of Research and Demonstrations in Modifying the Benefit Package

A significant amount of research related to the structure of the Medicare benefit structure has been conducted or is ongoing. This research has had (or may have) some effect in modifying Medicare benefits. In this section, I briefly review some of the research that has been conducted to examine the optimum structure of insurance programs, as well as some of the research conducted on specific coverage issues.

The structure of insurance

A number of economists have developed theoretical models of the demand for insurance to determine the optimum structure of an insurance program (Zeckhauser 1970; Mossin 1968). The optimum insurance package has been shown to have three characteristics: a deductible to decrease administrative costs of processing a large number of small claims, coinsurance designed to reduce moral hazard (insurance-induced demand), and a catastrophic cap on beneficiary liability.

Although many economists believe that this is an "ideal" model, some health services researchers point out that the purpose of health insurance is not only to insure against financial risk but is also to provide an incentive for people to use services (one person's moral hazard is another person's increased access). Also, some economists are concerned that a catastrophic cap could lead to a large increase in overall costs because of reimbursement-influenced system changes (Zook, Moore, and Zeckhauser 1980). This concern may be less relevant today because of changes in hospital payment methods and because of improved utilization review programs.

Against this ideal, Medicare gets a failing grade. The Part A deductible is not designed to decrease administrative costs. It may have been originally implemented to deter unnecessary hospitalization, but given the growth in outpatient surgery and preadmission review programs, that deterrent is probably no longer needed. The initial Part B cost sharing does follow the "ideal model." However, neither Part A nor Part B has a cap on Medicare beneficiary liability.

Before leaving this issue, it should be noted that there is some question as to whether Medicare should be evaluated as an insurance program. The Medicare program is usually described as a program designed to increase the access of the elderly to the health care system and to reduce the financial burden associated with being sick. It seems reasonable, therefore, to consider its effectiveness as an insurance program against the costs of covered services as a *de minimus* criterion for evaluating the program.

Coverage research (excluded services)

There have been a number of studies into specific coverage issues; that is, into assessing the implications of adding certain services to the Medicare benefit package (HCFA 1986a). Most of these studies ask, Is it feasible to cover these services; what would be the effect of covering this service on the cost of the Medicare program, on the cost to society of providing health care services, and on the health status of the beneficiary population? Some of these studies have been conducted at the direction of the Congress—often in response to pressure from specific groups (who argue that if only their services were covered, then the patients' condition would not worsen, and the need for acute care services would be reduced).

In recent years, Congress has directed HCFA to study the implications of adding orthopedic shoes, routine foot care, and home visits by registered dieticians and respiratory therapists to the benefit package. The first two studies have been completed with a recommendation of no change. In addition HCFA, along with the National Institutes of Health is doing a large study to determine whether commencement of nutritional therapy in early renal failure (utilizing controlled protein substances) can retard or arrest the progression of the disease. The coverage question is whether nutritional therapy should be a covered service. A final congressionally mandated demonstration, which was instigated more by the research community than by the provider community, is the social/health maintenance organization (HMO) demonstration.

In addition to the congressionally mandated studies, HCFA and other parts of the federal government have supported a number of major demonstrations to examine other coverage issues. For example, in 1978 HCFA was charged with developing a special research and demonstration study to examine the costs, benefits, and feasibility of having Medicare pay for hospice care. Although the hospice legislation was introduced before the demonstration results were made available, the fact that the demonstrations had shown such coverage was feasible may have facilitated the passage of the legislation (Mor et al. 1986).

The most important administration-initiated demonstrations are the long-term care demonstrations, which were undertaken to investigate the effect of changing the benefit package (usually of both Medicare and Medicaid) to include presently excluded long-term care types of service. The basic purpose of these demonstrations was to test the feasibility and cost-effectiveness of an alternative long-term care service delivery concept integrating health and social services. Advocates of the use of these services argued that their provision would be a lower-cost substitute for institutional services and would possibly prevent a deterioration of health status and hence lead to a decreased need for institutional care.

Many of these demonstrations have been completed and evaluated. While the addition of these social services has been shown to improve the quality of life of the beneficiaries, it has also been shown to add to the cost of the program (U.S. GAO 1982). HCFA has summarized the findings of the evaluation of the most recent set of demonstrations, the channelling demonstrations, as follows: "The evaluation of these demonstrations concluded that hospitalization rates, nursing home utilization rates and longevity were not different for clients enrolled in the demonstrations and the control clients. However, channelling did improve the well being of care-givers, reduced reported unmet needs and increased the social and psychological well-being of clients" (HCFA briefing notes 1986a). These findings will no doubt influence the direction of long-term care policy in some way.

There is one final demonstration activity to be mentioned. Medicare does not cover preventive services, and a number of physicians and policy analysts have argued that the result of this exclusion is that some lives are unnecessarily lost and problems are not found when they would be less costly to treat (Somers 1984). HCFA has funded two large demonstrations to assess the implications of adding a preventive benefit package to the Medicare plan. These demonstrations have just been started and are scheduled to run through September 1991 (HCFA 1986b).

Coverage issues: regulation

As explained above, many coverage decisions are made through the regulatory process. As new services become available, HCFA must decide if they are "reasonable and necessary" for the diagnosis and treatment of disease, where historically reasonable and necessary have been defined quite narrowly (Banta, Ruby, and Burns 1984). HCFA has used the results of literature reported in the medical research journals as input into its coverage decisions, and some of these decisions can be quite targeted. It is possible that much of the outcome-related research which is more familiar to health service researchers will be used to inform HCFA coverage decisions in the future.

There is, however, one coverage study that should be explicitly mentioned. In 1981 HCFA awarded a contract to the Battelle Memorial Institute to examine the implications of covering heart transplants. This study, which was to provide a model for making coverage decisions, included an analysis of the economic, ethical, and political implications of covering that procedure. Partly as a result of the study findings, the secretary of the Department of Health and Human Services (DHHS) recommended that heart transplants be a covered service.

Current Problems with the Medicare Benefit Package

Although the Medicare program is a popular government program, the benefit structure is not without major problems. In this section, the most important of those problems are discussed.

Lack of a catastrophic cap. Many policy analysts believe that the program is seriously flawed because it does not contain a limit on beneficiary liability for covered services. Table 1.2 presents information on the distribution of Medicare liability incurred by Medicare beneficiaries in using Medicare-covered services in 1983. These data slightly underestimate this liability because they do not include expenditures on services for which coverage ran out (i.e., expenditures over $500 for outpatient psychotherapy). As indicated by Table 1.2, beneficiary liability can be extensive: 7.2 percent and 3.1 percent of beneficiaries have potential out-of-pocket Medicare-related liabilities of between $1,000 and $2,000 and over $2,000, respectively. This means that nearly three million persons have Medicare liabilities of over $1,000. Part B liabilities, which include the liabilities on unassigned claims, account for about 72 percent of total liability.

Most Medicare beneficiaries, however, do not pay the full Medicare cost sharing out-of-pocket. Many Medicare beneficiaries have attempted to protect themselves against Medicare cost sharing and catastrophic medical expenses by buying additional medical insurance from the private sector, while other beneficiaries have their cost sharing paid for through the Medicaid program. Approximately 70 percent of people sixty-five and over have some private health insurance,

TABLE 1.2
Distribution of Aged Enrollee Liability Under Medicare
Part A and Part B, 1983

	Distribution of enrollees		
Total	Part A 100%	Part B 100%	Total 100%
0	75.1	32.9	19.6
1–99	1.6	8.4	22.5
100–299	0.4	34.9	28.0
300–499	17.9	9.1	7.5
500–699	3.5	4.6	6.4
700–999	0.6	3.9	5.7
1,000–1,999	0.4	4.5	7.2
2,000–4,999	0.3	1.5	2.7
5,000 and over	0.1	0.2	0.4
Total enrollees (thousands)	26,669	26,292	27,109
Total liability (millions)	$2,892	$7,414	$10,307

Source: Unpublished HCFA data.

which is either purchased directly or is part of a retirement benefit package,[3] while 17 percent have some support from the Medicaid program.

Most of the health insurance that is purchased from the private sector is "Medigap" insurance; that is, it covers some of the copayments and deductibles embedded in the Medicare program (Rice and McCall 1985). However, the Medigap policies are imperfect. They have administrative costs averaging about 40 to 50 percent of the premium (Harvard Medicare Group 1986); if not meeting "Baucus standards," they contain clauses excluding coverage of preexisting conditions, and they occasionally duplicate Medicare coverage. In addition, many economists argue that despite their high costs, Medigap premiums are subsidized by the Medicare program (Ginsberg 1981). The argument is the following: Medigap policies reduce cost sharing, and because Medicare beneficiaries now face a lower price, they increase their use of Medicare-covered services. As a result, the cost of the Medicare program itself is increased.

Out-of-pocket expenditures are high. Even with Medigap policies, people sixty-five and over pay a considerable amount for health care out-of-pocket. As shown in Table 1.3, out-of-pocket expenditures for the elderly are high. In 1980 the noninstitutionalized elderly had mean out-of-pocket expenditures of $332, while 5 percent of them had out-of-pocket expenditures of over $1,000. Large out-of-pocket payments are made for physician services, in particular for physician services received while one is an inpatient for physicians who bill in excess of the Medicare-allowed customary, prevailing, and reasonable (CPR) charges and for prescription drugs (Kasper 1986).

The Medicare program does not protect against long-term care costs. The Medicare program was designed to cover the costs of acute illness or the acute manifestations of chronic illness. It explicitly does not cover custodial care or other support services needed by the frail and impaired elderly. In addition, admission to nursing homes is often accompanied by catastrophic medical care expenses. The Select Committee on Aging found that in Massachusetts 63 percent of elderly persons aged sixty-six and older living alone would impoverish themselves after only thirteen weeks in a nursing home, while 37 percent of married couples would become impoverished within thirteen weeks (Chairman, Select Committee on Aging 1985).

Outlays on health care by people sixty-five and over remain high. In 1984 the elderly spent an average of $1,546 (for the Medicare premium, private insurance premiums, and out-of-pocket expenditures) or 14.6 percent of their income on health care services (Chairman, Select Committee on Aging 1985). This is the same percentage of their income that the elderly allocated to expenditures on

TABLE 1.3
Selected Data on Health Expenditures by Age of Individuals,
Noninstitutionalized Population, 1980

		Age	
Variable	Total elderly	65–74	75+
Number of people (thousands)	23,470	15,165	8,305
Out-of-pocket expense mean	$332	$302	$381
Distribution of out-of-pocket expenses			
$0		13.1%	10.2%
$0 < E < 250$		53.5%	52.6%
$250 < E < 500$		17.1%	21.1%
$500 < E < 999$		10.4%	9.6%
$1,000 < E < 2,500$		5.1%	5.3%
$E < 2,500$		<1.0%	<1.0%
SMI premium	$104	$104	$104
Percent with private insurance	70%	73.6%	63.6%
Percent supported by Medicaid	17%	15.0%	21.0%

Note: out-of-pocket expenditures do not include the SMI premium.
Source: J. D. Kasper (1986).

health care before the Medicare program began. It is difficult to know whether this simple comparison has any normative implications. Between 1966 and 1986 the income of the elderly has increased significantly. For example, in 1966, 29 percent of the elderly had incomes below the poverty level, whereas in 1984 only 12 percent of them did. As a group, the elderly are no longer disadvantaged and, on average, are as well off as the nonelderly (Grad 1984; Gornick et al. 1985). In addition, the types of services available have changed. Some of the services that are now purchased may have been produced at home in the early 1960s.

Outlays on health care by the poor and near-poor elderly are very high. Many health policy analysts are concerned that the cost sharing faced by the poor or near-poor elderly, not covered by Medicaid, may be too high. Since the purchase of Medigap policies is a positive function of health status, income, and high socio-economic status (SES) (Rice and McCall 1985; Long and Settle 1982), the elderly in poor health, with incomes just above the Medicaid eligibility level, are most likely to face Medicare cost sharing. It is possible that some low-income elderly may not obtain "needed" health care services. Overall, the poor and near-poor elderly spend a much higher proportion of their income on health services than do the rest of the elderly population. As shown in Table 1.4, the proportion of income spent on all health care (including long-term care) is strongly negatively related to income. The poor and near-poor spend 26.6 percent of their income on health care, while the elderly with incomes 200 percent above the poverty line spend 2.9 percent of their income on health care.

The Medicare program is confusing. The Medicare program is a very complicated program, and few Medicare beneficiaries really understand the nature of the program and the limits of coverage (McCall, Rice, and Sangle 1986). Some of the confusion arises from the cost-sharing and assignment rules. Confusion also arises because some benefits are not well defined. For example, the program covers an unlimited number of home health visits and up to 100 days in a nursing home. Yet beneficiaries who are receiving those services, and who believe that they still need those services, may find that they no longer meet the qualifying conditions. (Beneficiaries may no longer qualify for skilled care because they no longer need what Medicare defines as "skilled services." As noted earlier, these conditions are very strict.) The issue is even more complicated because HCFA regulations are often interpreted differently by different intermediaries (Smits, Feder, and Scanlon 1982; Loeser, Dickerstein, and Shiavone 1981). In addition, critics have argued that the regulations for home health have recently been tightened arbitrarily (Medicine and Health Perspectives 1986). Somers has commented bitterly on HCFA regulations: "More and more it appears that the difference be-

TABLE 1.4
Health Care Expenditure as Percent of Income

Percent of income spent	Income class			
	Poor[a]	Low income	Middle income	Upper income
Out-of-pocket	16.7%	5.1%	2.8%	1.4%
Medicare premium	3.1	1.1	0.7	0.4
Medigap	6.8	2.7	2.3	1.1
Total	26.6%	8.9%	5.8%	2.9%

[a]Poor: income less than 125% of poverty; low income: income between 125% and 200% of poverty; middle income: income between 125% and 200% of poverty.
Source: Adapted from Harvard Medicare Project (1986).

tween 'custodial care' and skilled nursing care has little to do with the degree of skill required, but a great deal to do with the patient's prognosis. The Medicare message to the seriously ill patient is clear. 'Get well fast, die or get lost—unless you can qualify for another acute episode'" (Somers 1983).

Options for Change

Defining options

Interest in restructuring Medicare benefits has intensified in recent years. In 1983, in response to the predicted deficit in the Part A trust fund, the Congressional Budget Office prepared a paper outlining various options for changing Medicare benefits (CB0 1983). Next, in November 1983, the staffs of both the Congressional Budget Office and the Health Subcommittee of the Ways and Means Committee held a conference on the future of Medicare (U.S. Congress 1984). Four of the participants (Davis, Rowland, Hsaio, and Kelly) proposed explicit changes in the benefit structure. In a major review of the Medicare program, the Advisory Council to the Social Security Program considered the benefit structure.[4] The twentieth anniversary of the Medicare program provided a stimulus for reflection and recommendations for reform (see, e.g., the 1985 Supplement to the *Health Care Financing Review*). Finally, the interest expressed in catastrophic medical insurance by Otis Bowen, secretary of the DHHS, has stimulated further thought on the issue.

Many of the proposals for change in the Medicare benefit structure have been stimulated by the problems listed above, although different "reformers" have attached different weights to them. The noun "reformers" has been placed in quotation marks because not all of the proposals for change should be considered reform. Some of the proposals would call for major changes in the program, whereas others make only modest changes. Nevertheless, at least as far as the

TABLE 1.5
Proposed Changes in the Medicare Benefit Structure

	Davis-Rowland	Harvard Medical Program	American Hospital Association	Bowen-Burke	Kelly-Hsaio
Combine A and B	Yes	Yes	Yes	No	No
Structure of cost sharing	Unchanged	Eliminate hospital and SNF copay; cut hospital deductibles by 50%; eliminate Part B deductible; reduce Part B cost sharing to 10%	Single deductible and same coinsurance rate across all services	Eliminate Part A copayments	Deductibles and cost sharing vary with cost of service
Catastrophic limit	$1,500 indexed to program expenditure	$1,000 indexed to Social Security payments	Limit tied to income	Maximum of two inpatient deductibles; limit Part B cost sharing	Maximum cost sharing tied to income
New services	Prescription drugs	Preventive physician visit; home health agencies for diagnostic visits; geriatric assessment; remove mental health limits	Relax home health and SNF guidelines; prescription drugs	None	None
Financing	"Premium" equal to 2.5% of income; limit of 50% of actuarial cost of total program	Level premium equal to 25% of cost of Part B type of services, plus earmarked income tax to supplement cost	Level premium set to cover cost of expanded service	Increase SMI premium to cover reduced Medicare liability	Unchanged
Mandated assignment	Yes—begin with inpatient	Yes—begin with inpatient	No	No	No

acute care benefit package is concerned, there is a fair degree of consistency with respect to the recommended directions for change. In this section, I first consider the proposals for changing the acute care package and then comment briefly on a few of the proposals for financing long-term care services.

Before discussing the options for reform, it is useful to digress and briefly discuss the current financing methods. Under current law, Part A is an entitlement, and people contribute to the Medicare trust fund over their working years. Part B is voluntary, and people enroll in Part B by paying a premium that covers approximately 25 percent of the cost of the program. Although there are extensive intergenerational and intragenerational transfers involved in Medicare financing (see Chapter 4), people view the program as providing services that they have earned over their lifetime. There can be no doubt but that this concept of earned benefits has contributed to the program's popularity. Major changes in the program may be viewed as violating a social contract that has been made with the aged.

The acute care package. Table 1.5 presents a description of five of the proposals that have been made for changing the benefit structure of the current Medicare program (a program that is not expected to cover long-term care services). With the exception of the American Medical Association (AMA) recommendations,[5] these proposals are representative of current recommendations for change (see also Ball 1985; Bromberg 1985).

Given the diverse backgrounds of the "reformers," there is considerable consistency in their recommendations. All proposals would eliminate the concept of the benefit period and the limit on the number of covered hospital days. All proposals would impose a catastrophic cap on beneficiary liability for covered services, although there is some difference in the nature of the cost sharing to be incurred before the cap is reached. The Hsaio-Kelly plan is the only plan designed to reduce the costs of the Medicare program itself; the other plans, because they add benefits (either through new services or reduced cost sharing) increase program costs. However, with the exception of the Harvard Medicare Project, all plans would pay for the cost of the additional benefits either through increased premiums or through increased taxes (either level premiums or increased taxes on the elderly—income-related premiums). The Bowen-Burke proposal is the only one that would make the benefit expansion voluntary (i.e., people could choose to purchase a catastrophic insurance policy from the government);[6] all of the other expansion proposals would make the expansion mandatory; thus, the premiums are really taxes. Four of the plans would decrease the expenditures on overall health care services by the poor elderly: two proposals make maximum out-of-pocket expenditures a function of income, while two would pay for the cost of the additional services through a tax on gross income of elders. Some of the "reformers" recommend that new services be added to the Medicare benefit package. Finally, two of the "reformers" would mandate assignment—beginning with inpatient care. This would lead to a decrease in out-of-pocket payments of all beneficiaries.

Some of the "reformers" have provided an estimate of the cost of the expanded benefits. The most reliable cost estimates are those made by HCFA's Office of the Actuary to determine the cost of having a cap on beneficiary liability on current covered services. HCFA actuaries estimate that if there is no adverse selection into the plan, the cost per Medicare enrollee in 1987 of the Bowen–Burke proposals would be $46.50 for the expanded Part A benefits and $181.50 to have a limit of $200 on Part B cost sharing.

In choosing among these proposals, the questions to be addressed are, What is the cost of the proposed changes? What are the benefits of the proposed changes in terms of increased beneficiary health status, decreased beneficiary cost sharing, and increases in program simplicity? To what extent will the proposal promote efficiency in the overall health delivery system? To what extent should the cost of health care services rendered to the elderly be borne by the elders themselves? Among the elderly, what proportion should be borne by the sick compared with the well and what proportion borne by the "rich" vis-à-vis the poor? To what extent should the expansion of benefits be voluntary? Finally, what should be the role of the private sector in limiting cost sharing?

This last question is very important. Since 70 percent of people sixty-five and over have purchased private health insurance, the Medicare beneficiaries have revealed themselves as preferring to pay for medical care through premiums rather than through cost sharing. If the cost-sharing limit is set high, as in the Hsaio–Kelly proposal, the private market in Medigap insurance will flourish. If Medicare cost sharing is reduced, then the Medigap market should diminish. Hence, any reform of the Medicare program will have a direct effect on the private insurance industry.

A proposed alternative

Among these proposals, I would recommend a combination of the American Hospital Association (AHA) and the Davis–Rowland proposal. I would recommend that maximum Medicare cost sharing be set at $1,750 but that it be composed of two separate limits: $1,000 for traditional services and $750 for drugs, with the first limit tied to the increase in expenditures on acute care services and the second to the increase in the price of prescription drugs. In addition, I would recommend that there be a single deductible (of about $150) for all services and then a 20 percent cost sharing on outpatient services, with a lower cost sharing on inpatient services. The cost sharing is deliberately set low enough to discourage the purchase of private-sector Medigap policies. I would recommend that the

SNF and home health benefits be simplified so that the beneficiaries can understand them and plan accordingly. The SMI premium should be replaced with a special income tax on the elderly (an income-related premium), which would cover the costs covered by the old SMI premiums plus the expanded benefits. This tax should be subject to both a minimum level and a maximum level. (The minimum level could actually be levied against the Social Security payment and retain the descriptor "premium.") I would recommend that those physicians whom the beneficiaries have little choice in selecting, such as hospital-based physicians (anesthesiologists, pathologists, and radiologists) and inpatient consultants, be obligated to take assignment. Finally, following the Harvard Medicare Project, I would recommend that the government sell a "Medigap" policy, where the premium is set at the actuarial value of the benefits, including any induced utilization of Medicare services caused by lower cost sharing. This Medigap policy would have a $150 deductible. This would be accompanied by a tax on Medigap policies sold by the private sector to cover the cost of induced Medicare utilization. The benefit expansion would not be voluntary.

The recommended plan has the characteristics of the "optimum" insurance plan: it has a deductible to screen out a large volume of small claims, a coinsurance range to limit moral hazard, and a catastrophic cap. The cost-sharing limits are set low enough to discourage beneficiaries from buying Medigap coverage. Thus, Medicare cost sharing will be real cost sharing and moral hazard should be reduced. By setting a low cap on beneficiary liability and by mandating assignment of most in-hospital physician claims, the plan will reduce out-of-pocket expenditures. Expenditures on health care by the poor elderly should be reduced because of the income-related premium and because of the mandatory assignment for most inpatient physician claims. At the same time, the cost of the new services are paid for by the elders as a group. The single deductible, cost sharing across covered services, and a modification of the home health and SNF benefit should simplify the program somewhat. I would not add an explicit preventive care benefit package until the preventive care demonstrations have been evaluated. I would also recommend a reevaluation of outpatient mental health coverage.

The recommendation on mandatory assignment needs further elaboration. Medicare has implemented a participating physician program—physicians who join this program must take assignment on each claim. If information is readily available on who is a participating physician, beneficiaries can reduce their expenditures on physician services by selecting a participating physician. As a result of competition among physicians for patients, the number of participating physicians should increase. However, once beneficiaries are hospitalized, they have no choice over the physicians from whom they receive services. Hence, it is unlikely that the "competitive" market could be effective in the inpatient setting.

This proposal, as are the ones on which it is based, represents a radical change.

Under this proposal, the distinction between Part A and Part B is eliminated, and the SMI premium is replaced by a tax on the elderly. But the basis of the social contract has changed—the elderly are no longer *entitled* to Medicare (Part A) without assessments. Although by and large this proposal substitutes taxes for privately paid premiums, the change will be controversial. If it is too controversial, then I would recommend that a modification of the Bowen-Burke proposal be implemented; that is, that the government sell a supplemental catastrophic medical insurance plan that limits beneficiary liability under Medicare.

Under this plan, the structure of the benefits package would be more rational. However, there is a major barrier to implementing this or any reform package and that is the private insurance industry. Because the Medicare program as originally designed contained more cost sharing than the Medicare beneficiaries were willing to face, and because that cost sharing became more onerous over time, the private insurance industry developed and sold a product, "reduced cost sharing," that people wanted. However, it is very expensive to produce reduced cost sharing through the private market; the government can produce it more efficiently. More importantly, the federal government can administer a fairer program. In order to control for adverse selection, many of the private policies have precondition clauses that limit the value of the policy. One implication of real Medicare reform (a reform for which the beneficiaries, as reflected by their actions in the private market, should be willing to pay for) would be the shrinking of the private insurance market.

Summary and Conclusion

The Medicare program was implemented in 1966 in order to decrease the financial burden the elderly incur in obtaining health care services and to reduce barriers to care. The program was designed to cover the cost of acute illness. Between 1966 and 1986 the structure of the Medicare benefit package, in terms of the listing of covered services and cost-sharing requirements, has remained essentially unchanged, although the nature of covered services has changed as a result of the regulatory process. Nevertheless, this has seen considerable stability despite the fact that the health care delivery system has changed markedly.

On the twentieth anniversary of the program, it is time to reconsider the program and to modify it. There appears to be a consensus about the direction of desired change for the acute care benefit package, which includes the elimination of the benefit period, removal of the limits on covered inpatient hospital days, reduced cost sharing, and the setting of a maximum beneficiary liability. There also appears to be a consensus that a considerable proportion of the cost of the increased benefits should be financed by increases in the amount that beneficiaries pay in either flat or income-related premiums (an increase in taxes). While most reformers would make these reforms mandatory, others would make them voluntary by allowing the beneficiaries to purchase a supplemental policy from the government that would provide for this expansion of benefits. Real reform should also include a simplification of the program, as well as the imposition of mandatory assignment for most inpatient physician claims. It will be very difficult to implement this set of reforms because of the probable opposition of the private insurance industry. Over 70 percent of Medicare beneficiaries have purchased private insurance policies, many of which are Medigap policies. Thus, Medicare reform would have a direct effect on that industry. However, this chapter argues that the government can provide reduced cost sharing more efficiently and equitably to the Medicare population than the private sector can.

The twentieth anniversary of the program would also seem to be a time to reassess the program's exclusion of long-term care services. Although long-term care is going to be the major health care financing problem facing this country in the future, I do not believe that there is yet any consensus about the appropriate roles of the private and public sectors in providing solutions to it.

Notes

I would like to express my gratitude to Marian Gornick, Jeanne Black, Lester Lave, and Ronald Vogel for helpful comments and criticisms on earlier drafts of this chapter. I would also like to thank Robert Rubin and Mark Schlesinger for their comments and criticisms, which were taken into account during the revision process.

1. The benefit period begins with the first day of hospitalization and ends when the beneficiary has not been an inpatient in a hospital or a SNF for sixty continuous days. There is no limit to the number of benefit periods that a person can use.

2. This estimate is based on unpublished data on the distribution of Medicare days by 1984 SNF total per diem costs that was made available by The Urban Institute. The basic data are presented below.

Distribution of Facilities and Medicare Days
by 1984 Facility Total Per Diem Cost

Total cost (dollars)	Facilities		Medicare days	
	Number	Percent	Number	Percent
1–29.99	6	0.17	3,904	0.05
30–39.99	235	6.73	262,078	3.56
40–49.99	634	18.16	846,217	11.50
50–59.99	858	24.57	1,435,465	19.51
60–69.99	656	18.79	1,348,223	18.32
70–79.99	388	11.11	950,334	12.91
80–89.99	247	7.07	615,288	8.36
90–99.99	160	4.58	468,672	6.37
100 and over	308	8.82	1,428,954	19.42
Total	3,492	100.00	7,359,135	100.00

3. Approximately 30 percent of private-sector insurance policies held by Medicare beneficiaries are made available through the employee benefit packages. However, given the current cost of providing health care benefits to retirees, the limitation of tax-exempt contributions to reserves under the Deficit Reduction Act, and current court decisions about employer responsibility, some analysts believe that employers may cut back on their coverage of retirees (Hosay 1985).

4. The 1982 Report of the Advisory Council on Social Security made a series of recommendations for reform. It recommended some modification in Part A cost sharing and recommended that a supplemental Part B policy be made available that provided a cap on beneficiary liability on covered services.

5. Not included in the proposals discussed in the text is the reform proposal by the AMA (AMA 1986). The AMA proposes that the current financing of Medicare be totally changed: the HI tax on employers would be retained, while that on employees would be replaced with a flat tax on gross income up to $100,000. These funds would be placed into a trust fund that would provide beneficiaries with vouchers. The vouchers would be used to purchase an adequate benefits policy from an approved insurance carrier or other health plan. The services covered include an augmented set of services. (Since no limits are given, the plan seems to represent a significant expansion of benefits.) The value of the vouchers would be based on a plan that has an income-related deductible of $500 or over and maximum coinsurance of $2,000. The AMA proposal is a combined financing and voucher proposal. The purpose of the proposal is to have each generation of elderly totally prepay the value of its own vouchers.

6. It is of historical interest to note that some of these proposals reflect the initial debate on Medicare. At that time, there were proposals to tie the deductible to income and to vary the SMI premium with the level of the individual's Social Security payment (Marmor 1973).

References

Advisory Council on Social Security, "Medicare Benefits and Financing: Report of 1982 Advisory Council on Social Security Executive Summary of Recommendations," reported in EBRI-EPF Policy Forum, *Medicare Reform: the Private Sector Impact,* Employee Benefit Research Institute, Washington, DC, 1985.

AMA, Report of the Board of Trustees, "Proposal for Financing Health Care of the Elderly," Chicago, IL, 1986.

American Hospital Association, "Statement of the AHA on Catastrophic Coverage Before the Private/Public Advisory Committee on Catastrophic Illness of the Department of Health and Human Services," Washington, DC, August 12, 1986.

Ball, R.M., "Medicare: A Strategy for Protecting and Improving It," *Generations:* 9–12, Summer 1985.

Banta, H.D., G. Ruby, and A. K. Burns, "Using Coverage Policy to Contain Costs," in U.S. Congress, House Committee on Ways and Means, Subcommittee on Health, *Proceedings of the Conference on the Future of Medicare,* Washington, DC: U.S. Government Printing Office, 1984.

Bowen, O. R., and T. R. Burke, "Cost Neutral Catastrophic Care Proposed for Medicare Recipients," *Federation of American Hospitals Review,* 42–45, November/ December 1985.

Bromberg, M. D., "Remarks on the Symposium of 20 Years of Medicare and Medicaid," *Health Care Financing Review,* Annual Supplement, 69–73, 1985.

Chairman, Select Committee on Aging, House of Representatives, "A Report: American Elderly at Risk," Washington, DC, July 1985.

Congressional Budget Office, *Changing the Structure of Medicare Benefits: Issues and Options,* Washington, DC, March 1983.

Davis, K., and D. Rowland, *Medicare Policy: New Directions for Health and Long-Term Care,* Baltimore, MD: Johns Hopkins University Press, 1986.

Ginsburg, P. B., "Altering the Tax Treatment of Employment Based Health Plans," *Milbank Memorial Fund Quarterly,* 224–255, Spring 1981.

Gornick, M., J. Beebe, and R. Prihoda, "Options for Change Under Medicare: Impact of a Cap on Catastrophic Illness Expense," *Health Care Financing Review,* 5(1): 33–43, Fall 1983.

Gornick, M., J. N. Greenberg, P. W. Eggers, and A. Dobson, "Twenty Years of Medicare and Medicaid: Covered Populations, Use of Benefits, and Program Expenditures," *Health Care Financing Review,* Annual Supplement, 13–59, 1985.

Grad, S., "Incomes of the Aged and Non-Aged 1950–1982," *Social Security Bulletin,* 47(6): 3–13, June 1984.

Harvard Medicare Project, *Medicare: Coming of Age, A Proposal for Reform,* Cambridge, MA: Center for Health Policy and Management, J. F. Kennedy School of Government, Harvard University, 1986.

Health Care Financing Administration, *Health Care Financing Status Report: Research and Demonstration in Health Care Financing,* Washington, DC: U.S. Government Printing Office, 1986a.

———, *Program Statistics Medicare Medicaid Data Book,* HCFA Publication No. 03110, Washington, DC: U.S. Government Printing Office, 1986b.

Hosay, C., "The Impact of Medicare Reform on the Private Sector,"in EBRI-EPF Policy Reform, *Medicare Reform, the Private Sector Impact,* Washington, DC: Employee Benefit Research Institute, 1985, pp. 65–76.

Hsiao, W. C., and N. L. Kelly, "Medicare Benefit: A Reassessment," *Milbank Memorial Fund Quarterly/Health and Society,* 62(2): 207–229, 1984.

Kasper, J. D., *Perspectives on Health Care: United States 1980 National Medical Care Utilization and Expenditure Survey.* Series B, Descriptive Report No. 14, Office of Research and Development, HCFA. Washington, DC: U.S. Government Printing Office, 1986.

Loeser, W. D., E. S. Dickerstein, and L. D. Schiavone, "Medicare Coverage in Nursing Homes—A Broken Promise," *New England Journal of Medicine,* 304: 353–354, 1981.

Long, S. H., and R. F. Settle, "Medicare Cost Sharing and Private Supplementary Health Insurance: Selected Research Findings," paper presented at the Medical Care Section, American Public Health Association Annual Meeting, Montreal, November 15, 1982.

Marmor, T., *The Politics of Medicare,* Chicago, IL: Aldine, 1973.

McCall, W., T. Rice, and J. Sangl, "Consumer Knowledge of Health Insurance Benefits," *Health Services Research* 20(6): 633–657, February 1986.

Medicine and Health Perspectives, "Hard Times for Home Health," *Medicine and Health,* Health Information Center, 40(33) McGraw-Hill Book Co., 1986.

Mor, V. with S. M. Allen, J. Ruddock, R. Kaufmann, and C. C. Borustrup-Jensen, *Medicare Hospice Benefit Program Evaluation: Literature Review and Synthesis, Phase I,* Center for Health Care Research, Brown University, 1986.

Mossin, J., "Aspects of Rational Insurance Purchasing," *Journal of Political Economy,* 553–568, March/August 1968.

Rice, D. P., "Coverage of the Aged and Their Hospital Utilization in 1962: Findings of the 1963 Survey of the Aged," *Social Security Bulletin* 27(7): 9–28, July 1964.

Rice, T., and N. McCall, "The Extent of Ownership and Characteristics of the Medicare Supplemental Policies," *Inquiry, the Journal of Health Care Organization, Provision, and Financing,* 22(2): 188–200, Summer 1985.

Ruby, G., H. D. Banta, and A. K. Burns, "Medicare Coverage, Medicare Costs and Medical Technology," *Journal of Health Politics, Policy and Law,* 10(1): 141–155, Spring 1985.

Smits, H. L., J. Feder, and W. J. Scanlon, "Medicare Nursing Home Benefit Variation in Interpretation," *New England Journal of Medicine,* 307(14): 855–862, 1982.

Somers, A. R., "Financing Long-Term Care for the Elderly: Institution, Incentive, Issues," unpublished paper prepared for National Academy of Sciences Institute of Medicine, Committee on an Aging Society, 82 pages, 1983.

————, "Why Not Try Preventing Illness as a Way of Controlling Medicare Costs?" *New England Journal of Medicine,* 311(13): 853–856, 1984.

U.S. Congress, Subcommittee on Ways and Means, U.S. House of Representatives, *Proceedings of the Conference on the Future of Medicare,* February 1, 1984.

U.S. General Accounting Office, *The Elderly Should Benefit From Expanded Home Care, But Increasing These Services Will Not Insure Cost Reductions,* Publication No. GAO-IPE -83-1, Washington, DC: U.S. Government Printing Office, 1982.

Vogel, R. J., "An Analysis of the Welfare Component and Intergenerational Transfers Under the Medicare Program," this volume, Chapter 4.

Zeckhauser, R., "Medical Insurance: A Case Study of the Tradeoff Between Risk Spreading and Appropriate Incentives," *Journal of Economic Theory* 2(1): 10–26, March 1970.

Zook, C. J., F. D. Moore, and R. J. Zeckhauser, "Catastrophic Health Insurance: A Misguided Prescription," *The Public Interest,* 60: 66–81, Winter 1980.

2. Vouchers for Medicare: The Impossible Dream?

❑ ❑ ❑

RANDALL R. BOVBJERG

The Voucher Concept

Are vouchers for Medicare beneficiaries an appealing reform finally ready to bear fruit in a newly competitive health sector? Or are they instead wholly impractical, an ideological pipe dream? Analysis can illuminate this question, but only experience can answer it. This chapter critiques the arguments about vouchers, pro and con, concluding that vouchers are worthy of a test that would provide needed practical experience.

The idea of vouchers is strikingly simple. In place of a single, standard version of publicly provided services, vouchers give consumers a chit with which to buy services to their own liking. The concept is hardly new. As Sloan (1982) points out, fully two centuries ago Adam Smith (1778) and Thomas Paine (1791) called for voucherlike entitlements for public education. Milton Friedman (1962) seems to have begun this era's policy discussions, and vouchers are generally seen as a "conservative" nostrum, a way of ending public monopoly on public services. Vouchers for housing and education have received the most attention, but many other services can be covered. The main goal is to make service providers compete for voucher payments. Individuals would then demand good value for money because they would "spend" vouchers much like their own money.

In health care, provision of services is already largely private, even under public insurance programs like Medicare, so insurance—or arranging for services—is what would be made subject to private decisions rather than public ones (Bovbjerg, Held, and Pauly 1987). Beneficiaries could use vouchers to buy privately designed and administered health plans to replace Medicare.

The word voucher calls to mind actual scrip, a food-stamp-like entitlement used in lieu of cash. But vouchers can function without such tangible certificates. All that matters is that consumers can control how government money is spent, rather than taking in-kind public benefits determined by the government.[1] Vouchers thus stand intermediate between cash redistribution of purchasing power and direct supply of in-kind benefits.

For health care, the basic idea of allowing Medicare beneficiaries to opt out of the federal program into a private plan first emerged around 1970, largely to encourage economizing through health maintenance organizations (HMOs). The situation changed after the Tax Equity and Fiscal Responsibility Act of 1982 (TEFRA) (U.S. Congress 1982). Under Health Care Financing Administration (HCFA) implementing regulations (HCFA 1985), Medicare has moved closer to vouchers but only for beneficiaries to choose HMOs or similarly organized prepaid plans. Numerous other choices are possible and desirable.

The Lengthy Gestation of Vouchers for Health Care

Early conceptions

Vouchers played a key role in the HMO strategy developed by Ellwood and his InterStudy colleagues at the beginning of the Nixon administration (Ellwood et al. 1971). Public vouchers were seen as the way to reform inefficient public plans by getting public beneficiaries into prepaid plans, alongside paying private customers. Throughout the 1970s various reformers—generally conservative ones—proposed versions of the public voucher theme, variously emphasizing HMOs and overall cost containment (e.g., Havighurst, Blumstein, and Bovbjerg 1976). This decade of theoretical development culminated with Enthoven's tax credit-voucher plan to restructure all of health care financing, not merely public plans (1980). Actual policy has not moved far toward vouchers, however.

Traditional Medicare inefficiencies

The litany of objections to Medicare as traditionally structured is well known. Medicare has come under increasing intellectual and political attack, both for its failures in cost containment and for its shortcomings in terms of benefit structure. A number of features are commonly blamed for federal difficulty in maintaining fiscal control. Briefly, as a result of political bargaining in the mid-1960s and the era's drive to improve access and quality almost without regard to costs, some pivotal early decisions made rapid increases in program spending almost inevitable (Harris 1966; Marmor 1973).

The program was enacted as an open-ended entitlement, with little cost sharing imposed on the patient at time of use and with definitions of need for care and level of payment left almost wholly outside federal control, so that the program had very few ways to protect itself from high and rising spending (Feder 1977). Medicare followed the "best practice" of provider-dominated private insurers. It accepted professionally determined standards of practice, through a promise to pay for all "medically necessary care" and not to interfere with "the private practice of medicine" (U.S. Congress 1965). At least until very recently, only *peer* review of individual physicians' treatment decisions was allowable, if that. Moreover, payment methods contemplated either reimbursing virtually all provider-incurred costs or passively accepting provider-set charges. These methods rewarded profligacy and penalized parsimony. The commitment to cost reimbursement also prevented Medicare from accommodating to the normal practice of prepaid group practices, or HMOs as they came to be known in the post-InterStudy 1970s.

Further, Medicare guaranteed every patient "free choice of provider" (U.S. Congress 1965). This guarantee was of considerable value to beneficiaries and providers, but it posed severe restrictions on Medicare's own administrative freedom of action. Very little change in operations is possible when all providers must be kept within the program. This one provision probably stood as the greatest single obstacle to constructive reforms of all types. As traditionally interpreted, freedom of choice meant that no administrator, public or private, could steer patients to low-cost physicians or hospitals—nor penalize high-cost ones. It also barred negotiation or bidding for good value because these methods require excluding at least some providers.

Finally, one major difficulty resulted not from specific program choices but rather from the general nature of public administration. Namely, political and legal constraints make it very difficult for public decisionmakers to effectuate discretionary changes. Finding the "right" approach to benefit levels, coverage, prices, and so on can require a lot of tinkering and some reliance on hunches and rules of thumb. Private actors can act much faster and more flexibly in this regard because they are subject only to market discipline, not to politicians or lawyers. The market can harshly punish mistakes in outcome but is undemanding in terms of process. Public actors, however, must carefully articulate their rationales well in advance and face legal requirements to operate through detailed written regulations.

Enter the HMO

HMOs were the first private plans to seek to compete with Medicare. Initially, Medicare refused to deal with HMOs on the voucherlike basis of monthly capitation—the latter's preferred way of doing business—but rather insisted on paying their costs or charges for each service, as for other providers. This barrier was reduced by the Social Security Amendments of 1972, which for the first time provided that certain large, mature, federally qualified HMOs could be paid on a "risk" basis. However, the risks and rewards were not balanced. Eligible HMOs could only retain half of any savings they achieved up to 20 percent below average expected spending and none of that above 20 percent. In contrast, HMOs had to absorb all losses (U.S. Congress 1972).

Not surprisingly, by the end of calendar 1979 only one plan with some 19,000 beneficiaries had taken advantage of these provisions (Langwell and Hadley 1986). The Social Security Amendments of 1976 (U.S. Congress 1976) made certain changes with regard to Medicaid, largely in response to scandals in California about prepaid plans there for the poor. With regard to Medicare, the next significant initiative was HCFA's demonstrations of capitation. Between 1980 and 1981 eight such demonstrations with various types of HMOs were undertaken. These tests showed that prepaid enrollment was indeed possible, although financial experience was mixed (Trieger, Galblum, and Riley 1981).

To this point, HMOs were generally seen as a means of promoting provider economizing through closed-end capitation in lieu of open-ended reimbursement. It was thus at least as much a provider-incentive model as a beneficiary- or patient-choice approach. To the extent that there were other goals, the main one was to promote comprehensive care for the elderly. Indeed, the federal model of HMOs emphasized comprehensiveness—in the fashion of mini-National Health Insurance—more than it did competition and consumer choice (U.S. Congress 1973; see discussion in Havighurst and Bovbjerg 1975). Arguably, the policy could also be seen as a way of helping a much discriminated against medical plan gain a foothold in an industry dominated by unconstrained fee-for-service practice. In some historical perspective, this early HMO period served mainly as a way station to other, more elaborate alternative plans.

TEFRA and today

The most significant recent development in the direction of vouchers has been the enactment of TEFRA (U.S. Congress 1982). In two main ways, TEFRA has gone well beyond prior law to promote availability of HMOs for the Medicaid and Medicare population.

First, it considerably broadens the type of entity that can be prepaid on a capitation basis. Capitation is no longer limited to traditional, federally qualified HMOs (whose services and rate making are regulated). Medicare will now also capitate other, somewhat less restrictively defined plans called competitive medical plans (CMPs) that would not meet the HMO Act's standards. CMPs can now serve the full spectrum of Medicare beneficiaries, with the sole exception of already institutionalized patients and patients with end-stage renal disease (ESRD).

Second, the statute permits prepayment without retroactive adjustment of the rate to reflect actual experience. However, CMP and risk-based HMO rates are regulated, as are the profits they may earn.[2] (See discussions in Ginsburg and Hackbarth 1987; Langwell and Hadley 1986; Iglehart 1985.)

Implementing the TEFRA requirements proved complex. Regulations did not appear until January 1985, with an effective date of April first of that year (HCFA 1985). After one year of operation, the TEFRA regime had signed up 119 CMPs with some 566,000 beneficiaries (Langwell and Hadley 1986), largely Independent Practice Association (IPA) HMOs, ones that offer beneficiaries greater choice of participating physicians than do closed-panel, group-style HMOs.

The second round of relevant HCFA demonstrations began just before TEFRA. These trial runs were called demonstrations of "competition," not of "capitation"—a subtle distinction, to be sure, but one showing a shift in emphasis within the HCFA. This time around, the emphasis was on examining the effects of the HMO as a competitive strategy. Some twenty-six plans were ultimately signed up between 1982 and 1984, covering 117,000 Medicare beneficiaries (Langwell and Hadley 1986). Results from the demonstrations are still being assessed.

On a parallel track, largely for Medicaid, attempts were begun during this period to test the viability and value of capitating, not HMOs, but rather primary care physicians. The theory has been that prepaid doctors will then act as case managers of all the care provided to beneficiaries (Evans 1980). Another voucher-like approach, called "intermediary at risk," received considerable attention for a time. The notion differs from previously described capitation in two main ways. First, the capitation would occur not by beneficiary but by area. Some intermediary between the government and the beneficiaries was to be put at risk for the entire population. This area approach eliminated the need to worry about selection factors adverse to Medicare—the possibility that capitated providers would enroll individuals whose expected spending was below the adjusted average per capita cost (AAPCC), leaving the public plan itself with mainly high spenders. It also eliminated competition at the program level, and probably in practice it would also have reduced beneficiaries' choices.

Second, the primary capitation incentive was to apply to an intermediary, more like a monopoly insurance carrier than like a provider of medical services. Removed from the actual delivery of services, this quasi-insurer was then expected to *manage* claims, spending its "own" money, instead of merely *paying* claims with Medicare's money. This concept takes one large step beyond even the practice of the Texas Medicaid program, which has long had an incentive-based contract for the fiscal intermediary that administers its Medicaid program.

This intermediary approach was never attempted for Medicare, although it was much discussed. Again, Medicaid has had more experience with this type of experiment. Massachusetts proposed to contract with an intermediary to run the entire state Medicaid program on a fully risk-based basis, but no satisfactory intermediary was found. And all Medicaid recipients in one section of Philadelphia are covered under one prepaid organization (Freund and Neuschler 1986).

The closest that actual vouchers have come to enactment for Medicare has been policy discussion (Committee on Ways and Means 1984) and the submission of congressional bills. Senator Durenberger (1985) recently authored one such voucher plan. Such bills have yet to receive serious legislative consideration.

Remaining concerns

In sum, Medicare and Medicaid have lately shown increased interest in using capitation payments to economize—along with other forms of prepayment, such as diagnosis-related groups (DRGs) for inpatient hospital care (U.S. Congress 1983). Simultaneously, voucherlike competition has increased as a result of TEFRA.

TEFRA constitutes a major step toward a voucher, but not all plans that consumers might desire can qualify. Notably, those that do not consist of a single prepaid entity are ineligible. So are plans that cover all or almost all providers in an area without prenegotiated agreements, rather than some organized subset of providers. In short, nothing very much like conventional insurance—still the most popular option in the private market—can qualify, no matter how promising it is in price or quality.

This start toward provider capitation without consumer vouchers clearly offers no panacea for all of Medicare's expenditure problems. Prepaid plans have suffered financial reverses that some observers think have threatened the HMO-CMP strategy.[3] Quality fears have also been voiced about HMOs. Moreover, Medicare spending continues to rise in worrisome fashion along with private costs, despite the growth of HMOs, as well as administratively imposed fee-for-service price constraints like hospital prospective payment and fee freezes for physicians (Hook 1986; Division of National Cost Estimates 1987; Causey 1987). Vouchers would open other pathways to economizing incentives, although economies would not necessarily always follow from decentralized consumer choices.

Furthermore, complaints remain about the structure and operations of the program. Both providers and patients complain about administrative problems, and many analysts consider Medicare inadequate in benefits design.[4] Vouchers could improve beneficiary welfare as well as program economy.

What new private sector approaches might be tried under vouchers? Only a trial could tell. But at a minimum, one would expect to see various preferred provider organizations (PPOs) emerge, some modified indemnity coverages, perhaps other types of large fee-for-service plans, and new capitated entities. These could operate under various kinds of administration and would presumably include innovative methods of cost control, benefits design, or both.

The Medicare Voucher: Prodigy or Problem Child?

How you see vouchers affects your view

Design matters. A voucher is not a voucher is not a voucher. And the precise features of any plan go a long way toward determining its likely accomplishments as well as political reactions to it, although ideology and practical expectations also play a role. This should not be too surprising, given that different versions of vouchers can be used either to privatize public medical programs altogether or to expand the public role to a kind of national health insurance.

Many different choices need to be made in designing vouchers, as in implementing any other deceptively simple theoretical notion. Among the major design options, a number deserve quick mention.

1. Is the voucher mandatory or voluntary? This may be the biggest decision of all. Does the system totally replace Medicare, leaving private plans competing only among themselves? Or do the private plans compete with Medicare itself? In general, this chapter covers only voluntary vouchers, on the assumption that totally privatizing Medicare is neither a good idea nor politically feasible.

2. How generous are the vouchers to be initially and over time? The answer here may well determine most attitudes about any proposal. Providing more than the current level of support through vouchers would engender a very different response than implementing cuts along with the vouchers.[5] Political reality in the post-Gramm Rudman era seems to require at least long-run savings. Whether the first year must already achieve some savings (as HMOs and CMPs must operate for 95 percent of otherwise anticipated Medicare spending) may be critical to the success of any new voucher initiative. Instant success is not to be expected of most innovations, public or private. Similarly, how predictable will the future increase in premiums be? Some stable expectations are probably needed to attract participating plans. In this regard, the continuance of Medicare itself as an option (and thus also as a benchmark for pricing vouchers) may be quite important. Under a universal mandatory voucher system, the ability of a future government to make rather arbitrary cuts would be much greater.[6]

3. How thoroughgoing is the voucher? Does it provide full capitation for all Medicare services or the actuarial equivalent or only partial capitation? What time period is involved? Partial or short-term vouchers—for outpatient care only, for inpatient care only, for a month, and so on—are seldom mentioned, but they are certainly possible.[7]

4. How will voucher values vary according to circumstances? No one expects flat-rate vouchers because one size clearly does not fit all, and TEFRA rates have already established the precedent of variable Medicare contribution. Possible adjustment factors include geographic area, characteristics of the beneficiary (e.g., demographics, history of spending, medical history or status), or even the amount that beneficiaries themselves are willing to spend (or perhaps their disposable income).

5. Does the voucher, like cash entitlements, allow a beneficiary to benefit financially from choosing a lower-price plan or are only in-kind inducements allowed? "Cash back" may be popular for selling cars, and the case for it under vouchers is conceptually strong, but Congress is leery of it for medical care, as the history of HMO-CMP payment shows.[8]

6. Are beneficiaries allowed or expected to supplement the public voucher with their own money (as through private Medigap policies now)? And what assistance, if any, will government make available to poor people for supplementation—aside from possible eligibility for Medicaid?

7. What is the anticipated relationship to other payers, especially Medicaid, which covers so many of the very needy elderly? Will cost sharing apply? On a sliding scale?

8. How many regulatory "strings" will be imposed on participating plans and on beneficiary choices among them? Any voucher arrangement necessarily turns over to beneficiaries, and to the private plans competing for their patronage, most responsibilities for making microlevel trade-offs in plan design and operations. But there remains considerable potential for a rather large public role. Possible provisions include conditions of participation for eligible plans—regulation of minimum benefits, open enrollment, quality of care, and so on—a role for government as the broker or market maker for private plans, and a role as a supplier of information. There exists a macrolevel tension here: the more that government tries to structure the market and protect its beneficiaries, the less scope there will be for significant innovation in cost containment and benefits design at the microlevel.

The case for vouchers

The voucher strategy is meant to bring three major benefits. The first and historically foremost is cost containment (Newhouse 1982; Friedman, LaTour, and Hughes 1984). Public spending will clearly be more predictable if entitlements are prepaid. Hence the love affair with capitation among the "green eyeshade" people in Washington. But would a practical voucher approach actually save money as opposed to cutting federal contributions surreptitiously?

Briefly, the answer is a definite "perhaps" (for more discussion, see the section entitled, Will Vouchers Undermine Public Support?). The main issue is whether the private sector can better control medical spending than the public sector. Private actors, after all, are closest to actual medical spending. And, as Sloan notes, vouchers effectively "engage recipients themselves in cost containment" by making beneficiaries bear the full marginal costs of their choices and their physicians' (Sloan 1982, p. 162).[9]

Whether long-run savings accrue to the government under vouchers, however, depends on many other factors, including how vouchers are priced to begin with, how values of vouchers are changed over time, what range of selection among plans is allowed, and so on. It is certainly possible that vouchers could result in a better or more efficient choices for beneficiaries, even if the government does not directly benefit compared with other cost-containment options.

The second main benefit of vouchers is less often advanced, namely that vouchers promote beneficiary preferences for medical benefits rather than bureaucratic ones. In today's budget-deficit Washington, improving beneficiary choice takes a back seat to improving federal fiscal status. Wrongly so. Vouchers could well allow the private sector to create a better product, or a better set of products, from the beneficiary viewpoint. Medical care is clearly quite personal. Both personal values and personal circumstances obviously differ, and many people might well want plans different from the standard Medicare model.

Certainly, all manner of different plans operate in the non-Medicare world, even in the same range of premium cost. Moreover, as already noted, many complaints exist about standard Medicare benefits. Some complain about the lack of catastrophic coverage;[10] others object to the failure to cover outpatient drugs, alternative, nonconventional providers, "wellness" benefits, and so on. In order to make public changes to a universal Medicare program, full collective consensus is needed, and everyone must agree at once. It thus takes a long time to put in a new hospice benefit, to add catastrophic stop-loss, to cover cyclosporine for transplant recipients, or to make any other change—as painful experience shows. Might it not be better to allow people to act on their own (within subgroupings), according to their interests or tastes, and thus to allow some experimentation, even though some failure might occur as well? Vouchers would surely allow plan designers and beneficiaries to make numerous trade-offs much more flexibly and quickly than a wholly public system. Moreover, new technologies could readily be added to coverage without the need for public cost-effectiveness analysis or complex political bargaining (on technology, see Office of Technology Assessment 1982).

What types of plans would emerge under vouchers? The main alternative not now available would presumably be some form of fee-for-service plan that differs from the organized IPA model of an HMO. New plans would need to establish either new cost controls that would make them more competitive or significantly improved benefits that would make them worth their extra cost. Fee-for-service has many attractive features, which along with professional dominance helps to explain its traditional popularity. Fee-for-service naturally encourages productivity—too much so under traditional open-access insurance. And, unlike capitation, it provides a steady and fiscally enforced stream of information about time, place, and nature of service. This type of information, although perhaps little used today, is essential not only for utilization reviews of many kinds but also for evaluating or influencing access to and quality of care, the next major challenge for all payment systems.

Some nontraditional controls would clearly be necessary. Current possibilities include at least forms of managed care, more sophisticated utilization review, direct negotiation of fees, and restructured cost sharing. Organizations accepting all or part of a voucher might include conventional indemnity insurers, PPOs, loose groupings of physicians (short of an IPA), specialty "HMOs" for chronic conditions, aggressive third-party payers, and large employment-based health plans. But it would be unwise to predict just what successful arrangements might evolve.

Ironically, the voucher idea began as a way to promote HMOs vis-à-vis traditional, unorganized fee-for-service. With cost-containing HMOs now widespread and growing rapidly, vouchers may offer the best way for restructured fee-for-service to survive under Medicare, with participants making their own quality-cost trade-offs rather than living with centrally imposed ones.

The third advantage, almost never articulated, overlaps the first two somewhat: vouchers and private plans would make government less intrusive in a very personal and sensitive area. This is attractive on its face, as anyone can attest who has tried to obtain exceptions to public rules. In an unappreciated way, keeping a lower government profile could improve cost containment in the long run, as savings increasingly must come from changing the style of care or rationing access rather than from relatively simple cutting of alleged "fat" in the system. Government will have a hard time openly saying no to a benefit or an identified patient in need. Private plans may be able to confront such trade-offs more successfully;[11] the PPO incentive of only partial coverage of disfavored providers shows one such approach.

These advantages must be argued mainly on a conceptual level at this point because there is so little experience with vouchers for public beneficiaries. Private workplace groups often operate on a voucherlike, multiple-choice basis, especially that supergroup known as the Federal Employees' Health Benefits Plan (FEHBP), after which Enthoven (1980) modeled his proposal for reform.[12] The FEHBP continues to function successfully, despite predictions of instability and insufficient cost control.[13] Public analogies come largely from housing and education. There is limited empirical evidence from those fields that vouchers do work, in the sense that consumers seem to be benefited vis-à-vis traditional providers, mainly teachers and public housing developers (Sloan 1982; MacRae 1986; Struyk 1981).

The case against

The commonly cited disadvantages of vouchers tend to be argued on a practical level (Luft 1984; Ginsburg 1981). Four concerns seem to predominate.

1. Will not adverse selection kill vouchers? Selection can occur not only in the original enrollment but also in disenrollment. The fear is that repeated cycles of "cream skimming" and "dumping" would make any system unstable or unfair. A particular fear is that government itself will lose if the public model of Medicare disproportionately keeps expensive beneficiaries, while inexpensive ones opt for private coverage.

2. How can private plans compete on the basis of price and quality with Medicare itself? Cited here are the administrative advantages of a single plan, the additional sales and informational costs associated with multiple plans, and the loss of large, centralized buying power.

3. Will not beneficiaries (at least a significant number of them) make bad mistakes when left on their own? This objection is flatly paternalistic but is a significant concern, especially for the most vulnerable population.

4. Will not a voucher plan be the first step on the slippery slope of destroying Medicare as we now know it? If only disadvantaged people are left in the public plan, say some, public support will erode. Alternatively, vouchers might serve as a smoke screen for across-the-board cuts not achievable through direct political action but only through the back door under the guise of improving choice.

The next four sections consider these objections, one at a time.

Risk Selection

How large a problem?

Under vouchers, both beneficiaries and plans that deal with them would have incentives to segment themselves according to expected spending levels. The policy objection is that with risk segmentation, differences in plan performance (and price) would reflect not success in achieving medical efficiency but rather success in attracting low-expense enrollees and shunning high-expense enrollees. Under these circumstances, one of a number of alternatives must occur, all of which are unacceptable to certain observers. Either the government must raise the general level of vouchers to cover high-expense enrollees in high-premium plans (thus, most likely also oversubsidizing the low-expense plans), or the high-expense persons must be left to bear the extra financial expense themselves, or the high-expense style of plan would be driven out of the market. In the case where Medicare itself is the residual option for Medicare beneficiaries, it itself might become the high-expense plan and could not be driven out of the market. It would instead incur much larger than expected spending, thus undercutting one of the goals of a voucher system.

Risk selection is as natural as self-interest. Any system offering multiple options is going to have selection effects. The real questions are how large they are and how significant. Unfortunately, evidence bearing on these issues seems quite mixed. The phenomenon of risk selection is easily described, but there is substantial disagreement over its extent and implications (see, e.g., Scheffler and Rossiter 1985; McClure 1984). Some analysts contend that selection problems are endemic to large multiple-option plans, such as the federal employees' plan (Price, Mays, and Trapnell 1983). There are also reports that employers are increasingly concerned that HMOs are cream skimming by charging community- rather than experienced-based rates for their employees, thus raising total costs to the employer because of selection (Luft, Trauner, and Maerki 1983; Jackson-Beeck and Kleinman 1983).[14]

It is notable, however, that the private market—whether for private or public sector employees—continues to offer a multiplicity of options. Employers and employees certainly seem to like choice. Despite claimed problems of adverse selection, these multiple options have been maintained, both in the federal plan and in almost all private plans.

A final note: it is difficult to separate adverse selection from moral hazard.[15] The type of plan that "loses" under selection is the high-benefits plan, such as the traditional Blue Cross/Blue Shield style of coverage, as opposed to the commercial plan; the high-option plan as opposed to the low; and, presumably, any residual federal Medicare plan compared with private entrants under a voucher system. The losing plans do attract and retain people who expect to have or who do have higher expenditures (also, those who are very risk averse, as many beneficiaries are). But it is difficult to disentangle how much of the difference is due to inherently higher risks and how much is due to a benefits and payment structure that encourages demand for care and fails to control utilization.

Thus, the true issue may not be empirical but normative—essentially that bad plans drive out good ones. Those who favor good plans with a high style of coverage do not like plans that reward low utilizers of care, including those who are willing to become low utilizers in response to the plans' incentives and controls.

Some responses to the problem

A number of responses exist to reduce selection or its consequences for federal taxpayers. The federal government could avoid the issue entirely by transferring the problem to the private sector through universal, mandatory vouchers. Then, only participating insurance companies or beneficiaries could lose through the process, not the government, whose contribution would be fixed by the voucher levels. This passing-the-buck response is conceptually unsatisfying and probably is politically unfeasible in any event.

Various design features could attack the extent to which risk selection could occur. One is to mandate certain minimum benefits in participating plans. For example, one could bar extremely high cost sharing (which would differentially attract persons with very low expectations for spending) or "cash-back" provisions. One could also require a balanced structure of benefits that would attract both low and high utilizers (such as high cost sharing plus coverage for chronic conditions). Mandatory open-enrollment periods in theory would allow even high-expense people to opt into low-priced plans and thus frustrate undue cream skimming, but such requirements are extremely difficult to enforce in practice.[16]

Two financial adjustments also address selection issues. One is the extent of premium borne by the beneficiary/employee, as opposed to that borne by the government/employer. Many or most employment-based plans do not charge the full actuarially accurate premium to each enrollee; rather, some amount of cross-subsidy is expected of the high-expense plans. Such a cross-subsidy might be preserved in Medicare. This cuts down on the incentive for low-expense utilizers to leave those plans.

Second, at least in theory, one could eliminate selection by pricing the vouchers to accurately reflect expected costs of each Medicare beneficiary. This would eliminate any incentive to select by type of plan. The practical difficulty is that existing methodologies only very imperfectly predict utilization. Perhaps these methods can be improved (Anderson and Knickman 1984; Lubitz, Beebe, and Riley 1985; Newhouse 1986), but the history of the HCFA's attempts to set a capitation rate for HMOs shows some of the problems (Trieger, Galblum, and Riley 1981; Hornbrook 1984).

A great deal of variation in spending exists that cannot be predicted in advance, at least by those distant from the actual medical care. Age, sex, race, medical diagnosis, and history of spending all influence the likelihood of future spending, but a great deal remains unexplained. The critical question is whether beneficiaries can predict those expenses, even when outside observers cannot. To the extent that variation is random from the viewpoint of the beneficiary, no rate adjustment is needed; and it has been argued that most high and low risks in one year in fact regress toward the mean (Welch 1985). There may also be political or legal problems with using certain actuarially accurate rating categories—including race and sex—as gauges to public entitlement.

An alternative to improved actuarial prediction is more rough-and-ready, after-the-fact adjustments. Rather than seeking precise advance rates, a viable system could set approximately correct rates and then observe the outcomes. For example, federal overseers could monitor plan performance on a group basis, which simplifies issues somewhat, taking action against what in hindsight seems to be cream skimming. Or individual beneficiaries' patterns of use could be followed before and after enrollment. Similarly, if observable categories of patients were seen to get insufficient service, their rate(s) could be raised, somewhat arbitrarily if no precise figure can be calculated.[17]

One recent development also bears on the risk-selection issue. Some employment groups now cover their own aged workers and retirees, thus acting as primary insurer for those still working and as secondary insurer for retirees primarily under Medicare. Negotiations are under way with some employment groups to run an integrated system (primary plus secondary) under a voucherlike arrangement. Specifically, both General Motors and Chrysler have proposed an arrangement whereby they would receive a lump sum payment for all of their beneficiaries from the government, which they would then supplement with monies they otherwise would have spent providing "Medigap" coverage (Scheier 1987; Rundle 1986).

Whether or not such arrangements are feasible and desirable remains to be seen. They would hold government harmless against any selection effects, which would be the problem of the employment plan(s). Beneficiaries would also gain by having continuity of insurance choices before and after retirement. And the actual plans might better meet their needs than Medicare would.

On the other hand, employees would receive fewer choices than they might in a broader voucher plan open to all beneficiaries. It could also prove quite difficult to establish the appropriate voucher amounts. That is, these populations may be quite different from Medicare at large—perhaps lower expense because they contain a disproportionately healthy long-time group of workers, perhaps higher because these workers have had a lifetime of high-style coverage. In any event, some companies seem convinced that they can achieve enough efficiencies through innovative controls and integration of benefits to make a profit.

Finally, it is notable that the real objection may not be selection adverse to the government but rather the inability of the poor to pay for the better-value coverage available to those with means. In short, the main problem is the spectre of a multi-tier system of insurance. Of course, a multi-tier system already exists, as many beneficiaries cannot afford to pay for higher-priced physicians or to buy Medigap. Vouchers might make these differences more overt, but they would also facilitate one obvious solution—income-related support—that is harder to achieve when no advance payment by beneficiaries is involved, as none is under today's Part A.

Cost Containment

The private sector cannot compete

The next most commonly heard objection to a voucher plan is that voucher plans cannot work because they cannot compete with Medicare on the basis of cost (Congressional Budget Office 1981). The argument is that private plans can no longer economize better than Medicare itself in the era of TEFRA and DRGs. There are two main reasons for supposing that Medicare is difficult to compete with. First, Medicare has very low administrative costs. As the main plan available to the elderly and disabled, it has no sales costs. Moreover, its claims settling and other administrative costs are low for a variety of reasons, especially the enormous volume of claims. In contrast, a voucher system would have additional costs of central administration—approving plans, monitoring them, explaining them to beneficiaries—plus the private administrative costs of the individual plans.

Second, Medicare receives a rather large "discount" below prevailing payment levels in the private sector, especially for hospitals but also for physicians. To what extent this discount is justified by lower costs and to what extent it imposes cost shifting on other payers is hotly debated. This discount existed even under so-called incurred-cost reimbursement, and it is often thought to have increased under prospective payment. Hospital discounts, of course, hold the beneficiary harmless, at least in the financial sense, because hospitals are required to accept the Medicare payment as full payment other than required cost sharing.

On the physician side, the Medicare economic index has for years held down the rate of increase in physician payments to a degree seldom matched by private payment arrangements. Here, however, the "savings" to the government have to be offset against the increase in expense passed on to the beneficiaries, who are not held financially harmless and must instead pay any difference between Medicare prices and prevailing market levels. The recent physician fee freeze moves toward using government buying power to protect beneficiaries from balance billing.

Even more savings may be possible, using Medicare's near-monopsony power as a very large purchaser. According to some observers, it would be unwise to break up this potential power by fragmenting beneficiaries.

Private cost containment

The first comment to make is that Medicare's purchasing leverage has hardly solved its fiscal problems (e.g., Hook 1986). There seems to be ample room for improvement. Indeed, in the long run, public Medicare may find it difficult directly to confront the hard trade-offs inherent in further economizing. And competition may be a better motivation than the public budgeting process.

With regard to medical spending, the cost question comes down to a kind of trade-off: can private plans through a variety of cost-sharing and other incentives, utilization controls, and restructuring of delivery vehicles achieve greater savings than can Medicare itself through exercise of large-purchaser power? Some are convinced that this is so (Califano 1986). It is also clear that under TEFRA, participating HMOs and CMPs at least think they can achieve such savings in a way acceptable to beneficiaries (leaving aside the cream-skimming argument).[18] This is an empirical question that can ultimately be resolved only through a market test or experiment.[19] Commercial payers and third-party administrators also successfully compete in the private market against Blue Cross/Blue Shield plans that get large discounts, apparently by offering more control over utilization and more tailored benefits structures.

Although Medicare's actions in the prepayment era superficially seem to demonstrate its superior clout in dealing with providers, the very price-cutting now imposed by Medicare has also tended to legitimize cost-containment devices once thought unthinkable. This new climate makes more active administration by private plans seem far more attractive than it might have a few years ago.[20] Moreover, integrating Medigap and Medicare administration could deal with the higher medical spending created by Medigap policies that normally fill in the cost sharing originally designed into Medicare, without substituting any utilization reviews or other cost-containment devices now common in integrated plans.

Finally, with regard to administrative costs, it is notable that many of the apparent disadvantages of vouchers come from simply internalizing costs that already exist but that are now borne by private parties. Beneficiary search costs are high in the Medigap market, and loss ratios (benefits paid as a percentage of premiums) are low. Integrating basic Medicare coverage plus Medigap under a voucher should improve overall administrative efficiency. It is also notable that a voucher scheme would at least eventually create a rather large market, under which principles of group sales and administration could begin to achieve economies relative to the largely individual Medigap market. This would also save individuals' search costs. Moreover, with integrated administration, groups could also begin to deal with gaps in benefits not reached even by the new catastrophic provisions of Medicare, such as balance billing by physicians for routine services.

Bad Consumer Choices

The problem

Offering choices raises the prospect that some people will make bad choices. And some Medicare beneficiaries are extremely vulnerable. There are many tales of abuse in the Medigap market, and the history of public HMOs is not without blemish. Vouchers will exacerbate this problem, goes this argument, because all choices will govern an entire plan (as for an HMO), not just a supplement to it.

A response

Voucher proponents can counter that good choices for improved value will outweigh mistakes. This is a value judgment based on a guess. More practically, they can note that beneficiaries are not so well off under the current regime. Beneficiary information in general is poor (LaTour, Friedman, and Hughes 1986). This is true with regard to choosing an individual provider, a Medigap policy, or an HMO or CMP.

Moreover, many or most Medicare beneficiaries are no more impecunious or less intelligent than the population at large in making insurance choices. It does seem somewhat disingenuous for federal policymakers, on the one hand, to promote choice among the federal workforce through the FEHBP and in the private market by mandating dual choice for HMOs and yet not to allow full choice under Medicare coverage. One wonders what magical threshold is passed when a retired worker becomes eligible for Medicare, although the need for paternalism must grow as some beneficiaries reach very advanced ages.

Furthermore, under any reasonable voucher system, including proposals to mimic the federal employees' plan, there should be considerable public efforts to structure the system of choice and to approve participating plans. There should also be greatly enhanced information given to consumers, not only about the choices available to them (which is not much now helped by the federal government) but also about their objective situation and likely need for coverage. Beneficiaries now have extremely little information about their likely needs, most obviously with regard to Medicare's failure to cover long-term care. That government allows such serious misinformation to persist, despite repeated documentation that people misperceive their situation, seems nothing short of a scandal.

A voucher system could also structure a safety net to protect people against bad choices. One such is the ability to revert to Medicare proper or to change from one plan to another at year's end. This protection could be made stronger by allowing transfer at any time, rather than only during a yearly open-enrollment period, but only at the cost of reducing the incentives for making good choices (reasonable quality-cost trade-offs) to begin with.

No doubt, quality of care will be difficult to monitor under a voucher arrangement. But it already is. Vouchers' advantages here are that they reward quality and price competition and allow more innovative approaches. Medicare's best-quality weapon is one not much used now—enormous amounts of utilization and outcome data maintained on a population basis (unlike that available to many private plans, except the very largest).

It is also possible that under a full voucher system, a true intermediary would emerge to help individuals make choices, rather than merely dealing with them at arm's length like a traditional insurer. The most obvious possibilities are private employers' continuing involvement for retirees and further growth of association-style coverage modeled on the American Association of Retired Persons (AARP) model for Medigap.

If bad choices were deemed totally unacceptable, vouchers could be limited to group-style operations (which is, after all, how most of those under sixty-five get their coverage today). Another design possibility would be to bar cash rebates so as to reduce the temptation to make improvident trade-offs of money against future medical need. One might also start any voucher system incrementally—beginning with those deemed most able to help themselves, the younger and the employed, and expanding only as success is demonstrated.

Will Vouchers Undermine Public Support?

Vouchers as a smokescreen for cuts

The fourth major argument against vouchers is that they would facilitate or encourage government economizers to make cuts that otherwise could not occur. There are at least two variants. One is that by making dollars the entitlement, rather than entitling beneficiaries to actual services, a voucher system would allow cuts to be made that would be unacceptable in a service program (e.g., Bovbjerg, Held, and Pauly 1982). A related argument is that once the elderly separate themselves into various subgroups (some of them better off under vouchers), the political coalition that supports very high Medicare spending for all would be weakened, and cuts would become more feasible. Either way, vouchers would be a first step down the slippery slope of abandoning the traditional Medicare goal of incorporating the needy elderly into a single-tier system of high-style medical care.

A contrary view

Vouchers obviously attract government economizers. But so do DRGs and other current approaches. Under DRGs and other administered prices, the price comes first and the standard of service available for that price is determined in the marketplace thereafter. These approaches differ from vouchers only in degree, in that only one hospital episode or one physician visit is affected at a time. In a way, any DRG cuts in service that occur (e.g., "quicker and sicker" hospital discharges) are even more surreptitious than cuts in the real dollar value of a voucher. The insurance market would quickly show the effects of voucher cuts, whereas program administrators cutting medical spending can always argue that only "fat" is being trimmed, whatever the merits of this contention.

Moreover, dollar programs are not necessarily easier to cut than medical ones. One may note that Social Security and Medicare have both been under economizing pressure, and that the former deals in dollars, the latter in services. Query which program more successfully has resisted direct and indirect cuts, if that is the concern.[21] It is even possible that relatively well-to-do beneficiaries may support vouchers more than they support the current system.[22]

Finally, if cuts or restructuring are going to occur anyway because of government deficits, vouchers at least get feedback from beneficiaries on how much they value different types of coverage. It is unknown whether patients would prefer, for example, to get outpatient drug coverage instead of such extensive inpatient coverage. Under a voucher system, plans might well be able to offer such trade-offs and thereby considerably improve the welfare of patients at any given price level.

Time for Testing

The $64 question in this area is whether beneficiaries want voucher-style choices. In the abstract, it is possible to argue that beneficiaries want very complete coverage under standard Medicare plus Medigap precisely so as to avoid having to make many choices. It seems premature to do so, however, because preferences may change, given the changing fiscal climate of the current program, as well as developments in health insurance generally. It is one thing to assert that the entire class of Medicare beneficiaries needs to be treated paternalistically and another to assert that they want to be. On the other hand, there are reasons to be cautious of assuming that particular vouchers would work as intended.

Such empirical issues deserve resolution now. Relatively controlled trials threaten little harm and offer significant potential gains. Going one step beyond TEFRA to promote PPOs and other new possibilities certainly seems worthy of a number of demonstrations, just as HMO demonstrations preceded and coincided with the TEFRA expansions. Experiments could be limited to certain regions and made subject to certain constraints.

Many innovations now commonplace were thought impractical when first proposed. Only time and a fair trial can determine what works and what does not. It is time for a trial.

Notes

This chapter was written with support from The Urban Institute and an honorarium from the University of Pennsylvania. It also draws upon earlier work done under an HCFA grant to develop competitive proposals for Medicare's ESRD program (no. 14-P-98275/3-01). I thank these funders for their support and also want to acknowledge my intellectual debt to Clark C. Havighurst (for whom I pinch-hit at the Leonard Davis Institute's conference), as well as to Philip J. Held, Mark V. Pauly,

Pete Welch, and the commentators at the conference. All opinions offered are, of course, my own responsibility.

1. Voucher as a term has gone out of favor, largely because of negative connotations. Many people see it as a code word for public abandonment of beneficiaries. So, many proponents of vouchers have abandoned the term itself. A very good paper by Ginsburg and Hackbarth (1987), for instance, creates the term private health plan options (PHPOs) to describe voucherlike choices allowable under TEFRA. This chapter continues to call a voucher a voucher. Voucher at least is both pronounceable and commonly understood and implies no reduction in government commitment to beneficiaries. Others are encouraged to develop a more palatable name for political usage.

2. The capitation amount cannot exceed 95 percent of the adjusted average per capita cost (AAPCC) for the region. (Adjustments deal with variations by age, sex, disability, as well as Medicaid and institutional status.) Moreover, if a prepaid plan's adjusted community rate (ACR) is less than 95 percent of AAPCC, it is paid only the ACR. The ACR is calculated from the HMO's or CMP's non-Medicare costs, adjusted upward to reflect the greater number of services used by Medicare populations. Alternatively, the HMO may "spend" the difference between the ACR and the AAPCC by upgrading services to beneficiaries, reducing their out-of-pocket payments.

3. The most publicized problems have occurred in the nation's largest Medicare HMO, International Medical Centers in Miami, which has been forced to suspend Medicare operations (Meyer 1987). At least twenty-four HMOs are said to believe that Medicare price-setting for HMOs results in unreasonably low payment and are expected to drop Medicare risk contracts at the end of 1987 (*Medicine and Health* 1987).

4. See, for instance, the chapters by Lave and Scheffler in this text.

5. Funding levels also crucially affect the actual impact of another economizing method for federal medical programs—"block grants" for states to operate formerly categorical programs of federal assistance. Depending on funding, they may expand state discretion and promote innovation or simply motivate cutbacks within the existing categorical structures (see, generally, Bovbjerg and Davis 1983).

6. The health sector is now witnessing what many hospitals perceive as a change in the ground rules they expected under Medicare prospective payment; rather than a yearly increase pegged to an inflation index, the actual changes have been politically determined and much influenced by evidence on hospital margins. Such greater budgetary control over spending growth is, of course, part of the appeal of a mandatory system.

7. One HCFA demonstration sought to create a voucherlike system under which kidney dialysis patients could shop for the best-value dialysis facility. The payment unit was not full capitation but rather the thrice weekly dialysis session only (see Bovbjerg, Held, and Diamond 1987).

8. Conceptually, allowing people to take the difference in cash is quite reasonable, where their voucher has been correctly priced. After all, if beneficiaries are willing to accept, say, high deductibles or stringent management of their medical care, should they not benefit from their self-imposed discipline? Perhaps the poor ought not be allowed to trade current cash for future cost sharing, but there are many well-to-do elderly. Pricing correctly is easier said than done, however, and policymakers worry about adverse selection, as discussed more below. Moreover, there is considerable political resistance to the appearance of any cash benefit in a medical program. (See Bovbjerg, Held, and Diamond [1987] for an analysis of a voucherlike demonstration that called for ESRD patients to share in the savings of their choosing a low-priced dialysis unit for care. The provision that patients receive cash proved a political weakness.)

9. Moreover, private plans would presumably combine the administration of the basic Medicare voucher benefits with the accompanying Medigap benefits, which would probably create economies.

10. Since this chapter was written, one version of catastrophic coverage was nearly enacted. Even getting serious consideration for this reform was a long time in coming.

11. See Havighurst, Blumstein, and Bovbjerg (1976) for a lengthy exposition of this possibility.

12. This plan stands as a striking counterexample to the fear that vouchers are promoted only by

people who want to cut coverage. Although the subtitle of his book emphasizes the cost-containment benefits of a voucherlike approach, the subtitle of an earlier article on the same topic indicated another theme, namely expanding health coverage into a full national health insurance scheme (compare Enthoven 1980 with 1978).

13. But large premium increases seem to be in the offing as this chapter is written (Causey 1987).

14. Another indication of growing employer concern about selection costs is the apparent attractiveness in many workplaces of the so-called triple-option approach to health plans. The three options are a traditional relatively open access plan, but with high cost sharing, one or more HMOs, plus a Preferred Provider Organization. Many employers are seeking to have triple-option plans all underwritten by a single insurance company, so as to make the insurer face any risk-selection costs that may arise.

15. Pauly makes this point most effectively.

16. Enthoven (1980) proposed to mandate such open enrollment.

17. The problem here is whether program administrators could operate in such discretionary fashion. The legal arguments are beyond the scope of this chapter, but I note that it would be appropriate to look to FEHBP precedents as well as regulatory ones. The market gives some protections that the law should recognize—compared, for instance, with purely regulatory federal provisions.

18. Almost all HMO savings compared with uncontrolled fee-for-service care, like traditional Medicare, seem to come from significantly reduced hospitalization rates (Luft 1981)—an area that well-run managed care systems seem capable of addressing.

19. It is, therefore, far from clear that cost concerns should block experimentation by would-be economizers. It hardly seems logical to object that an entrepreneur should not be allowed to try to fly just because the prediction is that he or she will not succeed. So long as the costs of failure are borne by the entrepreneur rather than the public and its beneficiaries, it seems insufficient reason for banning the attempt. Clearly, the Medicare population contains a high proportion of people commonly believed to be very vulnerable and deserving of public protection. In practice, this means assuring that they would not be injured in any crash by a high flier who failed. Such protection obviously can come in the form of entry requirements, requirements for reinsurance, and requirements of high capitalization to cover any loss during the voucher period. So long as Medicare itself, run by HCFA, remains an option at the close of the voucher period, clearly any beneficiary in a failed plan could revert to Medicare without long-term losses. Many of these ideas are standard insurance regulatory protections that have been applied for generations.

20. Moreover, it is conceivable that Medicare itself could use its clout to pass through price cuts under, say, DRGs to private plans bought by Medicare beneficiaries with vouchers. There is apparently precedent for this in experience with HCFA demonstrations.

21. Of course, it is also a concern that the program be able to economize successfully.

22. See, for example, Pauly's chapter in this book. The argument is that better-off beneficiaries can supplement Medicare more easily under vouchers than under DRGs and Medigap and hence will support the program better politically. Such people may have the most political clout of the elderly, as well.

References

Anderson, G., and J. Knickman, "Adverse Selection Under a Voucher System: Grouping Medicare Recipients by Level of Expenditure," *Inquiry* 21:135–143, Summer 1984.

Bovbjerg, R. R., and B. A. Davis, "States' Responses to Federal Health Care 'Block Grants': The First Year," *Milbank Memorial Fund Quarterly,* 61(4): 523–560, 1983.

Bovbjerg, R. R., P. J. Held, and L. H. Diamond, "Provider-Patient Relations and Treatment Choice in the Era of Fiscal Incentives: The Case of the End-Stage Renal Disease Program," *Milbank Memorial Fund Quarterly*, 65(2): 177–202, 1987.

Bovbjerg, R. R., P. J. Held, and M. V. Pauly, "Pro-Competitive Health Insurance Proposals and Their Implications for Medicare's End-Stage Renal Disease Program," *Seminars in Nephrology*, 2(2): 134–172, June 1982.

———, "Privatization and Bidding in the Health Care Sector," *Journal of Policy Analysis and Management*, 6(4): 648–666, 1987.

Califano, J. A., *America's Health Care Revolution: Who Lives? Who Dies? Who Pays?* New York, NY: Random House, Inc., 1986.

Causey, M., "U.S. Workers Face Insurance Premium Rise," *Washington Post*, A1, A10, September 5, 1987.

Committee on Ways and Means, U.S. House of Representatives, 98th Congress, 2d Session, Subcommittee on Health, *Proceedings of the Conference on the Future of Medicare*, Committee Print WMCP: 98–23, Washington, DC: U.S. Government Printing Office, 1984.

Congressional Budget Office, *An Analysis of the National Health Care Reform Act of 1981 (H.R. 850)*, Washington, DC: CBO (staff working paper), 1981.

Division of National Cost Estimates (Office of the Actuary, HCFA), "National Health Expenditures, 1986–2000," *Health Care Financing Review* 8(4): 1–36, Summer 1987.

Dowd, B., and R. Feldman, "Biased Selection in Twin Cities Health Plans," in Scheffler and Rossiter, eds., 1985.

Durenburger, D., "Medicare Voucher Act of 1986 (S. 1985)," *Congressional Record*, S 17991-96, December 18, 1985.

Ellwood, P. M. et al., *The Health Maintenance Strategy*, Excelsior, MN: InterStudy 1970; reprinted in *Medical Care* 9:291ff., 1971.

Enthoven, A. C., "Consumer-Choice Health Plan: A National Health Insurance Proposal Based on Regulated Competition in the Private Sector," *New England Journal of Medicine*, 298:709–720, March 30, 1978.

———, *Health Plan: The Only Practical Solution to the Soaring Cost of Medical Care*, Reading, MA: Addison-Wesley, 1980.

Evans, F. O., "Physician-based Group Insurance: A Proposal for Medical Cost Control," *New England Journal of Medicine* 302:1280–1283, 1980.

Feder, J. M., *Medicare: The Politics of Federal Hospital Insurance*, Lexington, MA: D.C. Heath, 1977.

Feder, J. M., and B. Spitz, "Hospital Payment," in J. Feder, J. Hadley, and J. Holahan, eds., *National Health Insurance: Conflicting Goals and Policy Choices*, Washington, DC: Urban Institute Press, 1980, pp. 301–347.

Freund, D., and E. Neuschler, "Overview of Medicaid Capitation and Case-Management Initiatives," *Health Care Financing Review*, 1986 Annual Supplement, 21–30, December 1986.

Friedman, B., S. A. LaTour, and E. F. X. Hughes, "A Medicare Voucher System: What Can It Offer?" 55–78 in Committee on Ways and Means, 1984.

Friedman, M., *Capitalism and Freedom*, Chicago, IL: University of Chicago Press, 1962.

Ginsburg, P. B., "Medicare Vouchers and the Procompetitive Strategy," *Health Affairs,* 1(1): 39–52, Winter 1981.

Ginsburg, P. B., and G. M. Hackbarth, *A Private Health Plan Option for Medicare,* R 3540 HCFA, Santa Monica, CA: Rand Corporation, July 1987.

Harris, R., *A Sacred Trust,* New York, NY: New America Library, 1966.

Havighurst, C. C., J. F. Blumstein, and R. Bovbjerg, "Strategies in Underwriting the Costs of Catastrophic Disease," *Law and Contemporary Problems,* 40(4): 122–195, Autumn 1976.

Havighurst, C. C., and R. Bovbjerg, "Professional Standards Review Organizations and Health Maintenance Organizations: Are They Compatible?" *Utah Law Review,* 1975(2): 381–421, Summer 1975.

HCFA (Health Care Financing Administration), "Medicare Program; Payment to Health Maintenance Organizations and Competitive Medical Plans" (final rule), (TEFRA) *Federal Register,* 50(7): 1314ff., January 10, 1985.

Hook, J., "Medicare Budget Facing 'Triple Jeopardy'," *Congressional Quarterly Weekly Report,* 44(3): 115–120, January 18, 1986.

Hornbrook, M. C., "Examination of the AAPCC Methodology in an HMO Prospective Payment Demonstration Project," *Group Health Journal,* 13–21, Spring 1984.

Iglehart, J. K., "Medicare Turns to HMOs," *New England Journal of Medicine* 312(2): 132–136, 1985.

Jackson-Beeck, M., and J. Kleinman, "Evidence for Self-Selection Among Health Maintenance Organization Enrollees," *Journal of the American Medical Association,* 250(20): 2826–2829, November 1983.

Langwell, K. M., and J. P. Hadley, "Capitation and the Medicare Program: History, Issues and Evidence," *Health Care Financing Review,* 1986 Annual Supplement, 9–20, December 1986.

LaTour, S. A., B. Friedman, and E. F. X. Hughes, "Medicare Beneficiary Decision Making About Health Insurance: Implications for a Voucher System," *Medical Care,* 24(7): 601–14, July 1986.

Lubitz, J., J. Beebe, and G. Riley, "Improving the Medicare HMO Payment Formula to Deal with Biased Selection," in Scheffler and Rossiter, eds., 1985.

Luft, H. S., *Health Maintenance Organizations: Dimensions of Performance,* New York, NY: Wiley-Interscience, 1981.

————, "On the Use of Vouchers for Medicare," *Milbank Memorial Fund Quarterly/ Health and Society,* 62(2): 237–250, 1984.

Luft, H. S., J. Trauner, and S. Maerki, "Rising Premiums in Multiple Option Health Insurance Plans: Causes and Potential Solutions," paper presented at the American Public Health Association Annual Meeting, Dallas, TX, November 15, 1983.

MacRae, N., "Education: The Most Important Choice So Few Can Make," *The Economist,* 19–24, September 20, 1986.

Marmor, T., *The Politics of Medicare,* Chicago, IL: Aldine, 1973.

McClure, W., "On the Research Status of Risk-Adjusted Capitation Rates," *Inquiry,* 21:205–213, Fall 1984.

Medicine and Health (newsletter), "Many HMOs Will Leave Medicare," Washington, DC: McGraw Hill, 41(41): 1, col. 1, October 19, 1987.

Meyer, H., "Biggest HMO Contract Pulled," *American Medical News,* 30(19): 1, 33, May 15, 1987.

Newhouse, J. P., "Is Competition the Answer?" *Journal of Health Economics,* 1: 109–116, May 1982.

———, "Rate Adjusters for Medicare under Capitation," *Health Care Financing Review,* 1986 Annual Supplement, 45–55, December 1986.

Office of Technology Assessment, *Medical Technology Under Proposals to Increase Competition in Health Care,* Appendix C: Federal Employees' Health Benefits Program, Washington, DC: OTA, 1982.

Paine, T., *The Rights of Man,* original edition, London: J. S. Jordon, 1791.

Price, J. R., J. W. Mays, and G. R. Trapnell, "Stability in the Federal Employees Health Benefits Program," *Journal of Health Economics,* 2(3): 207–224, December 1983.

Rundle, R. L., "Several Employers and Unions Propose To Administer Retirees' Medicare Plans," *Wall Street Journal,* 48, August 18, 1986.

Scheier, R. L., "HCFA Experiments with Paying Industry for Retirees Health Care," *American Medical News,* 30(2): 1, 36, May 15, 1987.

Scheffler, R., and L. Rossiter, eds., *Biased Selection in Health Care Markets,* vol. 6, *(Advances in Health Economics and Health Services Research),* Greenwich, CT: JAI Press, 1985.

Sloan, F. A., "Issuing Medicaid Vouchers," in R. J. Blendon and T. W. Moloney, eds., *New Approaches to the Medicaid Crisis,* New York, NY: FS Press, 1982, pp. 159–175.

Smith, A., *The Wealth of Nations,* original edition, London: W. Strahan and T. Cadell, 1778.

Struyk, R., *Housing Vouchers for the Poor,* Washington, DC: Urban Institute Press, 1981.

Thomas, J. W., R. Lichtenstein, L. Wyszewianski, et al., "Increasing Medicare Enrollment in HMOs: The Need for Capitation Rates Adjusted for Health Status," *Inquiry,* 20(3): 227–239, Fall 1983.

Trieger, S., T. Galblum, and G. Riley, "HMOs: Issues and Alternatives for Medicare and Medicaid," Baltimore, MD: HCFA, Office of Research, Demonstrations and Statistics, April 1981.

U.S. Congress, Social Security Amendments of 1965, Public Law 89-97, 79 *U.S. Statutes at Large,* 286–423, 1965.

———, Social Security Amendments of 1972, Public Law 92-603, 86 *U.S. Statutes at Large,* 1329–1493, 1972.

———, The Health Maintenance Organization Act of 1973, Public Law 93-222, 87 *U.S. Statutes at Large,* 914–936, 1973.

———, Social Security Amendments of 1976, Public Law 94-460, 90 *U.S. Statutes at Large,* 1945–1960, 1976.

———, The Tax Equity and Fiscal Responsibility Act of 1982 [TEFRA], Public Law 97-248, 96 *U.S. Statutes at Large,* 317, August 27, 1982.

Welch, W. P., "Regression Toward the Mean in Medical Care Costs," *Medical Care,* 23(11): 1234–1241, November 1985.

3. Positive Political Economy of Medicare, Past and Future

MARK V. PAULY

Introduction

Medicare was created in a political process, and its evolution is determined by political decisions. The purpose of this chapter is to offer some thoughts on why it took the form that it did, why it has changed over time in the way that it has, and how it is likely to change in the future.

Somewhat surprisingly, there has not been a very elaborate development of the positive political economy of Medicare. There has been extensive discussion of what Medicare ought to be or ought to have been, but little formal analysis of why it is as it is. There are at least two reasons, one suspects, why this is so. First, there is less demand for positive analysis. The Health Care Financing Administration (HCFA) itself or other special interests have funded or sponsored much of the research on Medicare, and there is usually little interest on the part of a decisionmaker in himself or herself being made the object of analysis. In addition, there is no fully satisfactory positive political theory in general, in the sense of a theory that links changes in exogenous influences with final outcomes. Thus, the process by which changes in underlying demands for activities of the public sector get translated into actions is just not well understood, and alternative theories are difficult to test.

Nevertheless, it seems useful to reconsider existing theories of the political economy of Medicare, both to see what we have learned and what might be expected for the future. As is discussed below, most existing theories explain the emergence and evolution of Medicare as a result of the interaction of various political pressure groups (Marmor 1973; Alford 1975). More recent models differ from earlier ones in supposing that new types of groups have somehow emerged, and that these new configurations help to explain why the Medicare program has changed (Brown 1985). This type of analysis is useful, but it is incomplete in two ways. It does not explain where these new groups come from; conversely, it does not relate changes in the Medicare program to the striking changes that have occurred in the broader environment in which political choices are made.

There have been significant changes in the economic and demographic characteristics of the elderly since 1966, changes that almost surely mean that anyone's preferred version of Medicare would be different now from what it was then. In addition, there have been substantial changes in relative prices and types of medical care. Moreover, at least some additional important changes can be forecast for the future. What do these kinds of changes in the environment say about the evolution of Medicare up to the present, and what do they suggest will happen in the future?

Here there are two contradictory explanations. Some see the increasing relative numbers of the elderly pushing the political process toward redistribution in favor of the elderly and, incidentally, away from children as the major rival age-related group (Preston 1984). Others note the possibility of a backlash by the young workers, who must bear the burden (Davis and Van den Oever 1981).

Compared with its situation in 1966, the over-sixty-five population today (1) is richer on average but with heterogeneity in economic resources; (2) is healthier on average but with a large share of frail persons; (3) is politically more potent but with some possibility of an under-sixty-five backlash; and (4) is buying higher-quality medical care, which improves health but costs many times more per unit and in total than it did when Medicare began. Although there is some room for exceptions, many of these trends are likely to continue for the next twenty years. What changes in Medicare have been or will be induced by these changes in the circumstances (and numbers) of the elderly relative to the rest of the population?

In this chapter, I explore some positive theories of political economy intended to answer those questions. I first try to summarize what I think are the important changes in the circumstances of the elderly, the circumstances of the rest of the population, and the "production possibilities" available for medical care that might be expected to cause people in the political process to want something different. I next develop a simplified base-case median voter model in which the decisive voter is not currently elderly but is concerned with his or her own old age, with the well-being of other elderly, current and future, and with the taxes that would be required for any level of support.

The *analytic* strategy examines separate models of (1) a selfish voter who cares only for his or her own welfare, (2) one who cares about the well-being of elderly family members (intrafamily externalities), and (3) one who cares about the well-being of unrelated elderly. This approach is done solely to make it easier to examine each of these different motivations—motivations that are all surely present for most voters. There is absolutely no intimation here that one type of motivation is more important or more praiseworthy than another.

I then add the possibility that the outcome is altered by the presence of various intense minorities, both on the demand side and on the production side. I finally consider how defined groups with defined interests might form and add an element of endogeneity in group formation to the model.

These three models—the simple median voter model, the model with exogenous pressure groups, and the model with endogenous groups—are applied to the history of the first twenty years of Medicare. Surprisingly, even the simple model seems to do fairly well in terms of its ability to explain. Then I apply these models to some forecasts in changes in the external environment in the next twenty years, and I use that to draw some conclusions about where Medicare is likely to go in the future.

Changes in the Circumstances of the Elderly

The economic, social, and demographic characteristics of the elderly population made eligible for Medicare on July 1, 1966, doubtless had some influence on the form the program took. While there was some attempt to foresee future demographic and economic developments, and while some aspects of program design may have anticipated this future, it is surely the case that there have been some important unexpected changes in the circumstances of the elderly and the rest of the population since 1965–66. Indeed, given the large changes that have occurred, the relative absence of major changes in Medicare until recently is a striking testimony to the power of political inertia. Nevertheless, there have been some changes in both the environment and in Medicare, and more may be anticipated for the future. Changes in demographics, increases in the prices of medical services, and changes in the rest of the economy are all likely to be influential.

Demographic changes

The most frequently noted change in the circumstances of the elderly is demographic. As shown in Table 3.1, the ratio of the number of the elderly relative to persons of working age has grown from 0.174 in 1965 to 0.193 in 1985. Virtually all of the growth has come from an increase in the proportion of persons seventy-five and over. The over-sixty-five ratio will increase only slightly until 2005 but then is forecasted to take a spectacular jump. Increased longevity among the elderly fuels the growth in all periods, and the leap after 2005 comes

TABLE 3.1
Ratio of Elderly Population to Other Adults, 1960–2025

Year	Persons 65–74/ persons 18–64	Persons 75+/ persons 18–64	Persons 65+/ persons 18–64	Persons 65+/ covered workers 18–64
1960	0.111	0.057	0.168	0.245
1965	0.112	0.062	0.174	0.225
1970	0.108	0.066	0.174	0.218
1975	0.110	0.070	0.180	0.217
1980	0.113	0.073	0.186	0.217
1985	0.115	0.078	0.193	0.227
1990[a]	0.117	0.089	0.206	0.251
1995	0.117	0.097	0.214	0.255
2000	0.107	0.104	0.211	0.252
2005	0.102	0.107	0.209	0.252
2010	0.113	0.105	0.218	0.268
2015	0.140	0.108	0.248	0.307
2020	0.167	0.120	0.287	0.344
2025	0.188	0.145	0.333	0.411

[a]U.S. Bureau of the Census, Projection (middle series), series P-25, number 952.

Source: U.S. Bureau of the Census, Current Population Reports, series P-25, nos. 519, 917, 985. The fourth column is from the U.S. Social Security Administration, Annual Statistical Supplement to the Social Security Bulletin, other reports, and unpublished data.

from the combined effect of this influence and the aging "echo" of the birth rate changes that brought on the baby boom. Even more striking is the growth in fraction of those seventy-five and over.

Income/wealth

Increases in Social Security payment levels, which have exceeded increases in incomes for the rest of the population, have resulted in improvement in the economic situation of the elderly both absolutely and relative to the rest of the population. As Boskin (1986, p. 23) notes, "the huge growth of Social Security benefits, their indexing, the expansion of private premiums, the availability of alternative means of support, and the nature of the inflation and growth performance of the U.S. economy from the late 1960s to the early 1980s rendered the elderly the group in the population with by far the largest relative gains in its standard of living." Table 3.2 compares the percentage and ratio of persons living at or below the poverty level and living at or below 125 percent of the poverty level. The number of elderly (sixty-five and over) in poverty began in 1966 at a much higher level than that for the total population, but the number has since fallen to a level below that for the rest of the population. If noncash benefits are taken into account, the percentage in poverty is even lower than the double-digit figures shown, as low as 3.5 percent, according to Census Bureau figures (1984).

While there is some ambiguity about exactly how to measure well-being, there is no doubt that welfare of the elderly relative to the rest of the population has improved considerably since 1966. Table 3.3 provides some measures of average income and consumption expenditures for persons in households headed by the elderly for selected years. Average household income for the elderly has improved relative to the nonelderly since 1972–73. This ratio changed because the real income of elderly households grew substantially, while the real income per household for the rest of the population was approximately constant. Relative income and expenditures per capita have not changed over the period, but the level is higher for the elderly than for the nonelderly. I do not mean to imply that there is no poverty among the elderly; widows in particular are especially likely

TABLE 3.2
Percent and Ratio of All Persons and Elderly Living at or Below Poverty Level and 125% of Poverty Level for 1966–85

	1966	1970	1975	1980	1985
Below poverty					
Total	14.7	12.6	12.3	13.0	14.4
65+	28.5	24.5	15.3	15.7	12.4
Ratio	1.94	1.94	1.24	1.21	0.86
Below 125% poverty					
Total	24.1	17.6	17.6	18.1	19.4
65+	NA	33.9	25.4	25.7	21.1
Ratio	NA	1.93	1.44	1.42	1.09

NA = not available.

Source: U.S. Bureau of the Census, Current Population Reports, series P-25, nos. 147, 149, and earlier reports.

TABLE 3.3
Average Per Capita and Household Income and Expenditures by Age of Head of Household for Selected Years 1972–83

		1972	1980	1983
Household income	Under 65	$13,767	$22,170	$25,478
(before tax)	65+	6,778	10,898	14,232
	Ratio 65+/under	0.49	0.49	0.56
Per capita income	Under 65	4,543	7,659	9,091
(before tax)	65+	4,236	6,411	8,372
	Ratio 65+/under	0.93	0.84	0.92
Household	Under 65	10,302	18,688	21,223
expenditures	65+	5,671	10,754	13,335
	Ratio 65+/under	0.55	0.58	0.63
Per capita	Under 65	3,416	6,482	7,643
expenditures	65+	3,544	6,326	7,844
	Ratio 65+/under	1.04	0.98	1.03

Source: U.S. Bureau of Labor Statistics.

to slip through the safety net. What is most relevant for the following discussion, however, is the indisputable conclusion that poverty is now much less characteristic of the elderly, as a whole, relative to the rest of the population than it was when Medicare was passed.

Living situation

Table 3.4 indicates that the elderly are less likely to be living with (and presumably dependent on) people other than their spouse. The percentage of elderly males living with their spouse has increased since 1965. In contrast, the percentage of females living independently has risen strikingly, as has the percentage of women living in institutions.

Medical care expenses

It almost goes without saying that total medical expenses for the elderly and expenses paid by Medicare have risen over time. Table 3.5 shows reimbursements per Medicare enrollee and expenditures per elderly person. As compared with

TABLE 3.4
Living Arrangements for the Elderly by Sex

		1965	1970	1975	1980
With spouse	M	67.9	69.9	74.0	71.8
	F	34.1	33.9	35.6	34.7
With others	M	15.2	11.5	7.4	10.1
	F	32.6	27.4	22.8	21.5
Independent	M	13.1	14.1	14.2	14.1
	F	28.6	33.8	36.0	36.9
Institution	M	3.8	4.5	4.4	4.0
	F	4.7	5.0	5.6	7.0

Source: U.S. Bureau of the Census, *1980 Census of the Population,* volume 1, chapter D, part 1, PC-80-1-D1-A, Washington, DC: U.S. Government Printing Office, March 1984.

TABLE 3.5
Per Capita Medical Expense and Medicare Reimbursements for the Elderly, 1977 and 1984

	1977	1984	Percent change 1977–84
Medicare reimbursements per elderly	$ 788	$2,051	+160
Total medical expenditure per elderly	$1,785	$4,202	+135
Medicare as a percent of total	44	49	+11.4

Source: *Health Care Financing Review,* Winter 1984, and unpublished data from the Bureau of Data Management and Strategy.

TABLE 3.6
Mean Out-of-Pocket Health Costs as a Percent of Income for
Persons 65 Years of Age and Over, Selected Years 1966–84

Year	Mean out-of-pocket expenditures	Mean personal income	Out-of-pocket as percent of income
1966	$ 300	$ 2,000	15
1977	690	5,592	12
1981	1,187	8,639	14
1984	1,575	10,615	15

Source: U.S. Senate, Special Committee on Aging, 1984.

expenditures per capita for those under sixty-five, both expenditures and Medicare payments have risen more rapidly. However, as Table 3.6 indicates, the percentage of income the elderly spent out-of-pocket was actually as high in 1981 as it was just before the passage of Medicare. Of course, because income has risen, the amount of real income spendable on other goods and services has also risen for the elderly over this period.

The picture then is one of ever-larger transfers of resources consumed in medical care for those sixty-five and over but with a modestly increasing burden borne by the elderly themselves. It is clear that the public sector has disproportionately shouldered the medical care burden of the elderly, as compared with the rest of the population.

Positive Models of Political Choice

Given such changes in circumstances, what alterations in the form of the Medicare program would one expect to occur? To answer this question, I sketch a simple model of the choice of Medicare benefits by a nonelderly median voter.

A base-case, selfish voter model of the choice of Medicare benefits
It is assumed that the voter with median preferences for Medicare is not elderly but expects to endure a period of tax payments before Medicare eligibility is obtained. Let us first examine any nonelderly individual's preferred level of benefits *if* he or she were only concerned about his or her welfare in the periods of work and retirement. We also initially assume that the population is stable, so that pay-as-you-go financing is equivalent to full funding.

The individual then faces a trade-off between the tax rate paid when working and the public medical insurance benefits he or she may expect to receive when retired. How would changes in this individual's external circumstances, either occurring in the present or forecasted for the future, be expected to change the form of the preferred postretirement medical insurance policy?

To begin to answer this question, we first need to say something about the extent of socialization of this decision. For the present, we simply assume that postretirement health insurance is to be provided uniformly, via taxation, to all persons sixty-five and over who are eligible for Social Security. Later, we offer some reasons for making this assumption, as well as a discussion of situations in which it will not hold.

There is, however, another critical assumption we need to make. The median voter in any period is decisive only for the level of Medicare taxes and benefits in that period. This means that there is no necessary connection between the level of benefits a nonelderly person supports when working and the level he or she will receive at age sixty-five. The optimal pattern of taxes and spending for any individual is, therefore, a zero level while working and a very large level after retirement. But the individual can be the median voter only when working. Hence, such a single-period, selfish model predicts zero benefits regardless of circumstances, as long as workers outnumber beneficiaries. Such a prediction is obviously not very satisfactory.

Sjoblom (1985) suggests that one assume instead that "commitment to the contract" is possible, so that the voter can make a commitment to pay taxes now for benefits that will persist when he or she retires. Sjoblom provides a game-theoretic rationale for this assumption. For purposes of this chapter, we need only assume that a change in the preferred postretirement benefit level of the median voter leads to a change in the current level of taxes and benefits, which in turn is positively related to a change in the level of benefits actually received.

Given that postretirement health insurance is socialized, what determines this selfish voter's desired level? Increases either in current income or the income he or she expects to receive when retired would usually lead the individual to desire less coverage against a given medical expense, since he or she would be better able to bear the risk of an out-of-pocket payment. However, since the level of medical care demanded—at a given out-of-pocket payment percentage—rises with income, higher income could induce purchase of smaller nominal benefits (measured by coinsurance percentages) but must lead to larger out-of-pocket payments. (This discussion ignores the tax subsidies that have warped private purchases of insurance.)

What would be the impact of an increase in longevity for this voter, when it is coupled with an increase in the number of years of elevated frailty at which one is at risk for higher expenditures? (The level of expected health at any age could rise, but the expected number of years in ages in which average health is low also rises.) If the marginal tax price per dollar of benefits is unchanged, the *total* amount of resources transferred for medical care in the retirement years would probably increase, but it is likely that the *annual* level of desired medical expense benefits at any given level of health would fall. That is, it is likely that desired payments out-of-pocket will be higher in any year at any level of health for a given level of post-sixty-five income. (Of course, since additional longevity also raises the cost of a given pension income, it is likely that the preferred annual level of such pension payments and, therefore, cash income will fall as well.) Thus, if the identity of the median voter was unchanged by an increase in average longevity, desired per year medical benefits would be likely to fall.

What about the impact of increasing medical care price levels? Even beginning an answer here requires an assumption about the nature of those increases. Are they increases in the price for a constant-quality product, caused either by more rapidly rising input prices or increasing inefficiency (with the word increasing being important), or do they represent improvements in quality, with higher expected benefit per unit? If we look at the relationship between medical care expenditure measures and indexes of the prices of specialized inputs to the production process, we find that such relative input prices represent only a fraction of the change in real expenditures—approximately one-fourth in the first decade of Medicare and about half in the next decade (Feldstein 1971). While there is a good deal of circumstantial evidence that health care and especially hospital care is not produced efficiently, it is difficult to believe that efficiency worsened over the period to so great an extent. So it seems safe to conclude that there has been a mixture of increases in real (quality-constant) unit price and in quality—somehow defined—per unit.

Demand for medical care is probably price-inelastic but probably rises with higher quality. Both of these causes suggest that total expenditures will rise when prices rise. Insurance theory suggests that desired coverage, as measured by the total premium, will also rise but the effect on nominal coverage, as measured by coinsurance, is ambiguous. We can say that the desired deductible and the desired average out-of-pocket payment will probably rise, regardless of the cause of the price increase.

Up to the present, it seems reasonable to assume that Medicare beneficiaries experienced approximately the same changes in quality and amenities as did other younger patients. The advent of diagnosis-related groups (DRGs) and physician fee freezes for Medicare alone suggest that this pattern need not continue. In theory, one could imagine a future system in which quality and amenity for Medicare beneficiaries is dictated by the level of spending the Congress and HCFA permit, rather than by the level of cost or charges incurred elsewhere in the privately financed system. How feasible it would be for doctors and hospitals to provide different levels of quality/amenity is unknown. But if separation is possible, then one would need to specify the quality level desired by the taxpayer. If real benefits are to be kept constant, expenditures will continue to rise with medical input prices but need no longer track marketwide service intensity.

In short, all these changes in the expected circumstances after retirement imply that an individual voter who pays a positive tax price for Medicare benefits will desire higher total out-of-pocket payments at a given tax price. The effect of changes in circumstances on nominal coverage is ambiguous, as is the effect on desired insurance premiums, but it would not be unlikely that desired premiums would rise as well.

That the payments are collected via a payroll tax also makes a difference, even for the median voter. The payroll tax, like any feasible tax, has incentive effects of its own; the tax can be avoided by working less for wages. This notion of increasing the marginal excess burden of taxation need not be taken as far as the Laffer curve; the idea that tax-induced distortions limit the desired size of public-sector spending holds even if tax rates are still in the range in which higher rates collect more. The excess burden cost of Medicare benefits depends on the level of *all* taxes on income from work, not just on those taxes earmarked for Medicare or Social Security. If the individual expects higher taxes to pay for a given level of Medicare benefits, this excess burden alone may dampen the demand for benefits, as well as pushing the individual to seek a non-tax-financed method for paying for them.

Identifying the median voter

To apply this demand model in a median voter context, we need to identify the median voter. We assume that the median voter anticipates a proportional increase in his or her (earmarked) Medicare taxes from increases in Medicare spending; all increases would take the form of a surcharge. A more critical assumption is that the median voter anticipates a positive net cost from payments to the elderly. For instance, an already elderly person who pays no payroll tax cannot be the median voter for Medicare Part A benefits.

The Medicare case differs from the Social Security case in that Medicare benefits are not cash. This means that even someone whose discounted future tax cost for an increase in Medicare spending is exceeded by the discounted dollar value of future Medicare spending may well not prefer the increased expenditure, since the dollars of cost may be worth less than equivalent dollars as cash. Of course, for younger workers every dollar of Medicare spending costs more than a dollar, so that these people will unequivocally oppose any increases in spending as long as they can purchase an equivalent private insurance for a premium less than the annual Medicare cost (including administration) per Medicare beneficiary. In effect, depending on the age of the taxpayer, it is as if there is a tax or subsidy on the cost of additional insurance benefits for oneself. Increases in longevity do not change the subsidy rate per additional dollar transferred to the over-sixty-five period.

Each taxpayer will have to decide how much he or she would want to spend per year after retirement. It was argued above that, at any given tax price, the desired amount paid out-of-pocket per year will rise, although the total amount provided by insurance over the whole period of retirement will also probably rise. The main conclusion then is that if the marginal tax price is unchanged, the level of real annual medical care costs desired to be paid out-of-pocket by those sixty-five and over will probably rise over time. Deductibles or coinsurance may well rise, or coverage may be cut in order to accomplish this objective. However, because total medical costs will also be rising, nominal coverage could remain unchanged or even rise. But increasing the cost burden on Medicare beneficiaries is the objective each voter desires, if faced with a constant tax price or share per dollar of the cost of the Medicare program.

Given that the median voter would prefer this change at a given tax price per dollar of Medicare benefits to himself or herself, the crucial question is the change in that tax price. Here there are two conflicting influences. As the age distribution of the population shifts toward older ages, the age of the median voter increases. Since the tax price (in terms of discounted value of taxes) of a dollar of postretirement Medicare benefits falls, the fewer the number of working years remaining, this shift coupled with the trend to earlier retirement reduces the price of a dollar of Medicare benefits to the worker-voter. However, the cohort that will become eligible when the median voter turns sixty-five is also growing, not just because of increasing longevity, which has already been taken into account, but because of the birth rate–induced demographic changes. It is possible that the increase in the numbers of the elderly will increase the burden on the median voter; if the tax rate must rise at all future ages, then this effect of higher taxes in any given year may well offset the effect of paying taxes over fewer years.

Suppose, for example, that a worker expects to earn a constant salary for all years in which he or she works. If there are N workers aged eighteen to sixty-five and M retirees, one can solve for the tax rate that yields enough revenues to pay a given benefit to retirees. Now suppose the age distribution shifts so that the number of retirees per worker rises; the tax rate in any one year must increase in proportion to the ratio of retirees to workers. In contrast, an increase in the age of the worker reduces the expected tax payment by the reduction in the present value of the future stream of tax payments. There is another issue here. In choosing a tax rate and benefit level for the current period, the voter must take account of the number of beneficiaries not only in the current period but also in the future. After all, if today's benefit level is likely to persist, it must be financed in future periods beyond the next one.

External benefits

Now we suppose that under-sixty-five voters do not make choices based only on their own future benefits. Instead, younger persons get utility from Medicare benefits to *today's* elderly, either because the elderly are related to them or because of altruistic feelings. Alternatively, we may suppose that ill health among the elderly is a kind of negative externality. Other things equal, altruistic concern should lead the median voter to support higher benefits to the elderly since additional benefits mitigate externalities, as well as paying for his or her own medical costs when the individual turns sixty-five.

What would be the impact of the changes in the circumstances of the elderly in the desired level of externality-motivated support? An increase in the number of elderly would be expected to decrease the desired level of benefits per elderly recipient since more recipients increases the cost of an increase in per recipient benefits, even while it increases the desired total level of support. Grannemann (1980) found that in a cross-sectional analysis of the Medicaid program, an increase in the number of potential recipients decreased the benefit level per recipient by a significant amount. An analogous story is likely to hold for the elderly, many of whom are on Medicaid in any case.

Other changes in the circumstances of the elderly will reinforce this predicted reduction in externality-motivated support. The proportion of the elderly living alone has also risen over time. Since it is likely that concern for one's relatives close by is greater than that for unrelated individuals or relatives at a distance, the expected effect is a reduction in the general level of support.

This prediction is not completely certain, however, because the distancing of the elderly from their families probably increases the demand for formal assistance, which the medical care system provides, because it makes providing informal assistance within the family more difficult.

Another relevant change in the circumstances of the elderly is the increase in cash income and assets among the elderly. (In part, this increase is probably related to the drop in the birth rate, which precipitated the demographic changes. Other things equal, the fewer the children, the greater the assets a spending unit can save to use in old age [and the greater the motive to do so since children cannot be expected to be available for support].) Whatever the reason, it is obvious that voter demand for publicly subsidized medical care for all elderly will be reduced by the apparent willingness of 60 to 70 percent of the nonpoor elderly to obtain Medigap insurance. Permitting deductibles to rise, or resisting extension of Medicare benefits to pharmaceuticals, is easier when Medigap insurance is expected to take up the financial burden for most of the elderly.

This observation suggests something even more dramatic than a failure of Medicare to keep pace with rising health care costs. Our earlier assumption of full socialization of Medicare may not continue to be valid. To understand more, we need to examine possible reasons for the "uniform benefit" nature of Medicare. There are two (not necessarily inconsistent) explanations of why public insurance for the elderly took the form of social insurance rather than means-tested welfare.

One explanation is that when being old was roughly synonymous with being needy, it was both administratively simpler and politically more palatable to base benefits only on age. Even here, the availability of Medicaid coverage for the poor for expenses that Medicare did not cover, and the purchase of Medigap coverage by the well off, meant that actual coverage was far from uniform. The easy integration of supplemental coverage, public or private, meant that there was less uniformity; the elderly not quite poor enough for Medicaid, but not well enough off to afford private coverage, had the lowest levels of both coverage and use/ expense. Nevertheless, the identification of age with need helped to rationalize the program.

The other influence for socialization, in the sense of uniform publicly provided levels of an excludable good, has been discussed by Usher (1977). He develops a median voter model to show that a commodity is more likely to be socialized the greater the inequality of income and the less diverse the tastes of individuals for the commodity. Usher's model is excessively restrictive in two ways. First, it implicitly prohibits supplementation of the social expenditure— which seems generally implausible for medical insurance, even though Usher developed his model for medical care. Second, it permits only full socialization or zero socialization, not socialization for subgroups of the population. Nevertheless, it may have some relevance.

Medicare did socialize only the elderly and did make supplementation easy. That the elderly were reasonably homogeneous probably served to ease this process. But now things are different. While the great bulk of the elderly have the money and the means to absorb part of the burden for their own care, there is also a sizable minority that cannot, that is even less able to cope with medical care costs than in 1966. Being over sixty-five is no longer a good proxy for being needy; but there are sizable numbers of elderly who are desperately needy, if only because of the poor level of health for this group.

The expected response to these changes of a nonelderly voter motivated by altruism is predictable: he or she will want to increase benefits to the poor and frail elderly but reduce the net benefits and transfers to the nonpoor, healthy elderly. The facade of "social insurance" may begin to crumble.

The push toward means-testing Medicare may be further fueled by some changes that have made or may make supplementation more difficult. The introduction of the DRG system not only introduced a new and more frugal payment method for hospital care for the elderly, relative to the types of coverage chosen by the rest of the population, but it also made supplementation of that coverage more difficult. It is administratively complex for a beneficiary to pay more for a Medicare admission, in order to stay longer or use an expensive hospital he or she prefers. (In contrast, it is easy to cover the deductible with private insurance.) Faced with a lower level of real hospital services per admission once they retire, reasonably well-off elderly may look with increasing disfavor on the Medicare program as their main source of care; they may prefer to continue to exercise choice. If physician payment is also changed to nonsupplementable fee schedules, this dissatisfaction with Medicare may increase among those who want to pay more for higher quality or amenities.

Medicare can be means tested in several different ways. The distributional impact of Medicare may be adjusted either by charging income-conditioned premiums for a uniform set of benefits, as Davis and Rowland (1984) have proposed, or it may be adjusted by varying the level of benefits. Probably some combination of the two elements is most likely.

Would consideration of means-testing Medicare premiums or benefits destine the program to the fate described by the English poor laws? Do means tests have to be demeaning? In an administrative sense, the answer is surely no. We do after all administer a means-tested taxation program, and no one regards it as shameful to report low income for purposes of an increase in one's disposable cash income. There would not seem to be insurmountable barriers to elevating the privilege of receiving more heavily subsidized medical care insurance to be a matter of right for lower-income elderly, something—just like lower taxes—to which they are entitled.

Who would lose in such an "increase-cutback" scenario? The answer is today's or a near-tomorrow's nonpoor elderly. The interesting thing is that this change could be sudden; it may require only a small jump in tax cost to make private insurance (even with high administrative cost and adverse selection) a better deal and, therefore, lead to a desire to replace all of Medicare. This kind of knife-edge behavior has already been exhibited in some cities' public school systems, and it could happen in Medicare, too. But the important thing to note is that a removal of the rigid social insurance linkage could actually lead to a higher level of benefit for the needy by preventing this collapse.

Pressure Group Politics

Would the conclusions about the future course of Medicare be changed if we recognize that public-sector resource allocation decisions are not made by referendum, and that organized intense minorities (pressure groups) often influence the outcome? The answer is probably negative.

First, we need to identify the relevant pressure groups that already exist. (We deal with endogenous pressure groups in the next section.) The most obvious group is the elderly themselves. To put things in perspective, it is useful to note that there was no elderly lobby at all when Social Security was passed and only a weak one when Medicare was passed. The elderly lobby flourished only when benefits once achieved were under threat of sizable cuts. The most obvious prediction then is that the elderly lobby will resist cuts.

However, as long as nothing happens to change the relative power of various lobbying groups, their existence should make little difference to predictions about changes in the level of support. The elderly lobby may have pushed the level of Medicare spending beyond what the median voter would desire, but a downward shift in preferences of that voter should still mean a reduction in spending. So long as the lobby has reached equilibrium, the change in that equilibrium should depend only on changes in external circumstances. Pressure groups may well just add a constant "margin."

The more interesting question is whether the relative power of lobbies has changed and will change over time. For the elderly lobby, there are two important developments. First, its membership will grow over time. Paradoxically, this development may actually result in reduced power since the interests of any single person will become more diffuse. The other question is whether there is some other political issue that is of little concern to the elderly but on which their pledge of support can be politically decisive. The answer here is always hard to judge, given the shifting nature of political currents. However, it does not appear that the elderly vote is one that is easily manipulable and deliverable on a particular issue; the elderly tend to vote on issues in much the same way as younger citizens.

The other major lobby is the provider lobby. In my view, the major turning point here has already occurred. It is conventional among analysts of Medicare policy to view providers as a crucial pressure group, decisive in many administrative decisions against the "true" wishes of public officials. The view comes from thinking of payments simply as transfers, rather than as payments for government-purchased goods. If we recognize that those goods have a cost that has to be covered if they are to be supplied, we see that any provider power can have meaning only insofar as payment levels are high enough to create rents (or quasi rents). For the largely nonprofit hospital sector, such rents in the form of excess profits seem unlikely but may exist in the form of inefficiency or shifting overhead costs to the Medicare program. Rents may exist for physician services, but the sizable number of physicians who reject assignment indicates that Medicare's payment schedule, limited since 1974, probably generates lower rents, although some rent is surely present.

Nevertheless, analysts have persisted in viewing the relationship between the Medicare program and providers as only a zero-sum tug-of-war. In Brown's (1985) view, for example, the Medicare program began by giving providers large concessions in order to buy support. Then it moved through a period of largely ineffective regulatory limits to an era of "technocratic cooperation," in which public officials and provider representatives negotiate budgets and prices, much like the European model of nationalized health systems.

We consider this argument in more detail below. For the present, we simply note that such an arrangement, if it were to exist, would require that both sides have the ability to make credible threats against the other.

Heterogeneity and endogenous political groups

The two major pressure groups for Medicare are the providers and the elderly. When age was synonymous with poverty, poor health, and dependency, and when all providers thought they could extract more resources from Medicare, each of these groups constituted roughly homogeneous lobbying units. But as Stigler (1974) has noted, not only are such lobbying organizations bedeviled by the free-rider problem, there is also the possibility that some subgroups will be taken on a "cheap ride" to a destination they do not prefer. In short, heterogeneous interests cause pressure groups to divide and recombine.

Let us first consider past and present heterogeneity of interests among providers. Hospitals and physicians do, of course, have different interests; the separation of Medicare into two parts was a way to deal with those differences. Within each part, a rough community of interest was maintained until recently, with only relatively minor complaints from specialty hospitals or nonphysician professionals who wanted to share in Medicare revenues.

Recent developments in Medicare policy suggest that this uniformity is eroding and is likely to continue to do so in the future, with the ultimate cause being the pressure on Medicare payment levels. On the physician side, the controversy over relative payment rates for "cognitive" versus "procedural" services has separated internists from surgeons. The split will only become more apparent over time since there is no noncontroversial way to settle the matter. With physician price levels for all physician services apparently in excess of the amount needed to bring forth an adequate supply of appropriate quality services, there is no economic point in trying to measure the relative costs of different services; equalizing the level of monopoly rents is only a matter of distribution, not of efficiency. But precisely because the issue is one of distribution of a fixed (or shrinking) sum, both game theory and common sense mean that there will not be unanimity of interest. Moreover, the movement of Medicare reimbursement policy toward a bidding model will also increase heterogeneity.

Hospitals have been more successful in maintaining uniform treatment. The obsession with "equity" in DRG policy—almost to the exclusion of considerations of willingness to supply—indicates that that uniformity may be fragile. It may well also fall under bidding and voucher-type models.

The most important kind of heterogeneity for Medicare policy is that among elderly beneficiaries. As noted above, the split of the elderly into "haves" and "have-nots" will make it difficult to maintain a united social insurance facade. On the one hand, the "adequate care" that taxpayers may feel is appropriate for the poor elderly may be insufficient in terms of quality, ease of access, or amenity for those well-educated, well-to-do elderly with strong preferences and the financial and social means to fulfill them. If, for example, the DRG payment mechanism continues to lead to financial stringency, it is unlikely that wealthy elderly will tolerate the standards of amenity and the hospital lengths of stay those payment levels imply. They would be willing to pay more if that is what it takes to get more, rather than be held to a "poor folks" standard. In contrast, the financial threat of high out-of-pocket payments or uninsured services is much more serious to low-income elderly. While both groups would prefer to maintain high levels of provider payment and quality and low levels of out-of-pocket costs, it is likely that they will differ in what they would prefer to sacrifice. Amenities are less valuable if you are poor, and out-of-pocket payments are less of a burden if you are not.

Applying the Models

This lengthy discussion of positive theories of Medicare policy formation yields some insights in interpreting past policy. The motives discussed above, both selfish concern for one's own welfare and concern for others, family members or not, were presumably the rationale for the enactment of Medicare. While no one would maintain that the poverty of the elderly was the sole reason for the passage of Medicare, it is equally foolish to suppose that their relative poverty in 1965, which was an undeniable fact, did not help to get Medicare enacted. Moreover, other reasons for passage, such as the possibility of adverse selection in the private market, have not worsened over the years to offset the erosion of altruistic motives.

After a year or two of adjustment, the history of the Medicare program has been one of extreme concern about cost, and a steady reluctance to expand nominal benefits beyond their 1966 levels. Some have argued that the story of this period is best represented as a continuous and ultimately fairly successful attempt by public-sector administrators to overcome unforeseen or politically unavoidable inflationary activities of providers. The initial failure, in this view, was a congressional oversight in not providing sufficiently robust administrative controls (Feder et al. 1980).

The story of congressional error is not especially persuasive since Congress may well have made the choices it did precisely because it wanted to buy high-quality care and a high level of access; it realized that limits on prices and restrictions on behavior would inhibit such a policy. What is not clear is whether politicians anticipated the future growth in prices that would be associated with such a blank check policy. But whether they anticipated but pretended not to notice in order to get Medicare passed, or whether they truly suffered from myopia, the pattern of Medicare policy over time has been quite consistent: an attempt to reduce costs while maintaining de jure benefits, except for increases in Part B premiums and Part A deductibles. For example, the extended care benefit was redefined administratively so as virtually to disappear, and the hospice and home health benefits have been severely restricted.

One result of this policy has already been discussed. Out-of-pocket payments for nonpoor elderly have risen more rapidly than inflation, at a rate sufficiently high that they represent the same average percentage of income as they did before Medicare was passed. At the same time, public expenditures per beneficiary have also been rising rapidly in real terms. All of this is consistent with the view that rising incomes, rising prices of specialized inputs, and rising medical quality mean higher expenses for the elderly and higher expenses for taxpayers.

In addition to the increase in monetary out-of-pocket payments, Medicare has shifted higher nonmonetary costs onto beneficiaries in order to reduce the cost to taxpayers. By limiting the rate of growth in physician payment since 1974, the program until recently caused fewer physicians to accept assignment, with a resulting reduction in access for those beneficiaries unwilling to pay any excess bill or to pay at the point of service and be reimbursed.

The most serious attempt to impose additional nonmonetary cost on beneficiaries is, of course, the DRG payment system for inpatient care. Hospitals predictably responded by shortening length of stay. But since earlier discharge does not mean earlier recovery, it is certain that this step has shifted the burden of caring for a convalescing patient onto the patient's family and friends. This action was probably economically efficient, in the sense that, on average, the real resource cost of the reduced days of stay exceeded what the family would have paid to avoid providing care itself. Nevertheless, it is also clear that even while total social costs may have been reduced, a larger share of cost has been shifted from the Medicare program (i.e., from taxpayers) and onto beneficiaries.

So much for the past and the present. What is likely to be politically feasible Medicare policy in the future? Forecasting the future as a response to exogenous influences obviously requires forecasting the movement of those influences. The demographic changes discussed earlier are predictable. We will assume continued growth in real income among the elderly. (To the extent that income growth has been due to Social Security benefit increases or other pay-as-you-go pensions, some slowdown might be expected, for the same demographic reasons discussed earlier.) We will also assume improving longevity. Finally, we will suppose that the heterogeneity in wealth and health among the elderly will not diminish.

Table 3.7 provides some data from which a rough idea of the strength of the conflicting demographic influences can be determined. The second column shows the median age of the voting age population. Since voter participation varies across age groups, the third column indicates the median age of the population that would have voted if the proportion of each age level voting was the same in all years as in the 1984 presidential election.

Table 3.8 shows the rate of change in the median voter age for three twenty-

TABLE 3.7
Median Age of Voting Population for Eligible Voters and Estimated Actual Voters, 1960–2030

Year	Median age of eligible voters (18+)	Estimated median age of actual voters (18+)
1960	41	47
1965	42	47
1970	42	47
1975	40	47
1980	39	47
1985	39	46
1990	40	46
1995	42	47
2000	43	48
2005	44	49
2010	46	50
2015	47	52
2020	48	53
2025	48	53
2030	48	53

Source: U.S. Bureau of the Census, Current Population Reports, series P-20, no. 397 and earlier reports; and unpublished data.

TABLE 3.8
Rates of Change (percent) for Median Voter Age (Eligible and Estimated Actual) and for the Ratio of Elderly to Younger Adults, 1965–2025

	1965–85	1985–2005	2005–25
Percent change in median age of eligible voter (18+)	−7.1	12.8	9.1
Percent change in median age of estimated actual voter	−3.2	6.5	8.2
Change in ratio 65+/18–64	10.9	8.3	59.3
Change in ratio of 65+ weighted[a]/ 18–64	14.1	13.7	54.1

[a]Over 65 weighted in three groups: 65–74, 75–84, 85+.

Source: U.S. Bureau of the Census, Current Population Reports, series P-25, nos. 397, 519, 917, 985; and unpublished data.

year periods for each of these measures. The bottom two rows show the rate of change in two measures of the elderly burden. The third row uses the simple ratio, while the final row weights age groups (sixty-five through seventy-four, seventy-five through eighty-five, and eighty-five and over) by their relative medical expense in 1981.

As can be seen, there was actually a fall in the age of the potentially decisive voter from the passage of Medicare up to the present; however, the worker tax burden of the elderly also grew at a relatively modest rate. For the next twenty years, the burden will grow at almost the same rate, but the voting population will shift more toward older ages. These changes suggest that on demographic grounds alone, there should be less pressure to cut Medicare in the relatively near future. But after the year 2005, the large increases in the dependency ratio, coupled with only modest growth in median voter age, suggest that strong pressure for cuts may begin soon after the turn of the century.

One critical assumption that is more difficult to make concerns the change in quality and real relative price of medical care services. The 1984 slowdown in the rate of growth in costs suggests that inflation is not inevitable, but the 1985 figures nevertheless suggest a continued rise in the real relative price.

The next decade or so, therefore, may bring something of a respite in pressures to cut or constrain Medicare; the crucial issue is what happens to the real price of medical services. If this price cannot be limited, even the respite may not occur. After this period, the picture is clearer. The predictable consequence of virtually all of these influences is a continued shifting of part of the cost of medical care onto the elderly, particularly after the year 2000.

The form that burden shifting will take is more difficult to predict, but one can expect that real deductibles and copayments could rise, along with premiums. If medical costs overall continue to rise, and if the acceptable level of quality for Medicare beneficiaries is not to fall appreciably, the increasing burden of health care costs on the elderly could be accompanied by a continuation of the trend toward growing transfers from the rest of the population toward the elderly. With rising prices, backlash and burden can coexist.

However, particularly after the turn of the century, the demographic trends, coupled with the other pressures toward low spending, suggest a real possibility that actual transfers could be reduced to the elderly as a group. Especially if Medicare continues to move toward payment mechanisms that are difficult to supplement privately, both the young and the nonpoor elderly may agree that a uniform universal insurance system for old people is no longer in their best interests.

It is not impossible that the improvements in service intensity and quality will not be missed by patients. If the private sector follows Medicare in changing payment levels and methods, this reduction will be less detectable. The pressure for this shift will intensify over time, as the age of the median voter stabilizes and he or she comes to anticipate the tax cost–increasing demographic changes early in the twenty-first century. All of the influences, except for the age of the median voter, point toward cutbacks.

Conclusion

What of the method of payment of providers, as opposed to benefit-level efforts? Brown has argued that the DRG innovation signifies a movement toward "more centralized and direct strategies, . . . initiating a period of 'technocratic corporatism' in which administrators and providers will engage in increasingly structured negotiations over the details of reimbursement policies." He hypothesizes that "the growth of the role of the central government in health care financing is leading to a stronger sense of a 'corporate' interest and agenda among bargainers for the public, which in turn is gradually inducing providers to clarify and unify their own positions in order to offer a more coherent and weighty corporate presence in dealing with their public sector interlocutors . . ." (Brown 1985, p. 579).

My view is rather different. I would not forecast a growing role for the central government. As large parts of the elderly population become capable of planning and financing their own health expenses at the margin, I foresee a reduction of the government insurance to a base catastrophic plan, possibly at rising cost but of less importance to the total. Moreover, I see the public sector increasingly adopting bidding or voucher models for both its poor clients and its nonpoor fallback coverage. While some negotiation always occurs in a bidding context, especially when the quality of the product is subject to variation, I see increasing movement toward an arrangement in which only some providers "win" the bids, with the bid then setting the value of a supplementable voucher. Rather than unity among providers, I see diversity. This diversity will be encouraged by voucher-type arrangements that permit those beneficiaries who do not prefer the winning bidder to transfer resources elsewhere.

This diversity, caused and facilitated by a voucher-type model, seems likely to continue regardless of the voter-equilibrium level of benefits. It seems unlikely that even in the 1990s, when the age of the median voter is increasing, the program will be willing to pay enough to keep up with the expenses and prices paid by fee-for-service medicine and conventional insurance. Although not all the elderly will benefit from this movement to exclusive contracting, at least for the next twenty years it seems likely that it can be maintained. After that, the demographic trends turn increasingly ominous.

This chapter has, it should be emphasized, been an exercise in *positive* theory. It is intended to predict what is likely to happen, not judge it as being desirable or undesirable. By conventional economic criteria of efficiency and equity based on income or wealth alone, many of the changes to be expected seem to be, if not desirable in themselves, at least the best accommodation that can be made to the demographic and economic changes that are sure to occur. There are some potential problems that from a normative viewpoint we might wish to guard against, especially the possibility that the truly needy elderly will be lumped together with the more numerous and more affluent elderly in a program of cutbacks. A moderately noncontroversial normative political economy theory would suggest, in contrast, that transfers continue to be made to these groups, even if some differentiation and means testing is required.

In contrast, if one adopts the normative view that the elderly have a right to transfers solely on the basis of age (and regardless of wealth) or that uniform social insurance programs are desirable per se, it will be more difficult to find a silver lining. Perhaps the major benefit is the fact that the upcoming pressures will cause all of us to rethink and reevaluate the way we think about the elderly or about age in general in the society of the future.

References

Alford, R., *Health Care Politics: Ideological and Interest Group Barriers to Reform,* Chicago, IL: University of Chicago Press, 1975.

Boskin, M., *Too Many Promises: the Uncertain Future of Social Security,* Homewood, IL: Dow Jones-Irwin for the Twentieth Century *Fund,* 1986.

Brown, L., "Technocratic Corporatism and Administrative Reform in Medicare," *Journal of Health Politics, Policy and Law,* 579–599, Fall 1985.

Browning, E. K., "Why the Social Insurance Budget is too Large in a Democratic Society," *Economic Inquiry,* 16:133–138, January 1978.

Davis, K., and D. Rowland, "Medicare Financing Reform: A New Medicare Premium," in *Proceedings of the Conference on the Future of Medicare,* Washington, DC: U.S. Government Printing Office, 1984, pp. 149–161.

Davis, K., and P. Van der Oever, "Age Relations and Public Policy in Advanced Industrial Societies," *Population and Development Review,* 1–18, March 1981.

Feder, J., J. Holahan, and T. Marmor, eds., *National Health Insurance: Conflicting Goals and Policy Choices,* Washington, DC: Urban Institute, 1980.

Feldstein, M., *The Rising Cost of Hospital Care,* Washington, DC: Information Resources Press, 1971.

Grannemann, T., "Reforming National Health Insurance Programs for the Poor," in M. Pauly, ed., *National Health Insurance,* Washington, DC: American Enterprise Institute, 1980, pp. 104–136.

Marmor, T., *The Politics of Medicare,* Chicago, IL: Aldine, 1973.

Preston, S., "Children and Elderly in the U.S.," *Scientific American,* 251 (6): 44–52, 1984.

Sjoblom, K., "Voting for Social Security," *Public Choice,* 45 (3): 225–240, 1985.

Stigler, G., "Free Riders and Collective Action: An Appendix to Theories of Economic Regulation," *Bell Journal of Economics,* Vol. 5 (2): 359–365, Autumn 1974.

U.S. Bureau of the Census, "Estimates of Poverty Including Noncash Benefits, 1979–91," Technical Paper No. 51, Washington, DC: U.S. Government Printing Office, 1984.

Usher, D., "The Welfare Economies of the Socialization of Commodities," *Journal of Public Economics,* 151–168, 1977.

4. An Analysis of the Welfare Component and Intergenerational Transfers Under the Medicare Program

□ □

RONALD J. VOGEL

Academics especially need to insist on the obvious in the face of its neglect or denial.

P. T. Bauer, *Reality and Rhetoric*
(Cambridge, MA: Harvard University Press, 1984)

Introduction

The Medicare program came into being on July 30, 1965, when Congress amended the Social Security Act (PL 89-97) by adding Title XVIII, "Health Insurance for the Aged." Medicare consists of two parts: Part A is Hospital Insurance (HI), and Part B is Supplementary Medical Insurance (SMI). Part B was principally designed to pay for physician and ancillary services for the elderly, while Part A, as its HI name implies, was designed to pay for hospital services.[1] The financing of HI was tied to the structure of the existing Old Age, Survivors, and Disability Insurance (OASDI) ("Social Security") with a similar trust fund, while the financing of SMI was to be partially done with premiums paid by the elderly, beginning at age sixty-five, and partially by contributions from the general fund into an SMI trust fund. Unlike OASDI, benefits under both HI and SMI were to bear no relation to past income and contributions into the program but were to be made according to the reasonable costs of an illness episode, no matter what the past income and past contributions of the ill elderly individual. Using insurance terminology, OASDI benefits are "indemnitylike benefits," based upon previous income and, thus, contributions (with a minimum benefit payment for lower incomes), while HI and SMI payments are "service benefits," intended to provide payment in full, based upon the cost of medical services rendered.

As its title implies, the purpose of this chapter is to address a public finance equity issue in Medicare that has been heretofore ignored, although the issue has been explored for Old Age and Survivors Insurance (OASI) (Munro 1976; Parsons and Munro 1978). In many respects, HI is large enough and is sufficiently different from OASI, in both the way its two components (HI and SMI) are financed and in the way that it pays benefits, to merit such an analysis in its own right.[2] Accordingly, this chapter first more fully describes and analyzes the tax and payment provisions of Medicare and the changes that have occurred in it since its inception.

Next follows an analysis of Medicare within a theoretical insurance context. Much analysis has already been done upon the structure and consequences of its deductible and coinsurance provisions; recently, some analytical misgivings have been expressed about the long-run solvency of its trust funds, given current financing arrangements (*Milbank Memorial Fund Quarterly* 1984 and the references contained in the papers therein). It is also common knowledge that Medicare is a subsidized health insurance scheme. What is lacking in the research literature is a careful conceptualization of the nature of this subsidy within an insurance context and quantified estimates of the extent of the subsidy. Any subsidy requires a transfer of resources from one group to another. Thus, the extent of the transfer subsidies in such public programs as Aid to Families with Dependent Children (AFDC) or Health Insurance for the Poor (Medicaid) may be measured by the amount of benefits that the target group receives over and above the taxes that the target group paid. For AFDC and Medicaid, we term this transfer "welfare." In a similar manner, one may estimate the present value of Medicare benefits to the aged relative to the present value of tax or premium contributions by the elderly into the Medicare program. The difference in values gives an estimate of the intergenerational transfer, or welfare component, of the Medicare program.[3] The Medicare program also entails intragenerational transfers that need analysis.

Medicare has also been characterized as an inefficient subsidy (Feldstein 1984). The principal measure of inefficiency is the relative cost of achieving a given objective. One course of action could be characterized as twice as inefficient as an alternative course of action for attaining a given objective if it cost twice as much, all other things being equal. The literature suggests that the primary purpose of Medicare was publicly to provide health insurance for the aged who could not otherwise obtain health insurance (Feder 1977; Long and Settle 1984). What is lacking in the research literature are estimates of the extent of the unnecessary subsidization in the Medicare program. Here, we define "unnecessary" subsidies as those given to the elderly who could and would pay the actuarially fair price of health insurance, had Medicare been less global and more selective in its target population. This analysis, therefore, ignores possible objectives of Medicare such as dealing with possible adverse selection or high private sector selling costs.

Finally, the implications of the above findings are explored with respect to the spectrum of public programs currently available to the elderly, with respect to the deficiencies seen in these programs as a total package for the alleviation of elderly economic need.[4]

The Structure of Taxes, Insurance Premiums, and Benefits Under Medicare

At its inception in 1966, the HI component of Medicare was closely tied to the already existing structure of OASI. They share the same annual maximum taxable earnings base, which was $6,600 in 1966 and which had risen to $42,000 by 1986. In 1966 the contribution rate for both employer and employee was 3.5 percent for OASI and 0.35 percent for HI; by 1986 these rates had increased to 5.2 percent and 1.45 percent, respectively.[5] Until 1984, when it doubled, the self-employed person contribution rate for HI was the same as the employee contribution rate; in 1984 the self-employed person contribution rate for OASI was increased to 10.4 percent. At age sixty-five, the eligible elderly person becomes entitled to both OASI and HI benefits and, if not working, makes no further tax contributions into either program. Tax collections or "contributions" from both HI and OASI are placed in separate trust funds from which the benefits under the respective programs are paid. By 1982 the OASI trust fund was reduced to $4.6 billion in assets and, under the interfund borrowing provisions of PL 97-123, was allowed to borrow $17.5 billion from the HI and Disability Insurance (DI) trust funds. After the HI loan of $12.4 billion, the HI trust fund had $8.2 billion remaining (Social Security Administration 1985). Although the HI trust fund is relatively healthier than the OASI trust fund, it too faces imminent insolvency, even when the OASI loan will have been repaid (Advisory Council on Social Security 1984), given current financing and benefit arrangements.

The SMI component of Medicare is financed in an entirely different manner than either OASI or HI. During their working years, neither employees nor employers directly contribute to SMI. At age sixty-five, the elderly are entitled to voluntarily join SMI and pay a monthly premium. This monthly premium is the conceptual equivalent of an ordinary health insurance premium paid for coverage of physician and ancillary services, except that it is subsidized by federal government contributions from the general fund. Between 1966 and 1974 the monthly general fund contribution exactly equaled the monthly premium paid by the elderly person, $3.00 in 1966 and $6.70 in 1974. Because medical care prices were increasing at such a rapid rate in the 1970s, it was thought that a one-for-one premium match into SMI by the elderly and the general fund would impose too heavy a financial burden upon the elderly (Feder 1977). Accordingly, the general fund monthly contribution increased from $8.30 in 1975 to $46.50 in 1986, while the elderly monthly premium amount increased from $6.70 to $15.50 between the two dates.[6] Premiums collected from the elderly and those paid by the general fund are placed in a separate SMI trust fund from which benefits are paid. Total assets in the SMI trust fund have increased from $122 million in 1966 to $4.9 billion in 1979 and to $9.7 billion in 1984. Unlike the HI trust fund, assets in the SMI trust fund have shown a steady increase, thanks to an increasing share of general fund contributions into it.

Until recently, the manner in which Medicare medical benefits were paid by both HI and SMI was similar to the manner in which the typical Blue Cross/Blue Shield plan paid medical care benefits.[7] That is to say, medical care providers, whether they be hospitals or physicians, were paid on a "reasonable cost" basis for the medical services rendered. With the inception of diagnosis-related groups (DRGs) in 1983, Medicare HI began paying hospitals according to "diagnosis-related groupings" on a fixed-fee per-diagnosis basis, rather than on a reasonable cost basis.[8] Prior to receiving HI benefits, the elderly individual is required to pay a hospital deductible per benefit period that had reached $492 by 1986; no coinsurance payments are required until the sixty-first day of hospitalization, when the daily coinsurance rate becomes 0.25 of the initial $492 deductible (or $123). After ninety days in the hospital, the elderly patient may draw upon a sixty-day lifetime reserve (the lifetime reserve can only be used once), and the daily coinsurance rate increases to 0.50 of the initial $492 deductible (or $246). In 1986 SMI required a $75 annual deductible for physician services and a 20 percent coinsurance rate. In order to obtain help (and further insurance) for the payment of these deductibles and these coinsurance rates, the elderly frequently purchase the so-called Medigap policies from Blue Cross/Blue Shield and the commercial health insurers. Depending upon the amount of premium paid, Medigap policies also cover catastrophic health care costs that Medicare does not cover, such as the expenses beyond the 120th day of hospitalization.

Thus, the total acute health care expenditures by and upon the elderly are greater than Medicare public expenditures upon the elderly. Indeed, much of the discussion about the "unfairness" of Medicare has concentrated upon the growing gap between total acute health care expenditures by and upon the elderly and Medicare expenditures upon them (Davis and Rowland 1986a). While it is true that the poor elderly pay a greater percentage of their incomes on their portion of this gap than do the better-off elderly, much of the discussion about the unfairness of this gap could equally well be applied to any of the consumer prices for the essentials of life that the elderly already have to face, such as those for food and housing.

By way of summary, the typical elderly person becomes entitled to HI benefits at age sixty-five and ceases to make HI tax contributions at that age. This entitlement endures until the person dies. The HI spending commitment bears no relation to prior earnings and, during the period of this analysis, was essentially open-ended, depending solely upon the length of periods of hospital treatment for the elderly person and the "reasonable cost" of each period of treatment, apart from the deductible per benefit period and coinsurance.[9] On the other hand, explicit voluntary SMI contributions (or premiums) do not begin until the person reaches age sixty-five;[10] these premiums are not related to prior earnings nor to income once past the age of sixty-five. As long as the elderly person pays the voluntary premium each month, he or she remains eligible for the essentially open-ended SMI physician and ancillary benefits that, apart from the deductible and coinsurance, are also paid on a "reasonable cost" basis. Total health care expenditures by and upon the elderly are greater than Medicare public expenditures upon them; here, we concentrate upon the value of Medicare public expenditures.

The Insurance Value of Medicare

The demand for insurance in general stems from the fact that there are certain events in the life cycle over which the individual has little or no control and that may strike on a random basis. The insurance literature indicates that most insurable events have three primary characteristics: (1) the probability that they will occur to any given individual is not close to one, (2) their occurrence would have catastrophic financial consequences for the individual or entity involved, and (3) the insurable event itself lies outside of the control of the insured individual. Most kinds of health insurance purchased and sold in the United States violate all three of these characteristics to a greater or lesser extent, when contrasted to, say, life or fire and casualty insurance. For any individual, the probability of incurring mild influenza is large but the probability of incurring liver cancer is small, especially for the young, and yet health insurance covers the treatment of both. The cost of a visit to a physician represents a small part of an individual's income, although many such visits might not represent such a small percentage. Finally, the individual can control how often he or she visits a physician, although the individual cannot legally admit himself or herself to the hospital. For these reasons, commercial insurers of other events were reluctant to sell health insurance before the creation and entry of Blue Cross/Blue Shield into this market (MacIntyre 1962).

Blue Cross/Blue Shield originally employed the concept of "community rating." In such a rating system, all insurees—regardless of health experience, age, sex, or any other distinguishing characteristic for health insurability purposes—pay the same premium into a common pool that is used to pay the health care bill for the collective experience of the covered population. The actual health care benefits received by any individual in this community-rated pool are independent of individual premiums paid in any given year. When the commercial insurers cautiously entered this field, they refined this concept of community rating to "experience rating," which is conceptually nothing more than taking subsets of the community pool, ranging the subsets from high to low incidence of average expenses, and charging a premium to each subset according to the units of its expected health care utilization times the expected price per unit of health care utilization.[11] Whether community or experience rating is used, a common principle underlies the insurability of the group: the pool of insurees has to be large enough so that the mean expenditure and standard deviations around it can be forecast with a sufficient degree of accuracy, so that a premium can be set that will ensure that the insurer can pay all the medical bills of its insurees and its own administrative costs (plus a return on equity for for-profit insurers). Experience rating minimizes, to a certain point, the extent of adverse selection; it also enables an insurer to target its product price in a competitive market. Experience raters have also attempted to minimize the risks of moral hazard by using deductibles and coinsurance. The purchase of health insurance itself is the result of an even bet among a pool of healthy persons that a certain percentage of them will become ill in any given year, assuming no adverse selection and no moral hazard. At the margin, deductibles and coinsurance minimize moral hazard. Whenever illness occurs, income is transferred from the well to the ill on an *ex post* basis. But, everyone within the group pays the same premium and has the same *ex ante* anticipation and probability of incurring losses. Premiums paid by, or on behalf of, individuals are never tied to specific services used by those individuals; if they were, then there would be no purpose for insurance. Presumably, the area under the aggregate experience-rated demand curve for health insurance measures its value to the experience-rated individuals who purchase it.

For purposes of quantification for the measurement of health insurance in the gross national product, we denote this value (which ignores consumers' surplus) as

$$V = \sum_{j=1}^{m} \sum_{i=1}^{n_j} P_{ij}$$

where P is the premium paid by the individuals $1, \ldots, n$, in the experience-rated groups, $1, \ldots, m$. The total value, V, goes to pay

$$V = \sum_{j=1}^{m} \sum_{i=1}^{n_j} p_{ij} q_{ij} + A$$

where p and q are, respectively, the price and quantity of medical services consumed by the $1, \ldots, n$ individuals, in the experience-rated groups, $1, \ldots, m$, and A is administrative costs (or the load factor). The premiums are collected *ex ante* and the medical bills are paid *ex post*. The annual *ex ante* value of the health insurance to any individual in any experience-rated group is simply V_j/N_j (where N is the number of individuals in the group) or the average cost of the experience-rated premium.

Title XVIII of the Social Security Act is specifically entitled "Health Insurance for the Aged." With respect to the previous discussion in this section, Medicare may be classified in insurance terminology according to the following taxonomy. First, the insurer (the entity at risk) is the federal government. Second, the "rating system" that is used would seem to be a hybrid of community and experience rating. Those aged sixty-five and over are singled out as the target group to be insured, and the SMI premium bears some relationship to the health experience of those sixty-five and over. Yet Medicare could also be characterized as a form of community rating. In its first year, Medicare had 18.9 million enrollees, and in 1986 it has 28.0 million (U.S. Department of Health and Human Services 1986). This is one of the largest insurance pools in the world. One of the strongest correlates is that between age and illness/debility (Scanlon 1980; Harrington et al. 1985). Clearly, this large group could have been broken down into smaller age subsets that could, nevertheless, continue to remain large subsets for insurability purposes. For many reasons, including the way that was chosen to finance it, Medicare did not experience rate beyond specifying the aged as its target pool of insurees (see Appendix 4.1). Third, Medicare is a health insurance plan that offers to its target group payment for the *expected value* of the medical services covered under it. Just as with the health insurance offered to the rest of the population under Blue Cross/Blue Shield and commercial health insurance, income is transferred from the well to the ill on an *ex post* basis, although this transfer under Medicare is much more complex due to the present pay-as-you-go financing of Medicare HI and due to the general fund subsidization of Medicare SMI. But, the population paying HI taxes and paying SMI general fund subsidies has approximately the same *ex ante* anticipation and probability of incurring losses, once they become elderly. Each elderly individual paying SMI premiums has the same *ex ante* anticipation of losses as members of the whole group aged sixty-five and over, but within the cohort itself, there may be transfers of income from the less aged to the more aged, to the extent that illness is correlated with advancing age. Fourth, Medicare also attempts to limit moral hazard with the use of deductibles and coinsurance.

As with Blue Cross/Blue Shield and commercial health insurance, the *ex post* experience of the Medicare program in any given year can be expressed as

$$M = \sum_{i=1}^{n} p_i q_i + A_i$$

where M is total Medicare expenditures, p and q are the prices and quantities of medical services consumed by Medicare enrollees $1, \ldots , n$, and A are Medicare administrative costs. The *ex ante* annual actuarial value of M to any given Medicare enrollee is simply M/N, where N is the number of Medicare enrollees. Table 4.1 contains the *ex ante* insurance value of Medicare HI and SMI per aged enrollee, using data for past years back to 1966 and Health Care Financing Administration (HCFA) projections into the year 2003. Once a person reaches the age of sixty-five and becomes eligible for Medicare, he or she will be eligible for Medicare Part A (HI) for the rest of his or her life. Likewise, when the elderly person reaches the age of sixty-five, he or she remains eligible for Medicare Part B (SMI) for the rest of his or her life, as long as the individual pays the monthly SMI premium. The *ex ante* present actuarial value of these benefits can be defined as

$$B_y = \sum_{i=y}^{E} \frac{b_i}{1 + r_i} (i - 1) \tag{1}$$

where

B_y = the present actuarial value of the Medicare benefit in year y;
E = the life expectancy;
r = the discount rate;
b = the actuarial value of the benefit in year y or M/N in the previous discussion.

In contrasting Medicare with conventional health insurance, as purchased by and sold to the under-sixty-five segment of the population, what is clear is that in any given year, for conventional forms of health insurance, premiums collected from the insured population must meet health care cost claims plus administrative expenses if the insurer is to remain solvent. On an *ex ante* basis, each insuree annually directly pays the expected costs of the average loss plus average administrative expenses, and this relationship of premium-to-loss should hold over

TABLE 4.1
Ex Ante Insurance Value of Medicare HI and SMI Per Aged Enrollee or Mean HI and SMI Benefits and Administrative Costs for the Elderly, 1966–2003

Year	Mean HI benefit and administrative cost ($)	Mean SMI benefit and administrative cost ($)
1966	71.22	36.65
1967	182.85	65.97
1968	225.55	81.13
1969	252.01	95.71
1970	269.90	107.50
1971	295.54	114.73
1972	320.33	124.16
1973	345.71	132.51
1974	401.47	145.80
1975	474.30	167.34
1976	550.01	195.82
1977	620.48	224.97
1978	698.44	261.25
1979	784.69	295.00
1980	927.01	339.36
1981	1,088.77	397.99
1982	1,242.41	457.87
1983	1,359.26	532.79
1984	1,480.37	615.80
1985	1,524.94	680.50
1986	1,581.24	763.11
1987	1,699.11	874.39
1988	1,854.43	972.84
1989	2,027.37	1,069.86
1990	2,211.98	1,179.76
1991	2,405.82	1,306.93
1992	2,608.06	1,448.72
1993	2,822.38	1,608.81
1994	3,051.11	1,788.06
1995	3,291.51	1,986.63
1996	3,538.05	2,213.02
1997	3,801.66	2,472.74
1998	4,085.19	2,763.57
1999	4,390.29	3,089.96
2000	4,708.92	3,453.92
2001	5,064.85	3,857.53
2002	5,440.53	4,309.72
2003	5,845.80	4,815.81

Source: Calculations based on data from the Office of the Actuary, HCFA.

time.[12] If *ex ante* premiums from each insured individual just equal expected *ex ante* average losses plus average administrative expenses, we cannot speak of subsidization (except in the sense of the second part of note 12). On the other hand, if the present value of premium payments for the insured group is less than the present value of expected losses (insurance benefits) and administrative expenses for the insured group, then this group must be subsidized if the financial viability of its insurer is to remain intact over time.

TABLE 4.2
Welfare Component of the HI Program Under Medicare, 1966–85 (dollar values in thousands)

Year	Annual present value of stream of HI benefits	Accumulated tax contributions at interest	Welfare component	Welfare ratio
1966	42,361,531	0	42,361,531	1.00
1967	5,036,582	21,391	5,015,191	1.00
1968	5,665,582	57,676	5,607,582	0.99
1969	6,572,258	104,776	6,467,482	0.98
1970	8,159,647	162,036	7,997,611	0.98
1971	9,282,552	225,766	9,056,785	0.98
1972	10,604,079	296,708	10,307,370	0.97
1973	12,664,028	389,413	12,274,616	0.97
1974	14,600,940	540,531	14,060,409	0.96
1975	18,309,433	749,372	17,560,061	0.96
1976	19,827,798	899,258	18,928,539	0.95
1977	22,815,506	1,103,997	21,711,509	0.95
1978	25,852,952	1,348,860	24,504,092	0.95
1979	29,280,959	1,659,111	27,621,848	0.94
1980	32,481,695	2,076,074	30,405,621	0.94
1981	35,322,948	2,548,087	32,774,862	0.93
1982	38,849,013	3,229,316	35,619,696	0.92
1983	43,436,652	3,982,853	39,453,800	0.91
1984	49,940,744	4,732,427	45,208,318	0.91
1985	54,534,974	5,572,012	48,962,962	0.90

Total value of HI benefits compounded forward to 1985: $962,818,235

Total value of HI taxes   compounded forward to 1985:   45,469,018

Total welfare: $917,349,217

Global welfare ratio: 0.95

Source: Calculated from data in Table 4.1.

Intergenerational and Intragenerational Welfare Aspects of the Medicare Program

The descriptive analysis of the structure of taxes, insurance premiums, and benefits under Medicare indicates that the financing of this program deviates in significant ways from the financing of the kind of health insurance provided by the nonprofit Blue Cross/Blue Shield Associations and the for-profit health insurers such as Aetna. To the extent that the present value of Medicare benefits for the aged, as a group, exceeds the present value of their past tax contributions or their past premium payments plus interest on them, as a group, the benefits of each age cohort of persons aged sixty-five and over must be subsidized by those currently in the labor force, if the pool of reserve funds (the trust funds) is not to become depleted and the program terminated. This is an intergenerational transfer and is conceptually no different from conventional forms of transfer, or welfare, such as that used for AFDC. Subsequent calculations in this chapter show that the size of this intergenerational transfer is substantial in both the HI and

TABLE 4.3
Welfare Component of the SMI Program Under Medicare, 1966–85
(dollar values in thousands)

Year	Annual present value of stream of SMI benefits	Annual present value of SMI premiums	Welfare component	Welfare ratio
1966	14,360,035	7,968,099	6,391,936	0.45
1967	1,726,660	828,903	897,756	0.52
1968	1,945,049	905,989	1,039,060	0.53
1969	2,339,342	1,016,848	1,322,494	0.57
1970	3,017,318	1,204,581	1,812,737	0.60
1971	3,510,761	1,309,010	2,201,751	0.63
1972	4,127,706	1,456,571	2,671,135	0.65
1973	5,055,507	1,690,203	3,365,304	0.67
1974	6,009,405	1,902,218	4,107,187	0.68
1975	7,930,557	2,316,297	5,614,260	0.71
1976	8,858,747	2,464,377	6,394,369	0.72
1977	10,433,955	2,779,940	7,654,014	0.73
1978	12,143,343	3,103,562	9,039,782	0.74
1979	14,043,292	3,468,666	10,574,626	0.75
1980	16,104,505	3,828,988	12,275,517	0.76
1981	18,079,710	4,154,832	13,924,878	0.77
1982	20,495,903	4,560,873	15,935,030	0.78
1983	24,503,805	5,115,776	19,388,030	0.79
1984	28,883,129	5,907,443	22,975,686	0.80
1985	32,474,239	6,412,910	26,061,329	0.80

Total value of SMI benefits   compounded forward to 1985: $433,580,878

Total value of SMI premiums compounded forward to 1985:   131,690,199

Total welfare: $301,890,679

Global welfare ratio: 0.70

Source: Calculated from data in Table 4.1.

SMI components of Medicare. Intragenerational transfers take place when tax contributions or premium payments are a function of income or earnings within the generation, rather than upon the actuarial price of the HI benefits. Because SMI monthly premiums, beginning at age sixty-five, are not a function of income, there is no direct SMI intragenerational transfer, or redistribution, of income.[13] The general fund taxes people pay before and after they retire, which then are used for SMI benefits, are ignored in this analysis. On the other hand, HI tax contributions are based upon earnings prior to age sixty-five, while the expected value of HI benefits after age sixty-five is the same across all earnings classes. Therefore, intragenerational transfers do occur within this component of the Medicare program.

Tables 4.2 and 4.3 contain estimates of the intergenerational transfers that have taken place for the elderly age groups that became eligible for Medicare between the years 1966 and 1985. Table 4.2 contains the estimates for HI, and Table 4.3 contains the estimates for SMI. Appendix 4.1 gives a detailed account of how the estimates in both tables were derived, and Appendix Tables 4.1.1 and 4.1.2 show the data from which they were derived.

Column 2 in Table 4.2 gives the estimates of the annual present value of the stream of HI benefits. Using equation (1), the stream of expected benefits over the life expectancy was discounted down to the year of becoming eligible for Medicare for each age group. Thus, on July 1, 1966, 18,926,000 persons received a promise that for the rest of their remaining lives, they would receive a stream of HI health benefits. Some of the persons in this initial Medicare cohort were age sixty-five, and others were older. If we adjust this initial cohort for its age distribution and its consequent differing life expectancies in 1966 (as explained in greater detail in Appendix 4.1) and discount the adjusted annual *ex ante* actuarial value of Medicare HI benefits down to 1966, we arrive at a present value of $42.4 billion for this 1966 cohort. (See the Appendix for details on the discounting procedure.) In subsequent years, we only need to concern ourselves with the "new" (or marginal) elderly, because the 1966 calculation has already taken into account the initial age distribution of the Medicare elderly. In 1966 there were 1.5 million persons who were sixty-four years old (see Appendix Table 4.1.2). For purposes of the calculations, these 1.5 million turned age sixty-five on January 1, 1967, and thereby became eligible for a stream of *ex ante* HI benefits throughout their life expectancy of 14.8 years (see Appendix Table 4.1.2). When discounted to 1967, this stream of benefits had a present value of a little more than $5 billion. In turn, each group of new elderly from 1968 to 1985 could expect an *ex ante* stream of HI benefits, whose present value ranged from $5.7 billion for the 1,524,000 new elderly in 1968 to $54.4 billion for the 2,000,000 new elderly in 1985.[14]

Column 3 of Table 4.2 contains the estimates of the accumulated amount of tax contributions, plus interest, of each age grouping. The formula used for these calculations was

$$T_n = \left(\sum_{i=1}^{n-1} T_i \right) + (2 \cdot tM)(1 + r_n) \tag{2}$$

where

T_n = the present value of HI tax contributions;
t = the HI tax rate;
M = the adjusted median earnings each year (see Appendix 4.1 and Appendix Table 4.1.2);
r = the interest rate on three-month treasury bills.

Because economic theory predicts and the empirical evidence shows that the employer portion of payroll taxes is shifted onto the employee (Aaron 1982; Feldstein 1974; Brittain 1972), the amounts in column 3 represent a doubling of the employee contribution. In the accumulated tax contributions, the groupings of the elderly were treated exactly as in the benefit calculations. Thus, for example, the 18,926,000 elderly who became eligible for Medicare in 1966 paid no Medicare taxes. On the other hand, the two million new elderly in 1985 had worked and had paid HI taxes for the 19 years between 1966 and 1985; their accumulated tax contributions totaled $5.6 billion by January 1, 1985, when, for the next 17.4 years of their life expectancies, they became eligible for the *ex ante* stream of Medicare HI benefits, whose present value was $54.5 billion in 1985.

Column 4 gives the estimates of the welfare component, which is the annual present value of the *ex ante* stream of HI benefits minus the accumulated tax contributions at interest. Column 5 presents the welfare ratios, which are the annual present value of the welfare component divided by the annual present values of the *ex ante* stream of HI benefits (column 4 ÷ column 2). Because the initial cohort of elderly paid no HI taxes, their welfare component is the full $42.4 billion *ex ante* present value of the stream of benefits; their welfare ratio is, consequently, 100 percent.[15] The 1967 group of 1.5 million new elderly paid only some $21 million in HI taxes, so the present value of their welfare component is almost as large as their *ex ante* present value stream of HI benefits, and their welfare ratio is 100 percent due to rounding. Over time, for groups of new elderly, the amount of accumulated HI taxes increases, so that it reaches $5.6 billion for the group of new elderly in 1985. As a result, the welfare ratio falls to 0.90 by 1985, even though the absolute value of the welfare component has risen from $5 billion for the 1.5 million new elderly in 1967 to $49 billion for the 2 million new elderly in 1985. Finally, the bottom portion of Table 4.2 shows the 1985 present value of the stream of *ex ante* benefits and taxes paid by all of these Medicare HI beneficiaries and the 1985 welfare component and global welfare ratio. According to these calculations, the 1985 present value of the welfare component in the first twenty years of the Medicare HI program was $917 billion, and the global welfare ratio was 0.95.

Table 4.3 contains essentially the same kinds of calculations for the SMI component of Medicare as were done for the HI component. The only difference is that because premiums are paid into SMI *after* age sixty-five and not before, the time stream of premium payments for SMI is different from the time stream of HI tax contributions.

The present values of SMI premium payments were calculated, using the following formula:

$$P_y = \sum_{i=y}^{E} \frac{P_i}{1 + r_i} (i - 1) \tag{3}$$

where

> P_y = present value of premium payments in year y;
> E = life expectancy;
> p = annual premium payment; and
> r = the interest rate on three-month treasury bills.

The present actuarial value of the stream of SMI benefit payments was calculated using Equation (1).

The two major differences between the results of the welfare computations in Tables 4.2 and 4.3 are that (1) although constantly increasing after the first year, the absolute value of the SMI welfare component is smaller in SMI than in HI for any given year and (2) the welfare ratio for SMI, rather than declining as with HI, increased from 0.45 percent in 1966 to 0.80 percent in 1985. The first difference stems from the fact that hospital expenditures occupy a greater weight in total health care expenditures than do physician expenditures.[16] The second difference arises from the increasing share of SMI premiums being financed from the general fund (55 percent in 1975 and 75 percent by 1985), rather than from premium contributions by the elderly. As a further result, the absolute value of the welfare component in SMI has been increasing at a much more rapid rate than in HI (2,800 percent vs. 878 percent). The bottom portion of Table 4.3 shows the 1985

TABLE 4.4
Present Value of Mean HI and SMI Welfare Payments, 1966–85

Year	HI	SMI
1966	$ 2,238	$ 376
1967	3,757	728
1968	4,043	810
1969	4,639	997
1970	5,646	1,332
1971	6,293	1,589
1972	7,013	1,883
1973	7,865	2,234
1974	8,829	2,652
1975	10,228	3,356
1976	11,301	3,898
1977	12,684	4,564
1978	13,963	5,253
1979	15,581	6,087
1980	16,795	6,897
1981	18,264	7,874
1982	19,871	9,011
1983	21,669	10,799
1984	24,426	12,539
1985	26,044	14,097

Source: Calculated from data in Table 4.1.

TABLE 4.5
Intragenerational Welfare Effects of Medicare HI, Males

Present actuarial value of HI benefits, 1980	Present value of tax contributions at 1.00, 0.75, 0.50 and 0.25 of maximum tax base to and including 1979	Ratio of benefits to taxes
$11,200.10	$3,861.70	2.90
11,200.10	2,896.28	3.87
11,200.10	1,930.85	5.80
11,200.10	965.43	11.60

Source: Author's working paper.

present values of the *ex ante* stream of Medicare SMI benefits, premiums paid, and the welfare component. For SMI, the 1985 total welfare value was $302 billion, and the global welfare ratio was 0.70, as opposed to the 0.95 for HI. Because the financing of SMI more closely approximates the financing of conventional health insurance, it creates less of an intergenerational transfer than does HI.

Table 4.1 showed the mean annual *ex ante* actuarial value of HI and SMI benefits. Table 4.4 shows the *ex ante* present value of the mean HI and SMI welfare payments that an elderly individual could expect to receive upon becoming eligible for Medicare. For the elderly who became eligible for Medicare benefits on July 1, 1966, the mean present welfare HI and SMI values were $2,238 and $376, respectively; for the new elderly who became eligible for Medicare on January 1, 1985, the respective values were $26,044 and $14,097 or a mean total *ex ante* present value of $40,141.

The above values are mean values, and, as such, they mask the *intra*generational transfers that also occur on an *ex ante* basis in the HI component of Medicare. Many of the elderly earned less than the maximum tax base for Medicare HI tax contributions during their working years, and another smaller group of elderly who were self-employed during their working years paid only half the tax rate that the employed person paid (until a change in the law in 1984). Table 4.5 contains data that illustrate this aspect of HI. For a male, reaching the age of sixty-five on January 1, 1980, the present value of the future stream of HI benefits until death was $11,200.10. The maximum amount of HI tax contributions that he and his employer would have paid plus interest on them, between January 1, 1966, and December 31, 1979, would have been $3,861.70. Thus, the ratio of the present value of benefits to HI taxes is 2.90. Those earning less than the maximum taxable earnings base are subject to a lesser amount of taxes. Because HI benefits are not tied to taxes paid and can thus be expressed as a present-value actuarial calculation, they have the same *ex ante* value for every person aged sixty-five and older and are dependent only upon what year they turned age sixty-five. Table 4.5 shows what the ratio of benefits to taxes paid was for males who turned age sixty-five on January 1, 1980, depending upon whether their previous earnings had been 1.00, 0.75, 0.50, 0.25, or the HI maximum taxable earnings base; for these parameters, the ratio ranges from 2.90 to 11.60. A self-employed person, even at the maximum taxable earnings base, would have contributed only (relative to an employed person) $1,930.85, with interest, for the $11,200.10 present value of *ex ante* benefits, whereas an employed person at the maximum taxable earnings base would have contributed two times as much, or $3,861.70, with interest.

The Relationship Between Medicare and Medicaid Benefit Payments for Medical Care

The calculations in Tables 4.2 and 4.3 show the size and extent of subsidization of public health care expenditures for those aged sixty-five and over, who over the course of their working years paid HI taxes, and for those elderly who had the financial wherewithal to pay SMI premiums, after they reached age sixty-five. At the other end of the income spectrum, there is a group of elderly who qualify for HI coverage because they are eligible for some minimal amount of OASI benefits but who are too poor to pay either deductibles or coinsurance under HI and too poor to pay premiums, deductibles, or coinsurance under SMI. Many states make Medicaid payments for these persons that cover their premiums, deductibles, and coinsurance. These so-called "buy-in" agreements establish Medicare as having primary responsibility for the payment of medical bills, and the states receive federal matching funds under their Medicaid programs for the payments of premiums under SMI and deductibles and coinsurance under both HI and SMI for cash-assistance recipients (Health Care Financing Administration 1983). For these persons, Medicaid supplements Medicare. Unlike with the automatic entitlement to Medicare, persons can be eligible for Medicaid only after they have undergone a means test, in order for the state to determine whether they are medically needy or in need of cash assistance. In effect, these persons are the "poor" who are in need of "welfare" payments for daily living expenses and acute medical care. The latest Medicare/Medicaid data for this group indicate that of the 26,011,000 aged persons enrolled in HI and/or SMI in 1981, 3,367,000 aged persons, or 12.9 percent, were Medicaid recipients, and thus "buy-in" beneficiaries (Social Security Administration 1985; Health Care Financing Administration 1983).[17] Data for 1980 indicate that the states spent $269.3 million for SMI "buy-in" premiums for this group and $1,832.6 million for SMI deductibles and coinsurance (Health Care Financing Administration 1983). The state Medicaid programs themselves spent a total of $8,686.7 million on care for those sixty-five and over; of this amount, $7,485.8 million (or 87.2 percent) went for long-term care, and the remaining $1,200.4 million paid for acute medical care (Health Care Financing Administration 1983).[18] Total buy-in expenditures and Medicaid expenditures were, thus, $10,788.6 million; of this amount, total Medicaid acute care expenditures for the poor elderly were $3,302.3 million.

Therefore, Medicare and Medicaid establish the bounds of subsidization of total public payments for acute medical care for the elderly. At the lower bound of the elderly income distribution, Medicare SMI, supplemented by Medicaid, provides a 100 percent public subsidy of acute physician and ancillary medical care for the poor elderly.[19] At the median of the elderly preretirement earnings distribution, a global 70 percent of public monies spent on SMI and a global 95 percent of public monies spent on HI can be regarded as subsidies.

"Unnecessary" subsidy payments under Medicare

Like beauty, the margins of poverty may be in the eye of the beholder. In the past, there has been some debate about what constitutes the level of poverty (Orshansky 1965; Friedman 1965). Also, it is now widely recognized that official poverty statistics may be misleading about the extent of poverty among the population because these statistics do not include the substantial income in-kind that many of the poor and near-poor receive from food, housing, medical care, and transportation programs (Moon and Smeeding 1981; Smeeding 1982; Brecher, Knickman, and Vogel 1986a). Smeeding (1982) found that "in no subgroup of the population is the effect of the value of medical benefits greater than on the elderly." He showed that the poverty rate among the elderly in 1979 was reduced from 14.7 percent to 12.9 percent, when the in-kind market value of food and housing benefits were included in the analysis, and from 12.9 percent to 4.5 percent, when medical benefits with institutional care were included. However, he did not make any adjustments in real income for the presence of illness, so that by his measure someone with high medical costs (and Medicare benefits) would be "rich."

Thus, Medicare, the Medicaid buy-in provision under Medicare, and the Medicaid purchase of long-term institutional care for the elderly have made a significant contribution to the alleviation of poverty among the elderly, and very few people would argue that these funds had not been humanely spent. On the other hand, many would argue that some of these funds have been inefficiently spent. For example, Medicaid has a definite institutional bias in its long-term care provisions, and many poor elderly probably could have received care more suited to their preferences and at less public expense outside of an institutional setting (Palmer 1983). Because of its reasonable-cost method of payment, Medicare has sanctioned inefficiency in the provision of physician and hospital services to the

TABLE 4.6
Distribution of Noninstitutionalized Elderly Enrollees and Their Income by
Family Income Category, 1977 (in 1984 dollars) and Distribution of Family
Income, All Families, 1984

Family income category (dollars)	Percent of Medicare enrollees		Percent of *all* families	Average Medicare family
5,000 and less	12.6			$ 3,659
Under 5,000			5.0	
5,001–10,000	22.0			7,312
5,000–9,999			9.4	
10,001–15,000	19.4			12,334
10,000–14,999			10.8	
15,001–20,000	11.9			17,412
15,000–19,999			10.8	
20,001–30,000	14.7			24,503
20,000–24,999		34.1	10.7	
30,001 and above	19.4			58,306
25,000 and above			53.2	
All noninstitutionalized elderly enrollees	100.0			$21,358
All families			100.0	

Source: National Medical Care Expenditure Survey, as given in M. Moon (1983, 22) and U.S. Bureau of the Census (1985, 450).

elderly. As expressed in the introductory section of this chapter, Medicare may also be characterized as an inefficient subsidy if it provides health insurance for those elderly who could and would have purchased their own health insurance had Medicare been more selective in its target population. Here, we make some estimates of the possible magnitude of the costs of this excessive, or "unnecessary," subsidization. We do not adjust for family size since there is no unequivocally correct way to do so.

Table 4.6 presents an interesting picture of the distribution of income of the noninstitutionalized elderly Medicare enrollees in 1977, brought forward to 1984 dollars. In 1984, the median family income of *all* families was $26,433 (U.S. Bureau of the Census 1985), and the average income of all families was $28,638 in 1983 (the latest data available). The distribution of family income for all families has been added to Table 4.6; up until an income of $20,000, the income interval of the two series of distributions match, except for $1 at each end of the intervals. Table 4.6 shows that Medicare families were poorer than all families. At the upper end of the distribution, only 34.1 percent of Medicare families had family incomes above $20,000, while 63.9 percent of all families had family incomes above that level. At the lower end of the income distribution, 34.6 percent of Medicare families had family incomes below $10,000, whereas only 13.4 percent of all families had family incomes below that amount. The contrast in these two sets of income distribution suggests that depending on one's definition of "afford," many elderly families would not be able to afford health insurance if Medicare did not exist. However, the upper end of the Medicare family income distribution also indicates that at least 19.4 percent of Medicare elderly families probably could afford to purchase their own health insurance if they were not covered by Medicare; even the 34.1 percent of the Medicare elderly families with incomes above $20,001 might be able to pay for some portion of their health insurance premium.

Appendix Tables 4.1.3 through 4.1.6 present four alternative definitions of the poor elderly for the years of this analysis. The first definition is the percentage of the elderly with income below 125 percent of the official poverty level (U.S. Bureau of the Census Series P-60); the next definition is a permutation of the first, with the percentage of the elderly with income below 250 percent of the official poverty level. The last two definitions have their basis in Table 4.6; although it is not possible to derive a time series from Table 4.6, the 14.7 percent and 19.4 percent of Medicare elderly families with family incomes above $20,001 and $30,001, respectively, does give some notion of those Medicare elderly who might be financially able to purchase their own health insurance. Thus, 65.9 percent and 80.6 percent[20] of the Medicare elderly were assumed to be Medicare poor for the purposes of calculating the unnecessary subsidy payments under the Medicare program over the last twenty years, for the last two columns in Appendix Tables 4.1.3 through 4.1.6. Here, by unnecessary subsidy, we mean those amounts that could be subtracted from the total welfare amounts in Tables 4.2 and 4.3 if Medicare had only been available to the poor elderly, depending upon the four definitions of elderly poverty. Table 4.7 contains the estimates of the 1985 present value of these unnecessary subsidy payments, and the section on

TABLE 4.7
Present 1985 Value of "Unnecessary" HI and SMI Subsidy Payments, Using Alternative Definitions of the Poor Elderly (dollars in thousands)

	Percent of elderly with income below 125% of poverty level (census)	Percent of elderly with income below 250% of poverty level (census)	65.9% of Medicare families considered poor	80.6% of Medicare families considered poor
HI	$664,129,980	$410,910,744	$312,816,083	$177,965,748
SMI	223,498,872	145,107,066	102,944,722	58,566,792
Total	$887,628,852	$556,017,810	$415,760,805	$236,532,540

Source: Author's calculations.

the estimation of unnecessary subsidy payments in Appendix 4.1 explains how these estimates were derived. For HI and SMI combined, the range of their present values goes from $888 billion to $237 billion. Depending upon one's definition of poverty, these values represent a kind of opportunity cost of the Medicare program in its present form. During the first twenty years of the program, the annual present values of these monies (see Appendix Table 4.1.6) could have been spent upon other social "needs."

Medicare Within the Context of Other Public Programs for the Elderly

Public programs for the elderly may be divided into three categories for analytical purposes: (1) those that meet basic food and shelter needs; (2) those that meet acute medical care needs; and (3) those that meet chronic care needs, such as long-term care (Brecher, Knickman, and Vogel 1986a). At one extreme of the income distribution are those elderly who have substantial private resources (see column 4 of Table 4.6) that are supplemented by entitlements to OASI that were originally meant, at the inception of that program, to take care of basic food and shelter needs; this same group of elderly are also entitled to HI and SMI benefits that meet their needs for acute medical care.[21] Here and elsewhere (Parsons and Munro 1978), it has been shown that for this segment of the elderly population, HI/SMI and OASI contain substantial welfare components.[22] At the other end of the elderly income distribution, it would appear that increases in OASI benefits, together with an ever-increasing prevalence of private pensions and in-kind public benefits, have sharply reduced the percentage of elderly living in poverty. Meanwhile, Medicare made it possible for this group to have what some would regard as adequate access to acute medical care for the first time (Long and Settle 1984), albeit with deductibles and coinsurance that consume a relatively large percentage of their income (Moon 1983; Berk and Wilensky 1985). Despite substantial public expenditure, some feel that the chronic/long-term care needs of this group of elderly are inadequately met by current public programs (Brecher and Knickman 1985; Brecher, Knickman, and Vogel 1986a).

There are many examples of ostensibly redistributive public expenditure programs that subsidize the upper end of the income distribution more than the lower end.[23] Beginning January 1, 1984, up to one-half of Social Security (OASI) benefits have been subject to the personal income tax if the modified adjusted gross income of OASI recipients exceeds $25,000 for single taxpayers and $32,000 for married couples. Thus, a precedent for using a form of means testing for OASI benefits has been established. These two cut-offs were not indexed for inflation or for economic growth; if they remain constant into the future, an increasingly larger percentage of the elderly will become liable for the tax, and the OASI intergenerational/intragenerational transfers will diminish at an even more rapid rate. The proceeds from this tax will revert to the general fund and will, presumably, be used to finance, among other things, HI and SMI and long-term care for the elderly. Given the relatively large HI and SMI subsidies to the relatively well-to-do elderly that currently exist in the Medicare program and, given the gaps that exist in social services, particularly in long-term care for the poor elderly, symmetry of treatment, as well as equity considerations would indicate that some form of means testing also be applied to both HI and SMI. In this way, the three basic sets of human needs, outlined at the beginning of this section, could be financed in a more consistent and equitable manner.

The term "means testing" has a particularly negative connotation in the United States, as does the word welfare. In the political realm, the meaning of words can easily become tangled and twisted. In popular parlance and in official documents, OASI and Medicare are designated as "entitlements." If OASI and Medicare were fully funded insurance mechanisms, they would, indeed, deserve the title of entitlements, but they are not fully funded. Given the rate of benefit increases in both programs, and the reluctance of politicians to raise payroll taxes to keep up with the rate of benefit increases that they have legislated for OASI and that have caught them by force of circumstances in the Medicare program, these two programs probably never will be fully funded in their present form. The recently enacted, subtle introduction of means testing into the OASI program is at once a response to the "crisis" in the OASI trust fund and a tacit admission that the form of that program has to change if OASI is to remain viable and equitable into future years. But, nowhere do official documents refer to this recent change in OASI as means testing, even though it is means testing, only in a different form than that used for AFDC or Medicaid.

Likewise, means testing for the Medicare entitlement could involve an equally subtle introduction. In fact, Medicare HI already has a means test for those who do not qualify for HI under OASI eligibility rules or who are not "deemed" into the program (for the deeming provision, see U.S. Department of Health and Human Services 1986). These persons may become eligible for Medicare HI (and then by extension into SMI) simply by voluntarily paying a monthly HI premium that approaches one-twelfth of the *ex ante* insurance value of Medicare HI in Table 4.1. One among many possible means tests for both HI and SMI for all Medicare beneficiaries could be similar to the new taxing provision for OASI benefits and similar to the means test now used by Medicare for the select few HI voluntary entrants who do not qualify for HI eligibility by virtue of having OASI eligibility. Each year at tax time, elderly family income, elderly family taxable income, or the elderly family tax bracket would determine what percentage of the annual *ex ante* insurance value of both Medicare HI and SMI would be paid as the health insurance premium "tax" for the preceding year. This amount could be added as a surcharge to the tax due to the IRS on April 15 and could be remitted to the HI and SMI trust funds, respectively, or used for long-term and chronic care purposes. As in the income tax system itself, the premium "tax" rate could even be made progressive. Because of the regular exemptions now in the tax law, those elderly at lower income levels would not have to pay this Medicare tax.[24] Besides enhancing equity in Medicare and shoring up the HI and SMI trust funds, such a Medicare tax might also create an interesting form of health insurance selection out of the Medicare program itself. There would be some upper-income elderly who, having paid the full Medicare premium "tax" for one or two years, might conclude that they could obtain similar or better health insurance coverage elsewhere at a lower premium, such as with an HMO or with Blue Cross/Blue Shield or with the commercial health insurers. Indeed, just as with Medigap health insurance, a lively competition among insurers might develop for this market. Of course, the ultimate conclusion of such a chain of events might be the kind of "spiraling" that took place out of the old Blue Cross/Blue Shield comprehensive community-rated plans. Upper-income, healthy, elderly persons would enter non-Medicare experience-rated health insurance plans offered by Blue Cross/Blue Shield or commercial health insurers or would enter HMOs. Medicare would then become the residual insurer of those elderly who could not obtain health insurance elsewhere—which it theoretically was to be in the first place.

Adoption of such a policy or a variant of it would do away with some of the present anomalies in Medicare finance. For example, lower- and middle-income nonaged family workers would no longer be paying payroll taxes for HI—from income that has not increased in real terms over the last decade—for the health insurance of the relatively well-to-do elderly, who could pay for their own health insurance. While these families would still have to pay payroll taxes, at the margin, the Medicare-financing mechanism would be perceived as being more equitable. From an *intra*generational perspective, the financing of HI would also become even more progressive because the ratio of benefits to taxes paid before retirement would decline even further for the upper-income elderly (see Table 4.5). Efficiency in the health care system would be improved to the extent that a progressive Medicare tax on upper-income elderly benefits provides incentives to seek private-sector insurance that provides care more efficiently, such as in HMOs. Finally, depending upon the elderly income level at which a Medicare premium tax began, a fairly substantial amount of funds could be generated that could be used for the long-term care of the poorest elderly, and this again would enhance the equity of public programs for the elderly.

Conclusion

In the last twenty years, a large body of literature has accumulated on the Medicare program. This literature, especially of late, has mainly concentrated on the cost and budget implications of the program. Another part of the Medicare literature has focused on the equity aspects of SMI premiums and on the equity aspects of deductibles and coinsurance in both HI and SMI; this kind of analysis has universally concentrated upon the burdens of low-income Medicare enrollees. Until now, no research has concentrated upon broader equity aspects of the program such as (1) how well do the affluent and even relatively affluent elderly fare under its provisions and (2) what is the nature and magnitude of the intergenerational transfers involved in the program.

Analysis of the tax, premium, and benefit streams of both HI and SMI under Medicare reveals that the relatively well-to-do elderly have enjoyed a large intergenerational welfare transfer because of the manner in which this program has been publicly financed.[26] If the current method of finance were to continue on into the future, the welfare ratio in HI might gradually diminish to zero; but, in the meantime, further large absolute intergenerational transfers would have taken place. On the other hand, the absolute amount of SMI welfare payments has continued to increase, as has the welfare ratio of the payments. Given current financing arrangements for SMI, there is no reason why the absolute value of the welfare component should ever diminish, and the welfare ratio could asymptotically approach 100 percent. Although it is generally recognized that any pay-as-you-go social insurance system, such as OASDHI, will contain elements of both a fully funded system and transfer elements, the transfer elements in Medicare would appear to be extreme for upper-income groups of the elderly.

When viewed within the context of the spectrum of public programs that have been established to meet the needs of the elderly, SMI and particularly HI presently contain a high welfare ratio for the well-to-do elderly. Now that OASI will be subjected to a form of progressive means testing into the future,[27] its means-tested aspect will conceptually approach that of the Medicaid program and the other so-called welfare programs.[28] Thus, basic food and shelter public expenditures and long-term care public expenditures will be financed in a more progressive fashion. All needs will not be met in the long-term and chronic care sector, simply because demographic and epidemiological factors will increase the elderly as a percentage of the population, will make the "old-old" a larger percentage of the elderly population, and will make chronic care assume a greater importance in the mix of acute care/chronic care (Rice and Feldman 1983). By way of contrast, the Medicare program will be the only one of the three programs attempting to meet the three basic human needs of the elderly that will not be progressively financed, and whose expenditures upon the acute care of the relatively well-to-do elderly could conceivably be used to fill in the gaps and expand long-term care and other chronic care services for the poor and near-poor elderly.

APPENDIX 4.1

The Estimation of the Present Actuarial Value of HI Health Insurance Benefits and of the Present Value of HI Tax Contributions

As shown in the text, the *ex ante* insurance value of Medicare to any enrollee is simply M/N, where M is total Medicare and administrative expenditures in the year and N is the number of Medicare enrollees. The program's title, "Health Insurance for the Aged" implies that Medicare may be viewed as a community-rated health insurance program for all of its aged eligibles. Except for the subsidization from the general fund, Medicare Part B is similar to the health insurance sold in any of the old Blue Shield community-rated health insurance plans. The rules and regulations for benefit payments and for premium payments under SMI are the same for everyone in the program regardless of age and/or sex. It is true that *ex ante* benefit payments can be anticipated for a longer period of time for females, given the relatively greater difference in life expectancy at any given age. However, in any one of the old Blue Shield community-rated health insurance plans a similar phenomenon occurred; at any given age, females lived longer than did males, and thus could expect to receive benefits for a longer period of time. But, given that Blue Shield premiums were paid on an annual basis, females also paid premiums during their full lifetimes. Thus, in an actuarial sense, annual premiums paid and benefits received were exactly equal (abstracting from administrative costs) for both males and females. Medicare Part B, where annual premiums-paid begin at age sixty-five and continue until death, shares this common actuarial characteristic with the old Blue Shield community-rating system. In contrast, Medicare Part A is an anomaly, or more properly speaking, a hybrid. *Ex ante* benefits under Part A are the same for every person of the same sex as they turn age sixty-five. But, because Medicare Part A is not financed by premiums, the actuarial equivalence of premiums-benefits does not hold. In the case of Part A, females do have a financial advantage, all other things being equal. For example, consider a male and female, both of whom turned sixty-five on December 31, 1981, and began paying the HI tax contribution on January 1, 1966. Assuming equal annual earnings, both would have contributed the same amount of tax contributions. However, on January 1, 1982, for example, the female could expect 18.8 years of HI benefits, whereas the male could expect only 14.5 years of the same. In this respect, there is no premium-benefit actuarial equivalence in Medicare Part A, although the present value of the HI tax contributions paid, plus interest paid, before retirement may be viewed as a form of single-premium health insurance payment. Here, in this chapter, we view Medicare HI and SMI as the equivalent of a community-rated program for all of the elderly.

In order to estimate the present actuarial value of the health insurance benefits of Medicare HI for each year, and also in order to estimate a total present actuarial value of HI benefits for all of the years up to 1985, it is first necessary to consider the time stream of *ex ante* benefits[29] relative to the elderly age distribution in 1966. On July 1, 1966, the 18,926,000 elderly persons who became immediately eligible for HI had differing life expectancies. Those who were aged sixty-five on that date could expect to live 14.6 more years, whereas those who were aged eighty-five could only expect to live 4.7 more years. Consider the age distribution of all sixty-five and over HI enrollees in 1966.

Age bracket	Percent of elderly	Midpoint of age bracket	Life expectancy at midpoint of age bracket (years)
65–69	35.3	67	14.8
70–74	28.7	72	11.5
75–79	19.2	77	8.6
80–84	10.9	82	6.1
85+	6.0	87	4.8

In order to make the estimates manageable, the midpoints of the age brackets were used. Thus, 35.3 percent had a midpoint age of sixty-seven, and so on. Given the protocol chosen for estimation purposes, this group could expect, on average, 14.8 years of HI benefits. The 6 percent of the elderly in that year who were at midpoint age eighty-seven could expect only 4.8 years of HI benefits. The present actuarial value of benefits for HI in 1966 would be the percentage-weighted total of the annual actuarial value of benefits discounted to 1966 for each of the five life expectancies for the midpoint of age brackets sixty-seven, seventy-two, seventy-seven, eighty-two, and eighty-seven. The discount rate used was the interest rate on three-month treasury bills for 1966–83 (Tax Foundation 1983) and the mean of that rate forecasted for 1984–2000.

That calculation, then, captures *all* of the benefits received by this initial group of elderly. As one moves chronologically from 1966 to 1985, all of the persons in this initial group of Medicare beneficiaries will have died statistically, but these deaths will have been taken into account by the use of the life expectancies for discounting purposes because the life expectancies are average life expectancies. As a consequence, estimates of actuarial benefits for 1967 and the years thereafter need to take into account only those new (marginal) elderly who were, for example, aged sixty-four in 1966 but became sixty-five in 1967. Again, for purposes of the manageability of estimation, it was assumed that all individuals became HI beneficiaries on January 1 of each year. Thus, the 1.5 million elderly who were aged sixty-four in 1966, as reported in the census (Series P-25, 1965–85) became, for purposes of this analysis, sixty-five on January 1, 1967, and had a life expectancy of 14.8 years (National Center for Health Statistics 1966–85). The yearly actuarial value of HI benefits was then discounted to 1967 for each of the 14.8 years and then multiplied times the number of new elderly adjusted for Medicare eligibility. The same procedure was used for each new group of elderly for each year in the time series for column 2 in Table 4.2. For each year, the number of new elderly were taken from census data, and their life expectancies at age sixty-five were taken from National Center for Health Statistics data. The census new elderly for each year were adjusted downward, using Social Security Administration (1985) data on the percentage of those aged sixty-five and over eligible for OASI and HI. The total present actuarial value of HI benefits for all of the years at the bottom of Table 4.2 is simply the sum of the yearly accumulated values compounded to 1985, using the interest rate on three-month treasury bills. The HI expenditures used for the 1966–82 estimates were the total, incurred, calendar year expenditures for the aged, supplied by the Office of the Actuary, HCFA; expenditure data used for the years 1983–2003 were those from Alternative II-B (the middle range) of projections in the 1986 Annual Report of the Medicare Board of Trustees (U.S. Department of Health and Human Services 1986). We next turn to the estimation procedure used for HI payroll tax contributions.

Payroll tax contributions into the HI trust fund began on January 1, 1966. As with all other tax revenue collected, HI tax revenue is a function of both the tax base and the tax rate. In 1966 the annual maximum taxable earnings base was $6,600, and by 1986 the maximum base had risen to $42,000 (Social Security Administration 1985). It has been estimated that 75.8 percent of all workers in 1966 had total annual earnings below this annual maximum; the comparable figure for 1982, the latest date for which data were available, was 93.0 percent of all workers (Social Security Administration 1985). In 1966 the HI tax contribution rate was 0.35 percent and had risen to 1.45 percent by 1986; the rate is projected to remain at 1.45 percent for the remainder of this century (Social Security Administration 1985). This tax rate is paid by both employer and employee on all wages and salaries up to the point where the employee wage or salary reaches the annual maximum taxable earnings base; after that point, no payroll taxes are paid. Self-employed persons paid only the employee rate until changes in the law, beginning in 1984, mandated that self-employed persons pay at the employer-employee combined rate of 2.6 percent (2.9 percent in 1986).

For the purpose of estimating the present value of the yearly tax contribution and the present value of total tax contributions into the HI trust fund by those aged sixty-five and over eligible for Medicare benefits during the period 1966–85, annual median earnings for all wage and salary workers were used as the wage and salary base.[30] These data come from the Social Security Administration (1985). It was assumed that for each calendar year (including 1966), all individuals paid taxes throughout the year until December 31, and that year-ages changed, and individuals moved from being taxpayers to HI beneficiaries on January 1 of the next immediate calendar year. In addition, an adjustment had to be made in the median earnings data for female labor force participation. The total median earnings data used for each year (as given by the Social Security Administration 1985) are the weighted median for males and females who actually worked full time in any given year. If these total median earnings data were used as the tax base for the calculation of the tax contribution, the total tax contribution in any given year would be overstated because not all of the elderly female HI enrollees had worked full time before having become HI enrollees. Therefore, the total annual tax contribution data were weighted downward each year by 1 minus the female labor force factor.[31]

Most of those elderly who became eligible for HI benefits on July 1, 1966, had not paid any taxes into the HI trust fund, simply because most of them were already beyond the working age and had already retired. Some few paid taxes between January 1 and July 1, 1966.

As with the HI actuarial benefit estimates, the present value of the yearly tax contribution estimates had to take into account the time stream of tax contributions relative to the initial age distribution in 1966. Again, however, for years after 1966, the relevant group of aged were the new, or marginal, aged—only those turning sixty-five as of January 1 of each year. As an example of how these estimates were made, consider the two million new aged who became sixty-five on January 1, 1985. Given their life expectancy of 17.4 more years in 1985, they would receive benefits until the middle of the year 2002. They would have paid HI tax contributions between January 1, 1966, and December 31, 1984, or nineteen years. The present value of their accumulated tax contribution of $5.6 billion, as of December 31, 1984, is the result of doubling each year's employee contribution (the median earnings in the relevant year[32] times the HI tax contribution rate in the relevant year), in order to take into account the employer's shifted tax contribution (see chapter text), and each year's contribution was compounded forward, using the interest rate on three-month treasury bills. The accumulated tax contributions for each year in column 3 of Table 4.2 is the previously estimated value times the number of new sixty-five-year-olds in that year. This value is the present value of the yearly tax contribution. To derive the 1985 present value of total tax contributions at the bottom of Table 4.2, each yearly accumulated tax contribution was compounded forward to 1985, using the interest rate on three-month treasury bills.

The Estimation of the Present Actuarial Value of SMI Health Insurance Benefits and the Present Value of SMI Premium Payments

The procedure used to estimate the present actuarial value of SMI health insurance benefits was similar to that used for HI benefits. A present actuarial value of benefits was estimated for each year (the entries for each year in column 2 of Table 4.3), and then a total present actuarial value was derived by compounding each yearly entry to 1985, using the interest rate on three-month treasury bills. Because the time stream of benefits for SMI is conceptually the same as for HI benefits vis-à-vis the age distribution of the aged in 1966 and their life expectancies, and because the concept of the new elderly is the same for each subsequent year after 1966, the treatment of the SMI benefit data was the same as that done for the HI benefit data. The data used for SMI benefits and enrollees were fiscal year data that were interpolated to fit calendar years; these data come from the Office of the Actuary, HCFA, and, in the case of the benefit figures, are total, incurred expenditures for the aged. Beyond the year 1985, both the benefit and enrollment data are based upon Alternative II-B in the 1986 Annual Report of the Medicare Board of Trustees (U.S. Department of Health and Human Services 1986).

The estimation of the present value of SMI premium payments was much more straightforward than the estimation of the HI tax contributions, simply because SMI premiums are conceptually the same as any other health insurance premium paid. For the initial entry group of elderly into Medicare in 1966, future SMI premiums were discounted back to 1966, according to the life expectancies of the five midpoints of bracket ages. For the new elderly in each subsequent year, future premiums were discounted to the relevant year, according to the life expectancy for a sixty-five-year-old in the relevant year. The premium data came from the Office of the Actuary, HCFA. As noted in the text, there is no calculation of prior (general revenue) taxes for SMI, since these taxes are not earmarked for SMI.

The Estimation of "Unnecessary" Subsidy Payments

Table 4.1.3 contains alternative definitions of the percentage of the elderly living in poverty. Columns 2 and 3 give the percentage of the elderly with income below 125 and 250 percent of the official poverty level as reported by the census for the years 1966–85. Columns 4 and 5 are based on the elderly income data contained in Table 4.6. The number of poor Medicare elderly for each year, given in

Table 4.1.4, is the result of multiplying the poverty percentages contained in Table 4.1.3 times the initial 1966 cohort of Medicare eligibles and times the number of new elderly in subsequent years in both HI and SMI. The census new elderly in column 4 of Table 4.1.2 were adjusted downward in order to eliminate those new census elderly who were not eligible for Medicare. In 1985, for example, the adjustment factor was 0.06. As an example of how the calculations were done for Table 4.1.5, the two million new elderly in 1985 were multiplied times 0.96 and then multiplied times 0.462 (the percentage of the elderly with income below 250 percent of the official poverty level); that calculation yielded an estimate of 868,560 new HI enrollees who were poor in 1985 in Table 4.1.4 (at the 250 percent definition of poverty). The estimated dollar values in Table 4.1.5 were derived by multiplying the mean present welfare values in Table 4.4 times the number of poor elderly people in both HI and SMI in Table 4.1.4. Again, for example, the $22.6 billion figure for HI in Table 4.1.5, using the percentage of the elderly with income below 250 percent of the official poverty level in 1985, is the result of multiplying the $26,044 average present value of the HI welfare payment in 1985 (Table 4.4) times the 868,560 elderly poor in Table 4.1.4. These "real" subsidies rightfully went to elderly people who were too poor to afford the purchase of health insurance for themselves. The unnecessary subsidy payments in Table 4.1.6 are the result of subtracting the real subsidies contained in Table 4.1.5 from the welfare component in column 4 of Tables 4.2 and 4.3. For example, in 1985, the present value of the HI welfare component for the new elderly in that year was $48.963 billion (Table 4.2); the present value of the real subsidy for the truly poor, at the 250 percent definition of poverty, was $22.621 billion (Table 4.1.5). Therefore, the present value of the unnecessary subsidy to the nonpoor Medicare elderly was $26.342 billion in 1985 (Table 4.1.6).

APPENDIX TABLE 4.1.1
HI and SMI Expenditures, Expenditures Plus Administrative Costs and Enrollees, Actual and Forecasted, 1966–2003 (dollars)

Calendar year	HI expenditures (millions)	HI expenditures and administrative costs (millions)	HI enrollees (thousands)	SMI expenditures (millions)	SMI expenditures and administrative costs (millions)	SMI enrollees (thousands)
1966	1,240	1,348	18,926	554	623	17,000
1967	3,435	3,512	19,207	1,054	1,171	17,750
1968	4,301	4,400	19,508	1,276	1,464	18,038
1969	4,870	4,988	19,793	1,605	1,803	18,833
1970	5,269	5,426	20,104	1,848	2,076	19,312
1971	5,887	6,037	20,427	2,010	2,256	19,664
1972	6,467	6,652	20,766	2,190	2,489	20,043
1973	7,108	7,317	21,165	2,394	2,707	20,428
1974	8,420	8,665	21,583	2,660	3,060	20,988
1975	10,227	10,466	22,066	3,134	3,599	21,504
1976	12,101	12,406	22,556	3,806	4,326	22,089
1977	14,060	14,315	23,071	4,585	5,086	22,605
1978	16,031	16,477	23,591	5,443	6,044	23,133
1979	18,568	18,973	24,179	6,370	6,990	23,693
1980	22,439	22,900	24,703	7,567	8,242	24,287
1981	27,080	27,426	25,190	9,154	9,881	24,826
1982	31,479	31,941	25,709	10,868	11,613	25,363
1983	35,181	35,667	26,240	12,981	13,785	25,873
1984	38,960	39,526	26,700	15,405	16,278	26,433
1985	40,985	41,736	27,369	17,382	18,315	26,914
1986	43,581	44,251	27,985	20,074	21,034	27,563
1987	47,872	48,598	28,602	23,640	24,649	28,190
1988	53,319	54,101	29,174	26,898	27,961	28,741
1989	59,431	60,290	29,738	30,235	31,371	29,322
1990	66,076	67,014	30,296	34,053	35,260	29,887
1991	73,097	74,116	30,807	38,431	39,707	30,382
1992	80,455	81,554	31,270	43,373	44,722	30,870
1993	88,312	89,495	31,709	48,915	50,351	31,297

Year						
1994	96,701	97,971	32,110	55,145	56,669	31,693
1995	105,656	107,017	32,513	62,135	63,751	32,090
1996	114,724	116,179	32,837	60,010	71,724	32,410
1997	124,150	125,702	33,065	78,880	80,698	32,635
1998	134,350	136,004	33,292	88,880	90,808	32,859
1999	145,338	147,101	33,506	100,140	102,185	33,070
2000	157,001	158,879	33,740	112,850	115,019	33,301
2001	170,200	172,205	34,000	127,150	129,451	33,558
2002	184,200	186,338	34,250	143,250	145,690	33,805
2003	199,400	201,680	34,500	161,400	163,988	34,052

Source: Office of the Actuary, HCFA.

APPENDIX TABLE 4.1.2
Life Expectancies at Age 65, Median Earnings, and the Number of "New"
65-Year-Olds

Year	Life expectancy[a] (years)	Median earnings[b] (dollars)	Number of "new" 65-year-olds[c] (thousands)
1965	14.6	—	—
1966	14.6	3,414	1,476
1967	14.8	3,566	1,500
1968	14.6	3,716	1,524
1969	14.8	3,945	1,549
1970	15.2	4,173	1,574
1971	15.2	4,375	1,599
1972	15.2	4,605	1,633
1973	15.3	4,870	1,715
1974	15.5	5,184	1,750
1975	16.0	5,531	1,846
1976	16.0	5,803	1,801
1977	16.3	6,235	1,821
1978	16.3	6,630	1,867
1979	16.6	7,204	1,886
1980	16.4	7,930	1,926
1981	16.5	8,547	1,909
1982	16.8	9,344	1,907
1983	17.1	9,795	1,937
1984	17.3	10,000	1,969
1985	17.4	10,000	2,000

Source: [a]National Center for Health Statistics (1966–85). [b]Social Security Administration (1985). [c]U.S. Bureau of the Census, Current Population Reports, series P-25.

APPENDIX TABLE 4.1.3
Alternative Definitions of the Poor Elderly, 1966–85

Year	Percent of elderly with income below 125% of poverty level (census)	Percent of elderly with income below 250% of poverty level (census)	65.9% of Medicare families considered poor	80.6% of Medicare families considered poor
1966	35.2	70.4	65.9	80.6
1967	33.0	66.0	65.9	80.6
1968	34.7	69.4	65.9	80.6
1969	35.2	70.4	65.9	80.6
1970	33.9	67.8	65.9	80.6
1971	31.6	63.2	65.9	80.6
1972	28.5	57.0	65.9	80.6
1973	26.8	53.6	65.9	80.6
1974	24.8	49.6	65.9	80.6
1975	25.4	50.8	65.9	80.6
1976	24.9	49.8	65.9	80.6
1977	24.5	49.0	65.9	80.6
1978	23.4	46.8	65.9	80.6
1979	24.7	49.4	65.9	80.6
1980	25.7	51.4	65.9	80.6
1981	25.2	50.4	65.9	80.6
1982	23.7	47.4	65.9	80.6
1983	22.4	44.8	65.9	80.6
1984	23.3	46.6	65.9	80.6
1985	23.1	46.2	65.9	80.6

Source: U.S. Bureau of the Census, Current Population Reports: Consumer Income, series P-60. Social Security Administration (1980; 1985), Tax Foundation, Inc. (1986), and Table 4.6 of this chapter.

APPENDIX TABLE 4.1.4
Number of Poor "New" Medicare Elderly, Using Alternative Definitions of the Poor Elderly, 1966–85 (thousands)

Year	Elderly with income below 125% of poverty level (census)	Elderly with income below 250% of poverty level (census)	65.9% of Medicare families considered poor	80.6% of Medicare families considered poor
Number of poor elderly (HI)				
1966	6,662	13,323	12,472	15,254
1967	440	881	879	1,076
1968	481	962	913	1,117
1969	490	981	918	1,123
1970	480	960	933	1,141
1971	454	909	948	1,159
1972	418	837	968	1,184
1973	418	836	1,028	1,257
1974	394	789	1,049	1,283
1975	436	872	1,131	1,383
1976	417	834	1,103	1,350
1977	419	838	1,128	1,379
1978	410	821	1,156	1,414
1979	437	875	1,168	1,428
1980	465	930	1,193	1,459
1981	452	904	1,182	1,446
1982	424	849	1,181	1,444
1983	407	815	1,199	1,467
1984	431	862	1,219	1,491
1985	434	869	1,238	1,515
Number of poor elderly (SMI)				
1966	5,984	11,968	11,203	13,702
1967	407	814	813	994
1968	445	889	845	1,033
1969	466	933	874	1,069
1970	461	922	896	1,096
1971	437	875	912	1,116
1972	404	808	934	1,143
1973	403	807	992	1,214
1974	384	768	1,020	1,248
1975	425	849	1,102	1,348
1976	408	816	1,080	1,322
1977	410	821	1,105	1,351
1978	402	805	1,134	1,387
1979	429	858	1,144	1,400
1980	457	914	1,173	1,434
1981	445	891	1,165	1,425
1982	419	838	1,165	1,425
1983	402	804	1,183	1,447
1984	426	853	1,207	1,476
1985	427	854	1,218	1,490

Source: Author's calculations.

APPENDIX TABLE 4.1.5
Total Amount of "Real" Subsidies Paid Under HI and SMI, Using Alternative Definitions of the Poor Elderly, 1966–85 (thousands)

Year	Elderly with income below 125% of poverty level (census)	Elderly with income below 250% of poverty level (census)	65.9% of Medicare families considered poor	80.6% of Medicare families considered poor
HI				
1966	$14,911,259	$29,822,518	$27,916,249	$34,143,394
1967	1,655,013	3,310,026	3,305,011	4,042,244
1968	1,945,831	3,891,662	3,695,397	4,519,711
1969	2,276,554	4,553,107	4,262,071	5,212,790
1970	2,711,190	5,422,380	5,270,426	6,446,074
1971	2,861,944	5,723,888	5,968,422	7,299,769
1972	2,937,601	5,875,201	6,792,557	8,307,741
1973	3,289,597	6,579,194	8,088,972	9,893,340
1974	3,486,981	6,973,963	9,265,810	11,332,690
1975	4,460,256	8,920,511	11,572,080	14,153,409
1976	4,713,206	9,426,413	12,473,908	15,256,403
1977	5,319,320	10,638,640	14,307,885	17,499,477
1978	5,733,958	11,467,915	16,148,197	19,750,298
1979	6,822,597	13,645,193	18,202,798	22,263,210
1980	7,814,245	15,628,489	20,037,304	24,506,931
1981	8,259,265	16,518,530	21,598,634	26,416,539
1982	8,441,868	16,883,736	23,473,380	28,709,475
1983	8,837,651	17,675,302	26,000,054	31,799,763
1984	10,533,538	21,067,076	29,792,281	36,437,904
1985	11,310,444	22,620,889	32,266,592	39,464,147
SMI				
1966	$2,249,962	$ 4,499,923	$ 4,212,286	$ 5,151,901
1967	296,260	592,519	591,622	723,592
1968	360,554	721,107	684,740	837,482
1969	465,518	931,036	871,523	1,065,930
1970	614,518	1,229,035	1,194,593	1,461,066
1971	695,753	1,391,507	1,450,954	1,774,612
1972	761,273	1,522,547	1,760,278	2,152,935
1973	901,902	1,803,803	2,217,735	2,712,435
1974	1,018,582	2,037,165	2,706,636	3,310,393
1975	1,426,022	2,852,044	3,699,797	4,525,093
1976	1,592,198	3,184,396	4,213,889	5,153,862
1977	1,875,234	3,750,467	5,043,995	6,169,136
1978	2,115,309	4,230,618	5,957,216	7,286,064
1979	2,611,933	5,223,865	6,968,679	8,523,149
1980	3,154,808	6,309,615	8,089,565	9,894,066
1981	3,509,069	7,018,138	9,176,494	11,223,451
1982	3,776,602	7,553,204	10,501,185	12,843,634
1983	4,342,919	8,685,837	12,776,711	15,626,752
1984	5,353,335	10,706,669	15,140,977	18,518,403
1985	6,020,167	12,040,334	17,174,416	21,005,431

Source: Author's calculations.

APPENDIX TABLE 4.1.6
Total Amount of "Unnecessary" Subsidies Paid Under HI and SMI, Using Alternative Definitions of the Poor Elderly, 1966–85 (dollars in thousands)

Year	Elderly with income below 125% of poverty level (census)	Elderly with income below 250% of poverty level (census)	65.9% of Medicare families considered poor	80.6% of Medicare families considered poor
HI				
1966	27,450,272	12,539,013	14,445,282	8,218,137
1967	3,360,178	1,705,165	1,710,180	972,947
1968	3,661,751	1,715,920	1,912,186	1,087,871
1969	4,190,928	1,914,375	2,205,411	1,254,691
1970	5,286,421	2,575,231	2,727,185	1,551,537
1971	6,194,841	3,332,897	3,088,364	1,757,016
1972	7,369,770	4,432,169	3,514,813	1,999,630
1973	8,985,019	5,695,422	4,185,644	2,381,275
1974	10,573,428	7,086,446	4,794,600	2,727,719
1975	13,099,806	8,639,550	5,987,981	3,406,652
1976	14,215,333	9,502,127	6,454,632	3,672,137
1977	16,392,190	11,072,870	7,403,625	4,212,033
1978	18,770,135	13,036,177	8,355,895	4,753,794
1979	20,799,252	13,976,655	9,419,050	5,358,639
1980	22,591,377	14,777,132	10,368,317	5,898,691
1981	24,515,597	16,256,331	11,176,228	6,358,323
1982	27,177,828	18,735,960	12,146,316	6,910,221
1983	30,616,149	21,778,498	13,453,746	7,654,037
1984	34,674,780	24,141,242	15,416,036	8,770,414
1985	37,652,518	26,342,074	16,696,370	9,498,815
SMI				
1966	4,141,975	1,892,013	2,179,650	1,240,036
1967	601,497	305,237	306,135	174,165
1968	678,506	317,952	354,319	201,578
1969	856,976	391,458	450,970	256,564
1970	1,198,219	583,701	618,143	351,671
1971	1,505,998	810,244	750,797	427,140
1972	1,909,862	1,148,588	910,857	518,200
1973	2,463,403	1,561,501	1,147,569	652,869
1974	3,088,605	2,070,022	1,400,551	796,794
1975	4,188,238	2,762,216	1,914,463	1,089,166
1976	4,802,171	3,209,973	2,180,480	1,240,508
1977	5,778,781	3,903,547	2,610,019	1,484,879
1978	6,924,473	4,809,164	3,082,566	1,753,718
1979	7,962,694	5,350,761	3,605,948	2,051,478
1980	9,120,709	5,965,901	4,185,951	2,381,450
1981	10,415,809	6,906,739	4,748,383	2,701,426
1982	12,158,428	8,381,826	5,433,845	3,091,396
1983	15,045,111	10,702,192	6,611,318	3,761,278
1984	17,622,351	12,269,016	7,834,709	4,457,283
1985	20,041,162	14,020,995	8,886,913	5,055,898

Source: Author's calculations.

Notes

Without implicating them in the results or conclusions, the author gratefully acknowledges the yeoman service in computational assistance from Linda B. Vogel; the helpful comments of Bernard S. Bloom, Jon B. Christianson, and Judith R. Lave on previous drafts of this chapter; advice on the demographic aspects of the chapter from Korbin Liu; and aid in obtaining the Medicare data from Barbara S. Klees.

1. The acronyms used for Social Security can be confusing. The *total* program is designated as Old Age, Survivors, Disability, and Hospital Insurance (OASDHI), which consists of (1) Old Age and Survivors Insurance (OASI); (2) Disability Insurance (DI), and (3) Hospital Insurance (HI) (Medicare). The two components of Medicare are then called HI (Part A) and SMI (Part B). Thus, the designation HI can refer to either the whole Medicare program, as part of the acronym OASDHI, or to Medicare Part A. As used hereafter in this chapter, HI refers to Part A of the program (Hospital Insurance). Also, OASDHI covers other groups besides the elderly, such as nonelderly end-stage renal disease patients under Medicare. The discussion in this chapter and all of the data used pertain only to elderly Medicare enrollees and beneficiaries (those aged sixty-five and over). Otherwise, the data problems would have been insurmountable.

2. Medicare benefits are large and are growing at a more rapid rate than OASI benefits. In 1984, the latest year for which comparable data are available, OASI paid $157.8 billion in benefits, while Medicare paid $61.0 billion or a ratio of 0.387 between benefits in the two programs (Social Security Administration 1985). In 1978 this ratio was 0.310 and in 1973, 0.209. Thus, the Medicare benefit ratio nearly doubled in the ten-year period. Indeed, Medicare health benefits are expected to exceed Social Security payments in the next century (Etheredge 1984).

3. The term welfare used here and in portions of this paper refers to transfers that are pure transfers in the same sense that AFDC or Medicaid transfers are considered welfare, that is, governmental benefits that are received over and above taxes paid. As such, the word is less general than the welfare in "Welfare Economics." Another transfer aspect of the Medicare program that is not further discussed in this chapter but that should be noted is the regressivity of the payroll taxes used to finance Medicare HI. In comparing income data for 1966 and 1985, Pechman (1985) found that the two before-tax distributions of income were the same, but a decline in the progressivity of the tax system led to a more unequal distribution of income after taxes in 1985. He shows that this decline in progressivity was the result of the rise in payroll taxes and the reduction in corporate and property taxes between the two years. While the HI tax rate is now low relative to the OASI rate, it has been growing rapidly relative to it (also, see note 5), and, at the margin, contributes to the loss in progressivity of the tax system. Neither AFDC nor Medicaid is financed by means of payroll taxes.

4. Although widely used in the health literature, "need" is not a concept in positive economics. Rather, it is a normative concept, the definition of which is achieved by some Delphic group. Those living below the poverty level, as defined by societal consensus through the intermediary of the U.S. Department of Labor, are one group considered to be in need in the United States.

5. As with benefits under both programs (noted in note two), the HI contribution rate has increased at a more rapid rate than the OASI contribution rate. In 1966 the HI rate was 0.100 of the OASI rate; by 1986 it had become 0.279.

6. Thus, the general fund paid 55 percent of the total monthly SMI premiums cost in 1975 and 75 percent by 1986.

7. The benefit payments were deliberately designed to imitate those of Blue Cross/Blue Shield. At the time, it was thought that any other less generous system of benefit payments would relegate the elderly to second-class treatment status in the view of the medical care providers (see Feder 1977).

8. The HI expenditure data used in this chapter reflect Office of the Actuary, HCFA estimates of the effects of DRGs on HI expenditures after 1983 and into the future (see U.S. Department of Health and Human Services 1986).

9. For example, an elderly person who was in the hospital twenty days per year, at $492 per day,

over a ten-year period would cost the HI program an undiscounted $93,480 [(20 × $492) − $492] × 10, whether his or her prior-to-age sixty-five HI tax contributions with interest had been a hypothetical $750 or $7,500.

10. In 1982 (the latest date for which such data are available) voluntary SMI enrollment was 98.4 percent of HI enrollment (Social Security Administration 1985).

11. Prior to the great health insurance sales competition of the late 1960s and the 1970s between Blue Cross/Blue Shield and the commercial for-profit and mutual insurance companies, Blue Cross/Blue Shield's method was that of comprehensive community rating. Sales competition between Blue Cross/Blue Shield and the commercial insurers forced Blue Cross/Blue Shield to use "modified" community rating, which is, in essence, experience rating (see Greenspan and Vogel 1982).

12. Here we assume, as does economic theory, that over the long run the employer portion of the health insurance premium is passed onto the employee in the form of foregone money wages and salaries. We ignore the tax subsidies to employer-provided health insurance that have been analyzed elsewhere (Mitchell and Vogel 1975; Phelps 1986).

13. The SMI premiums are proportional with respect to expected benefits and regressive to income, in the same sense that any price is regressive to income. Because the general fund contribution to SMI premiums is constant across all income classes, it is progressive to income (i.e., it is a higher percentage of a low income than it is of a high income). For the poor elderly, for whom Medicaid pays all of the premiums plus deductibles and coinsurance under SMI, it is even more progressive to income. To the extent that the elderly continue to pay taxes into the general fund, after age sixty-five they do contribute indirectly to SMI.

14. The present value of the benefit stream increases at such a rapid rate because of the rapid rate of price and quantity increase in the hospital sector, and because the discount rate (the three-month treasury bill rate—see Appendix 4.1) is lower than the rate of increase in hospital prices and quantities.

15. One way of thinking about this is that it is as though the 1966 aged cohort had won a lottery for which they did not have to buy the ticket, and that it had a varying payoff, depending upon one's age in 1966. Clearly, the 1966 aged enjoyed a large windfall, as have all of the elderly between 1966–85, although at a declining rate in the case of HI (see column 5 of Table 4.2).

16. In 1983 hospital care expenditures were 43.3 percent of total health services and supplies expenditures; physician services were 20.3 percent (Gibson, Levit, Lazenby, and Waldo 1984).

17. For 1983 the Social Security Administration reported that 14.1 percent of those aged sixty-five and over were living below the official poverty level (Social Security Administration 1985).

18. The federal share of the $8.7 billion total was 56 percent. Although Medicare will pay for up to 100 days of skilled nursing facility care in a benefit period, it is primarily an acute medical care program. In 1980 Medicare spent only $331 million on skilled nursing facility care for the aged (Health Care Financing Administration 1983). The Medicaid program itself, which was originally designed to be an acute medical care program for *all* of the poor, has increasingly become a long-term care program for the poor elderly, by default (U.S. General Accounting Office 1983). As a result of limited state Medicaid budgets, this means that the poor *nonelderly* are increasingly being pushed out of the Medicaid program, either through increased income limits or through more exclusions and higher coinsurance or copayments. Given present Medicare-financing arrangements, the well-to-do elderly are indirect beneficiaries of this chain of events.

19. Because median earnings were used for the HI tax contribution calculations, the median earnings capture the amounts that the elderly poor would have contributed to the HI program during their working years.

20. The 65.9 percent is 100 − (14.7 + 19.4), and the 80.6 percent is 100 − 19.4.

21. While these elderly must still pay deductibles and coinsurance, these two items, including SMI premiums, amounted to only 0.6 percent and 1.6 percent of income for those elderly with incomes above $30,001 and with incomes between $20,001 and $30,000, respectively, in 1984 (Moon 1983).

22. If Medicare and Social Security were run on stricter insurance and pension principles, it might be possible to have a simpler, more efficient and still equitable solution to the long-run financing of these programs. Imaginative solutions to the problem for OASI have been put forth by Feldstein (1975, 1977), and Friedman and Friedman (1980); similar reasoning could be applied to the Medicare program.

23. For example, Mitchell and Vogel (1975) found that tax expenditures on upper-income groups under the medical deduction provisions of the federal personal income tax exceeded the amount that the federal government directly spent on Medicaid. Hansen and Weisbrod (1969) found that subsidies for higher public education varied directly with income in California and Wisconsin.

24. Blumenthal et al. (1986) and Davis and Rowland (1986b) have put forth Medicare taxing proposals that would *expand* the Medicare program.

25. Table 4.1 indicates that the total of the mean HI and the mean SMI benefit and administrative cost per elderly Medicare enrollee was $2,344.35 in 1986. Presumably, this is the amount that a national community-rating health insurer (other than government) would have had to charge each elderly person for health insurance in that year, if Medicare had not existed, in order for the health insurer to have broken even. However, the rate for 1986 does not differentiate by age or sex (as two of a number of experience-rating differentiating factors). Supposing that the health experience of female sixty-six-year-olds, for example, showed that an experience-rating health insurer could charge all female sixty-six-year-olds $1,500 per year for the equivalent of a promise of 1986 HI and SMI benefits. If there had been a Medicare tax of 64 percent or more on the 1986 *ex ante* benefits of $2,344.35 for the upper-income elderly, it would have been less expensive for all upper-income female sixty-six-year-olds to drop out of the Medicare program and pay the $1,500 to the private experience-rating insurer.

26. Parsons and Munro (1978) found similar effects for OASI, although it can be argued that the combination of Medicare financing and benefit provisions make it more "progressive" than OASI, in the sense that Medicare benefits are not tied to preretirement income, whereas OASI benefits partially are.

27. Assuming that the $25,000 and $32,000 cutoffs are not adjusted for inflation or economic growth.

28. The only difference will be one of administration. The IRS will administer the OASI means test, whereas social welfare agencies will probably continue to administer means tests for the other programs.

29. These benefits also include administrative costs because, when persons buy health insurance, they purchase a pure protection component and an administrative services component. Conceptually, these administrative services should be treated similarly to any other joint services that a consumer would purchase, such as, say, the services of the travel agent when buying an airline ticket (see Blair and Vogel 1975).

30. Mean earnings give an inaccurate measure of "true" earnings because the distribution of earnings tends to be skewed to the right, due to the existence of some high outliers on the earnings scale; the median of earnings gives a more representative picture of true earnings (see Neter and Wasserman 1961).

31. This factor is defined as the female labor force as a percentage of the female population sixteen years old and over (U.S. Bureau of the Census 1985). The factor ranged from 0.367 in 1965 to 0.532 in 1984. In 1980, for example, of the total 24,684,000 Medicare HI enrollees, 14,778,000 (or 59.9 percent) were females. Accordingly, 59.9 percent of the 1,926,000 new enrollees coming into HI in 1980, from the year 1979, were multiplied times the female labor force participation factor in 1979 of 0.511, in order to determine how many females of the total new elderly females in 1980 worked in 1979 and paid HI taxes in that year. This same procedure was followed for each year for the determination of the amount of male and female taxes paid into HI.

32. Median earnings never exceeded the maximum taxable earnings base in any of the years in question.

References

Aaron, H. J., *Economic Effects of Social Security,* Washington, DC: The Brookings Institution, 1982.

Advisory Council on Social Security, *Medicare: Benefits and Financing,* Washington, DC: U.S. Government Printing Office, 1984.

Berk, M. L., and G. R. Wilensky, "Health Care of the Poor Elderly: Supplementing Medicare," *The Gerontologist* 25:311–314, 1985.

Blair, R. D., and R. J. Vogel, *Health Insurance Administrative Costs: An Economic Analysis,* Lexington, MA: D.C. Heath, 1975.

Blumenthal, D., M. Schlesinger, P. B. Drumheller, and the Harvard Medical Project, "The Future of Medicare," *The New England Journal of Medicine,* 314(II):722–728, March 13, 1986.

Brecher, C., and J. R. Knickman, "A Reconsideration of Long-Term Care Policy," *Journal of Health Politics, Policy and Law,* 10:245–273, Summer 1985.

Brecher, C., J. R. Knickman, and R. J. Vogel, "Local Simulations of Alternative Policies for Financing Services to the Elderly," *Medical Care* 24:363–376, April 1986a.

———, "We Can Do Better for the Elderly," Working Paper, November 1986b.

Brittain, J. A., *The Payroll Tax for Social Security,* Washington, DC: The Brookings Institution, 1972.

Davis, K., and D. Rowland, *Medicare Policy: New Directions for Health and Long-Term Care,* Baltimore, MD: Johns Hopkins University Press, 1986a.

———, "Medicare Financing Reform: A New Medicare Premium," *Milbank Memorial Fund Quarterly: Health and Society,* 62:300–316, Spring 1986b.

Etheredge, L., "An Aging Society and the Federal Deficit," *Milbank Memorial Fund Quarterly: Health and Society,* 62:521–543, Fall 1984.

Feder, J., *Medicare: The Politics of Federal Hospital Insurance,* Lexington, MA: D.C. Heath, 1977.

Feldstein, M. S., "Tax Incidence in a Growing Economy with Variable Factor Supply," *Quarterly Journal of Economics,* 88:551–573, November 1974.

———, "Toward A Reform of Social Security," *The Public Interest,* 40:75–95, Summer 1975.

———, "Facing the Social Security Crisis," *The Public Interest,* 47:88–100, Spring 1977.

Feldstein, P. J., *Health Care Economics,* 2nd ed., New York, NY: Wiley, 1984.

Friedman, M., and R. Friedman, *Free to Choose,* New York, NY: Harcourt Brace Jovanovich, 1980.

Friedman, R., *Poverty: Definition and Perspective,* Washington, DC: American Enterprise Institute, 1965.

Gibson, R. M., K. R. Levit, H. Lazenby, and D. R. Waldo, "National Health Expenditures, 1983," *Health Care Financing Review,* 6:1–29, Winter 1984.

Greenspan, N. T., and R. J. Vogel, "An Econometric Analysis of the Effects of Regulation in the Private Health Insurance Market," *Journal of Risk and Insurance,* XLIX:39–58, March 1982.

Hansen, W. L., and B. A. Weisbrod, *Benefits, Costs and Finance of Public Higher Education,* Chicago, IL: Markham, 1969.

Harrington, C., et al. *Long-Term Care of the Elderly: Public Policy Issues*, Beverly Hills, CA: Sage Publications, 1985.

Health Care Financing Administration, *The Medicare and Medicaid Data Book 1983*, Baltimore, MD: Health Care Financing Administration, 1983.

Long, S. H., and R. F. Settle, "Medicare and the Disadvantaged Elderly: Objectives and Outcomes," *Milbank Memorial Fund Quarterly: Health and Society*, 62:609–656, Fall 1984.

MacIntyre, D. M., *Voluntary Health Insurance and Rate Making*, Ithaca, NY: Cornell University Press, 1962.

Milbank Memorial Fund Quarterly: Health and Society, Special Issue, "Financing Medicare: Explorations in Controlling Costs and Raising Revenues," 62, Spring 1984.

Mitchell, B. M., and R. J. Vogel, "Health and Taxes: An Assessment of the Medical Deduction," *Southern Economic Journal*, XLI:660–672, April 1975.

Moon, M., *Changing the Structure of Medicare Benefits: Issues and Options*, Washington, DC: Congressional Budget Office, 1983.

Moon, M., and T. Smeeding, "Medical Care Transfers, Poverty and the Aged," *Journal of Health Politics, Policy and Law*, 6:29–39, Spring 1981.

Munro, D. R., *Welfare Components and Labor Supply Effects of OASDHI*, unpublished Ph.D. dissertation, Ohio State University, 1976.

National Center for Health Statistics, *Vital Statistics of the United States*, 1966–1985, vol. II, *Mortality: Part A*, Washington, DC: NCHS, 1966 to 1985.

Neter, J., and W. Wasserman, *Fundamental Statistics for Business and Economics*, Boston, MA: Allyn & Bacon, 1961.

Orshansky, M., "Counting the Poor: Another Look at the Poverty Profile," *Social Security Bulletin*, 28:3–29, January 1965.

Palmer, H. C., "The Alternatives Question," in R. J. Vogel and H. C. Palmer, eds., *Long-Term Care: Perspectives from Research and Demonstrations*, Baltimore, MD: Health Care Financing Administration, 1983.

Parsons, D. O., and D. R. Munro, "Intergenerational Transfers in Social Security," in M. J. Boskin, ed., *The Crisis in Social Security*, San Francisco, CA: Institute for Contemporary Studies, 1978.

Pechman, J. A., *Who Paid The Taxes 1966–85?*, Washington, DC: The Brookings Institution, 1985.

Phelps, C. E., "Large-Scale Tax Reform: The Example of Employer-Paid Health Insurance Premiums," Working Paper No. 32, Rochester Center for Economic Research, March 26, 1986.

Rice, D. P., and J. J. Feldman, "Living Longer in the United States: Demographic Changes and Health Needs of the Elderly," *Milbank Memorial Fund Quarterly: Health and Society*, 61:362–376, Summer 1983.

Scanlon, W. J., "A Theory of the Nursing Home Market," *Inquiry* 17:25–41, Spring 1980.

Smeeding, T. R., *Alternative Methods for Valuing Selected In-Kind Transfer Benefits and Measuring Their Effect on Poverty*, Washington, DC: U.S. Government Printing Office, 1982.

Social Security Administration, *Social Security Bulletin, Annual Statistical Supplement, 1984–85*, Baltimore, MD: Social Security Administration, 1985.

Tax Foundation, Inc., *Facts and Figures on Government Finance, 1983,* Washington, DC: Tax Foundation, Inc., 1983.

U.S. Bureau of the Census, *Current Population Reports,* Series P-25, Washington, DC: U.S. Government Printing Office 1965 to 1985.

————, *Current Population Reports: Consumer Income,* Series P-60, Washington, DC: U.S. Government Printing Office 1966 to 1985.

————, *Statistical Abstract of the United States: 1985,* 105th ed., Washington, DC: U.S. Government Printing Office, 1985.

U.S. Department of Health and Human Services, Health Care Financing Administration, Office of the Actuary, *1986 Annual Report of the Board of Trustees of the Federal Hospital Insurance Trust Fund,* and *1986 Annual Report of the Board of Trustees of the Federal Supplementary Medical Insurance Trust Fund,* Washington, DC: USDHHS, 1986.

U.S. General Accounting Office, *Medicaid and Nursing Home Care: Cost Increases and the Need for Services Are Creating Problems for the Elderly,* Washington, DC: USGAO, October 21, 1983.

II ⊡⊡⊡
Medicare as
Insurance in
Insurance Markets

5. Unresolved Risk Under Medicare

CHARLES E. PHELPS

ANNE LENHARD REISINGER

Introduction

A brief history of Medicare

As health insurance expanded through the United States after World War II, employer group insurance became the primary source of coverage for most insured Americans. The use of this fringe benefit arose during the war in response to wartime wage controls. As the effective marginal tax rate for the economy increased in later years, the desirability of this fringe benefit expanded greatly, largely because the value of the health insurance premiums was not considered taxable income.[1]

As the labor force who had benefited from this employer group insurance grew to retirement age, it became increasingly apparent that this insurance mechanism was incomplete. Upon retirement, almost all of these insured persons lost their coverage. Ironically, this loss came at a time of life when both average expenditures for health care and the variance in expenditures increased due to the ravages of time and nature. Families accustomed to reasonably extensive health insurance, particularly for hospitalization, confronted a serious increase in financial risk.

Employer group insurance became attractive not only because of the tax subsidy, but also because the employer group structure minimized problems of self-selection of sickly people into better insurance plans. Both of these advantages of employer group insurance vanish upon retirement, leaving the prospects for private and individual purchase of health insurance much dimmer. The federal policy response to this issue in the early 1960s, the Kerr-Mills legislation, provided income-related health insurance for the elderly. While this provided considerable benefit to the lower-income segment of the retired population, it offered no assistance for the great bulk of the elderly.

Medicare was designed to remedy this problem. It offered, for the first time in the history of the United States, a health plan provided by the government that included an entire eligible population without a means test. As such, it was perhaps as revolutionary in health policy as was the Social Security Act for retirement policy.

Partly because of the universal coverage of the over-sixty-five population and partly because there was, in truth, little serious evidence with which to undertake programmatic planning, Medicare was structured with several features designed to limit overall programmatic expenditure. Our chapter reviews in the next section the potential financial risk to Medicare enrollees resulting from the structure of Medicare, using available data from various published sources and from Medicare's internal records. Where possible, we calculate the variance in financial outcomes arising from each feature of the Medicare policy. Under some assumptions, this allows calculation of an approximate measure of the amount a risk-averse person would pay to avoid each risk.[2]

We then use a simulation in the following section to better understand the lifetime risk imposed by certain features of the Part A (hospital) coverage, where existing data cannot provide a clear picture of the risk we seek to portray. This simulation contains acknowledged problems, but even with its limits it points out the large risks created by the failure of Part A insurance to cover more adequately the extended stays in the hospital confronting some Medicare recipients.

In the section on supplemental coverage, we review the insurance coverage people have purchased to offset the risk confronting them under Medicare's basic structure. As in other areas of insurance purchase, some of these choices seem not to conform with the usual expected utility maximizing model employed commonly by economists.

We discuss in the next section how recent changes in Medicare's structure have altered the risk confronting enrollees. Some of these changes, probably unintentionally, have reduced the apparent financial risk of enrollees considerably.

We conclude with discussions on the relationship between Medicare cost control efforts and consumers' desires to limit financial risk, and we point to some potential changes in Medicare that could reduce risk even further, with little fiscal effect on Medicare overall.

A note on lifetime versus annual perspective

Most of the calculations and discussion that follow deal with the risk on an annual basis. A prominent exception is the simulation of the risk imposed by the lifetime reserve (LR) features of Part A because this particular aspect of Medicare requires a lifetime perspective for analysis. However, each remaining feature of Medicare can be analyzed—as any insurance problem—with an annual time framework because (in simple analog) any person has the capability of insuring these events on an annual basis, and because all of the data we find present data on utilization and spending patterns on an annual basis.

The annual perspective creates two potentially deceiving features in the portrait of risk we wish to present. First, there is a known correlation of spending through time for individuals, so that high expenses in year i foretell abnormally high expenses in year $i + 1$ as well. This at least shifts the average expense facing the person; what might happen to the variance in risk is less clear. To the extent that the individual knows about or anticipates a higher mean expense but the insurance company does not, then any insurance policy will become more attractive. But since we generally focus on the risk premium—the amount people would pay to avoid the financial variance confronting them—these differences in information (consumers' vs. insurers') become less relevant.

The second consideration deals with the distinction between income and wealth. Most older people, compared with the remainder of their life cycle, have low incomes and high assets. The income available to an elderly person in any year is obviously a combination of past consumption and savings decisions, returns on any investments they have made, and economic fluctuations. For purposes of this chapter, however, we can think of the income stream, including possible asset depletion, available to an elderly person much as we would any other income stream, and we can think of the risk-avoiding problems confronting that person just as we would for any other person. Even the risk of running out of LR coverage on Part A (as we analyze later in this chapter) can be considered from this annual basis.

A note on normative criteria for analyzing insurance plans
In most of what follows, we implicitly accept the usual economics approach to analyzing a risky situation, that is, the expected utility maximizing model. Indeed, the calculation of risk premiums that we make hinges wholly on this assumption. We note that some of the decisions people actually *do* undertake in purchasing insurance may conflict with this model of behavior. We openly acknowledge the intellectual dilemma this creates, but because the expected utility model enjoys such wide use, we provide the summary measures (risk premiums) appropriate to this model throughout the paper.

The Structure of Medicare Payments and Resultant Risk

In this section, we characterize the financial risk arising from the various parts of Medicare coverage, concentrating first on Part A and then on Part B. This section reviews and uses evidence from previously published sources. This chapter later develops a simulation to expand upon available information.

Hospital care

Medicare separates insurance coverage into Part A (for hospital expenditure) and Part B (for physician and other expenditure). Within the hospital insurance plan, financial risk for any patient arises from three sources: (1) the first-day deductible, (2) the requirement of copayments for hospital days 61–90 in any hospital stay and during any of the 60 LR days used subsequently, and (3) the risk of running out of coverage under the LR program.[3] Each of these is discussed in further detail below.

An important concept in these discussions is the "spell of illness." All Part A benefits center on the spell of illness, which is equivalent to a single hospitalization in most cases. However, if a person is re-hospitalized within a week after being discharged from the hospital, the same spell of illness continues. For re-hospitalized patients, this means that the patient need not pay the first-day deductible a second time. However, as we discuss in more detail below, this administrative structure also creates added risk for extended stays, including those for which the patient is financially liable. This turns out to be a nontrivial issue; a goodly number of the people who must pay for some coinsurance days or use some LR days (see below) get into this situation through a repeat hospitalization within the same spell of illness.

The first-day deductible. Medicare requires that every patient pays for the first day of hospitalization of each spell of illness at a common rate throughout the United States. The law sets that rate at the average cost of a single day's hospitalization for the preceding year.[4] In Medicare's first year, the first-day deductible cost $56. The rate was set at $572 for 1987. Obviously, while some of this increase merely reflects background inflation (the consumer price index [CPI] has tripled in the intervening years), a substantial real increase in the deductible remains. Recent changes in the Medicare law place a cap on increases in this first-day deductible.

About one-quarter of the Medicare population faces at least one hospitalization each year.[5] Among this group, about 70 percent are hospitalized once, 20 percent are hospitalized twice, and 10 percent three or more times.[6] Only 6 percent of the Medicare population experiences more than one hospitalization, and hence the potential liability for more than one deductible per year. Thus, while there is some variation in risk from this first-day deductible, the variance in spending created by this feature of the plan is not extreme.

We can infer how often re-hospitalization occurs within the same spell of illness by comparing the number of hospitalizations with the number of benefit periods reported by Medicare. For example, during calendar year 1977—for which the most complete data on admissions are published—we calculate that three-eighths of all persons with multiple admissions have at least some of those admissions within the same benefit period.[7]

Based on these estimated frequencies of benefit periods occurring and using a first-day fee of $572, the expected loss in 1987 for an average Medicare beneficiary is $168, the coefficient of variation is about 2.5, and the variance in spending is approximately $183,500.

How much would we expect an individual to pay for insurance to remove this risk alone? Using the standard economist's approach, a risk averse person with a "moderate" level of risk aversion[8] would be willing to pay the actuarial value plus $18 for insurance to eliminate this risk if it were the *only* risk confronting the individual or if the risk were independent of other risks. That is, for an average risk of $168, the typical maximum insurance premium we would expect for such a decision-maker would be about $186.[9]

We can also calculate what the average and variance of spending on the first-day deductible would be if the spell-of-illness concept did not exist, so that each admission generated a separate deductible payment liability. In that case, the average payment would be $186 (vs. $168), and the variance in spending across the population would be about $230,500 (vs. $183,500). Thus, the spell-of-illness concept somewhat reduces risk on this dimension, with an associated risk premium reduction for our typical risk-averse persons of $1.50.

Coinsurance days. At the tail end of a spell of illness, a different type of risk emerges. For each spell of illness exceeding 60 days duration, the patient confronts additional financial risk. For days 61–90 of each spell of illness, the patient pays 25 percent of the current first-day deductible rate. In 1987 copayment days cost the patient $572/4 or $143 per day.

Aggregate data from Medicare records (HCFA undated) show that coinsurance days were used at a rate of about 140 per 1,000 enrollees in 1982 and 1983. Using data from the Health Care Financing Administration replicated in Table 5.1, we have calculated the variance in financial risk arising from the copayment day feature of Medicare. This empirical distribution tabulates the actual use of copayment days in 1983.

The average risk of hospital coinsurance days is $45 per year. The variance in financial risk arising from the coinsurance days feature is $53,000, using the 1983 frequencies and the 1987 daily fee of $143 per coinsurance day. Our prototypical risk-averse person would pay a risk premium of about $5 annually to avoid this risk, were it the only risk confronting the individual.

The risk is much larger than one would estimate if looking only at the distribution of hospital length of stay, because of the effect of multiple admissions

TABLE 5.1
Distribution of Copayment Days Incurred in Calendar Year 1983 Among Persons Hospitalized

Coinsurance days	Number (thousands)	Cumulative percent
0	11,239	
1	22	7.3
2	21	14.0
3	20	20.6
4	20	26.9
5	18	32.9
6	17	38.3
7	16	43.5
8	14	48.2
9	13	52.3
10	12	56.1
11	11	59.7
12	10	62.8
13	9	68.2
14	8	68.2
15	7	70.5
16	7	72.7
17	6	74.6
18	6	76.4
19	5	78.2
20	5	79.2
21	4	81.9
22	4	82.3
23	4	83.5
24	3	84.6
25	3	85.7
26	3	86.7
27	3	87.6
28	3	88.4
29	2	89.1
30	34	100.0

Source: HCFA (undated).

stacking into single benefit periods. Only 54,000 single admissions had lengths of stay that would have generated coinsurance days had they been the only admission within a benefit period, compared with an actual number of discharges of 309,000 requiring some coinsurance days. Making some necessary assumptions to compare data across years, we estimate that the average coinsurance day risk would be only $3, with a variance of about $10,000 if each hospitalization were a separate spell of illness.[10] Thus, while "saving" the prototypical individual a risk premium of $1.50 in avoiding payment of deductibles, the spell-of-illness feature generates an added risk for coinsurance days that the same individual would pay $4 to avoid.

This is a bad trade by any risk-averse person's standards, but it is not the end of the risk generated by the spell-of-illness concept. Because of the way admissions stack up within spells of illness, the risk of running out of coinsurance days (and hence needing to use LR days) also increases, as does the risk of running out of LR days as well. We address these risks more fully in a later section.

Lifetime reserve days. For patients experiencing a hospitalization over 90 days in length, coverage for the "spell of illness" ends, and the patient must then dip into an LR of 60 days of coverage, for which Medicare and the patient split the cost. For each of these LR days, the patient pays half of the first-day deductible, and Medicare pays the residual cost to the hospital. For 1987 the patient paid $286 per day for these days. After this coverage is used up, the patient must pay the full cost of any continued stay during that hospitalization.

Prior to 1984 an average of over 60 LR days were incurred annually per 1,000 enrollees. This rate fell to 37 LR days per 1,000 enrollees in 1984.

In 1985, 48,672 persons used at least one LR day (out of 28.2 million aged enrollees), or about 1 per 575 enrollees. During that year, 6,036 persons, or about 1 per 4,700 enrollees, exhausted their LR days, thereby becoming vulnerable to a large risk for hospital expenses (HCFA, undated).

Cumulative data over the history of Medicare show that 153,182 persons had exhausted their LR days by the end of 1985, and of those, 24,720 were still alive entering 1986. Thus, of all the Medicare recipients alive today, about 1 per 1,100 no longer can rely on Medicare to protect against very long hospitalization risk (i:e., those exceeding the 90-day spell-of-illness limit). Unfortunately, the very nature of Medicare data makes it difficult to know the extent of risk imposed by this lack of coverage. Since Medicare stops paying for care after the LR has been exhausted, little information is available on the distribution of lengths of stay in the range where the LR days would be used or for care after they are exhausted.

Simulations described later in this paper explore the nature of this risk more fully. At this point, we merely report the aggregate statistics, and note that the current rate of persons running out of LR days probably does not yet represent the eventual equilibrium.[11]

Physician care

While enrollment in Medicare Part A is compulsory for every person covered under the Social Security Act, coverage for physician services is voluntary. The name of the program, Supplementary Medical Insurance (SMI), reflects this official volunteerism. However, enrollment rates have been nearly 100%, partly due to the considerable subsidy in the premiums. For example, in 1987, the annual premium was $217, but Medicare paid charges almost four times that per patient.[12] Services covered under Part B (SMI) include virtually all physician services (MD and DO), laboratory and diagnostic tests they order, plus limited coverage of podiatry, chiropractic care, and other healers.

Financial risk to Medicare beneficiaries under Part B arises from two sources: (1) copayment of 20 percent and (2) fee variation and the fee schedule limit.

Copayment of 20 percent. The initial structure of Medicare physician payments closely matched contemporaneous private health insurance coverage, especially the newly growing major medical plans. The patient paid the first $50 annually of physician expenses ($50 deductible) and then 20 percent of all remaining charges. Even this coverage created considerable financial risk for patients since, unlike a growingly popular feature of private insurance plans, no "stop-loss" feature exists within Medicare. Patient risk grows unendingly at 20 percent of the rate at which resources are spent.

The large bulk of SMI payments occur within the hospital setting. In 1983, for example, 62 percent of payments to physicians were for services provided to hospitalized patients, 29 percent for patients treated in an office, 6 percent in a hospital outpatient department, and 3 percent for other settings. These data indicate that Part A and Part B risk will correlate quite highly for the Medicare population, which in turn implies that any measure of risk looking only at Part A or Part B alone will understate overall risk.

Fee variation and the fee schedule limit. Beginning in 1971 with the Nixon administration's wage-price freeze and subsequent economy-wide price controls, Medicare began to limit payments to physicians. First, physician fees were frozen nominally for three years, then they were allowed to grow according to an input-cost index that generally did not grow as rapidly as the CPI. While physicians were free to charge any fee they wished after the three-year price freeze ended, Medicare no longer paid 80 percent of billed charges but rather 80 percent of the "allowed fee" under the Medicare rules. Patients became at risk for any differences between physician charges and the Medicare payment.

Intimately connected with the fee schedule concept is the notion of "assignment of benefits" under Part B. Physicians can receive the Part B payment directly from Medicare, rather than channeled through the patient. This reduces risks of payment default, but in accepting assignment of benefits the physicians must agree to accept the Medicare-allowed fee as their full fee. They may still collect the 20 percent coinsurance for that fee directly from the patient. Willingness to accept assignment of benefits varies by specialty, region, and time, as well as the individual circumstances of the physician and patient. For our purposes here, we simply note that when physicians do accept assignment, they significantly reduce their patients' financial risks. Of course, we expect the physician to be more willing to accept assignment when his or her fee is relatively low in the fee profile, that is, when his or her charge is more likely to be covered fully (or nearly so) by the allowed fee.

The 1984 Deficit Reduction Act altered the incentives for a physician to accept assignment. We discuss these changes and their consequences in the section on recent changes in Medicare. Data on patient liability under Part B presented later in this chapter (unless otherwise noted) refer to actual physician charges incurred where assignment has not been accepted by the physician.

The risk-inducing effects of the Medicare Part B payment system can be considerable, particularly for in-hospital physician services. This risk arises because of the large variation of fees for a given procedure or medical activity, even within a small geographic area.

If consumer search is limited, variation in fees for a given procedure can arise even when quality is constant. The most useful conceptual modeling of this phenomenon arises from work by Schwartz and Wilde, Sadanand and Wilde. This work relies on a model of monopolistic competition and incomplete consumer search. Price variation arises because of varying fixed costs across producers, and it is sustained if consumer search is sufficiently incomplete. The variability in equilibrium prices increases (1) as the variability in fixed costs increases, (2) as the amount of search by consumers decreases, and (3) as the price elasticity of demand by consumers is smaller in absolute value.

The same conceptual approach remains valid when different qualities of a product or service coexist in the market. In concept, the markets separate by quality, with none of the original insights changing notably. Empirically, of course, when quality variation is not measured, the apparent variability in producer prices will increase as the product quality variance increases. Observed physician fee schedule distributions, for example, contain variation induced both by quality variation and by search-related issues as modeled by Wilde, Schwartz, and others.

An example of the effect of fee schedule limits on consumer risk appears in Table 5.2. This example considers a procedure with an average cost of $100 and a standard deviation from that average of $50 (so the coefficient of variation

TABLE 5.2
Medicare Payments, Patient Copayments, and Variability of Copayments for Hypothetical Fee Distribution

Fee cutoff	Average Medicare payment	Average copayment	Variance of copayment
50th percentile	$60	$40	$1,765
Average fee	66	34	1,521
75th percentile	70	30	1,156
90th percentile	76	24	484

Fee distribution: Mean = $100; standard deviation = 50; minimum = 16; maximum = 275.

[COV] is 0.5). This example shows a simulated fee distribution and the insurance payment arising from a plan that paid 80 percent of the lesser of the physician fee or an administratively prescribed cutoff (e.g., the 50th percentile of the fee distribution, the 75th percentile, and so on). The variance in payments arising from each type of payment constitutes the risk imposed on the insured population.

As the data in Table 5.2 show, the trade-off between risk and average payment is nontrivial. For example, if the insurer pays 80 percent of the median fee (or fee charged, whichever is less), the average payment is $60, and the variance of out-of-pocket expenses to the consumer is $1,765. Shifting payment to the 75th percentile raises the average payment (and presumably, the premium) by 17 percent, and the variance falls by 35 percent. Shifting to a 90th percentile cutoff raises the premium further by 8.6 percent (above that for the 75th percentile plan), and the variance falls by nearly 60 percent.

Actual COVs are much larger for many procedures than this example employs. Table 5.3 shows the average within-state COV in four separate states (New Jersey, North Carolina, Michigan, and Washington) for inpatient physician fees for the ten most common diagnosis-related groups (DRGs) in Medicare. In general, for nonsurgical procedures, the COV of physician charges centered near one for the four states studied by Mitchell et al. (1984). For surgical procedures, the COV was less but still nontrivial. These charges probably overstate the variation arising just from fee differences since there may be many different and separately

TABLE 5.3
Within-DRG Variability in Physician Fees for Four States for Most Common Medicare DRG Admissions

DRG	Hospital	Physician charges (average of 4 within-state variations)
		Coefficients of variation
Heart failure (DRG 127)	0.73	0.90
Angina (DRG 140)	0.68	0.98
Esophagitis (DRG 182)	0.78	0.92
Stroke (DRG 014)	0.81	0.84
Pneumonia (DRG 089)	0.61	0.97
Arrhythmia (DRG 138)	0.75	1.04
Metabolic disorders (DRG 296)	0.83	0.94
Joint reattachment (DRG 209)	0.46	0.27
Prostate removal (DRG 336)	0.62	0.27
Bronchitis (DRG 096)	0.68	0.92

Source: Medicare hospitalization rates (col. 1) from Callahan and Lawrence (1986). Physician DRG data (col. 2) from Mitchell et al. (1984).

TABLE 5.4
Average Out-of-Pocket Payments per Medicare Enrollee

	1975	1982
Total physician charges	$214	$664
Deductible	21	37
Coinsurance (20% of allowed charges)	30 (14% of fees)	91 (14% of fees)
Unassigned claims, additional fees	21 (10% of fees)	77 (12% of fees) ($43 in 1975 dollars)
Premium charged (percent of charges)	80 (37%)	139 (21%)

Source: McMillan, Lubitz, and Newton (1985) Table 1.

billable procedures or visits within a single DRG category. Inspection of the data in Mitchell et al. (1984) shows that the variability is less for most surgical procedures but greater for medical DRGs. Undoubtedly, this reflects in general the greater ambiguity of treatment for cognitive (vs. procedural) illnesses.

The tradeoff between average premium cost and risk portrayed in Table 5.2 suggests one reason why most private health insurance plans typically select a relatively high fee schedule cutoff, such as the 90th percentile of charges. Consumers who are risk averse will show preferences for higher average but lower variance expenditure patterns.[13] Higher fee cutoffs provide just such protection against risk.

Medicare Part B fee schedule reimburses the physician the smallest of (1) the actual fee charged, (2) the median fee charged by the physician to all his or her patients, and (3) the 75th percentile of the overall fee distribution for the locality. Thus, while this is certainly more generous than a 50th percentile cutoff, it is at the bottom end of a range of choices where risk falls rapidly with relatively small increases in program cost.

Table 5.4 portrays briefly the sources of financial liability arising under Part B for the average Medicare enrollee. Note that the premium has fallen, compared with actual costs of the Part B program. Thus, Medicare has systematically increased the subsidy to Part B from the (intended) 50 percent at the beginning of the program to now over 75 percent.

Table 5.5 shows the distribution of annual charges beyond those allowed by Medicare Part B and for which the patients retained liability. These data allow an approximation of the extent of risk generated by this feature of the Part B structure: the average excess liability among physician users was approximately $123 in 1982, with a standard deviation of $200, so the variance equals $40,000.[14]

TABLE 5.5
Distribution of Medicare Physician Payments above Medicare Fee Schedule (Population over Age 65, 1982)

Amount of fee above allowed fee (dollars)	Number of physician users (thousands)	Percent
0	3,305	21
1–99	8,635	54
100–299	2,387	15
300–499	724	4
500+	950	6

Source: McMillan, Lubitz, and Newton (1985) Table 10.

Adjusted to 1987 levels, assuming fee levels and assignment rates remain unchanged, this represents a risk of about $175, a standard deviation of $284, and a variance of $80,000. This, of course, represents only one source of Part B financial risk; the others include the deductible (now $75 per year) and the coinsurance payments of 20 percent of the allowed fee.

Using the same level of risk aversion as discussed previously (risk-aversion measure $= -0.0002$), the risk premium associated with this risk is $8 annually. Thus, the largest premium we would expect a risk-averse person to pay to avoid this risk is the expected value ($175) plus a risk premium of $8 or $183 total.

As Table 5.6 shows, the importance of the fee cutoff mechanisms rises with the realized amount of out-of-pocket liability. That is, the deductible and co-insurance payments account for a smaller percentage of total enrollee Part B liability as total expense rises. For that small fraction of the Medicare population facing large out-of-pocket risk ($1,500 or more annually), the role of the fee cutoff is considerable, with over half of patient liability arising because of the 75th percentile cutoff.

Finally, Table 5.7 portrays the overall resource use and risk, in more complete detail, for all spending under Part B. As noted earlier, of course, these risks are not independent but actually must be highly correlated. Thus, the overall financial risk confronting individuals under Parts A and B will be considerably larger than either component alone suggests.

In the distribution shown in Table 5.7, the expected Part B out-of-pocket liability for a typical Medicare enrollee was $146 per year in 1980 or about $200 per year in 1987 dollars. The COV is 1.76. Thus, the variance in personal expenditures under Medicare Part B in 1987 will be approximately $130,000.[15]

Adopting the same approach to measuring the risk premium as previously, we can calculate the risk premium associated with this facet of Medicare's structure at about $10 per person per year.

TABLE 5.6
Financial Risk from Part B Services, Aged Population, 1982

Amount of liability (dollars)	Percent of population	Source of liability		
		Deductible	Coinsurance	Fee above allowed
0	20	—	—	—
1–299	58	0.39	0.40	0.21
300–750	14	0.13	0.54	0.33
750–1,499	6	0.06	0.51	0.43
1,500+	2	0.02	0.44	0.54

Source: McMillan, Lubitz, and Newton (1985) Table 11.

TABLE 5.7
Distribution of Annual Out-of-Pocket Expenses for Physician Services for Medicare Aged Participants, 1980

Annual charges per person (dollars)	Percent of persons	Average liability in this category	Average liability
0–199	35.2	0.596	$ 64
200–399	22.4	0.450	119
400–699	14.2	0.377	180
700–999	7.1	0.342	256
1,000–1,499	7.0	0.324	355
1,500–1,999	4.3	0.319	495
2,000–2,499	2.9	0.311	615
2,500–2,999	1.9	0.310	752
3,000–3,999	2.2	0.309	927
4,000–5,000	1.1	0.299	1,143
5,000–6,000	0.6	0.305	1,424
6,000+	1.0	0.297	2,081
Total	100.0	0.348	$ 235

Source: Ruther and Helbing (1985) Tables 1 and 4.

Noncovered services

Nursing home and long-term care. Medicare deliberately avoided the coverage of long-term care, leaving that issue for other mechanisms to resolve. The long-term care financial risk is considerable and the mechanisms to resolve that risk only partial. The original Social Security Amendments of 1965 (Titles XVIII and XIX) that created Medicare and Medicaid left the coverage of long-term care to the federal/state Medicaid program, where eligibility and extent of long-term care benefits vary from state to state. Typically, eligibility for Medicaid requires a "spend-down" of assets of the family involved and restrictive limits on allowed income.

Admission into a nursing home is a rare event—much rarer than acute hospitalization—but the variation in risk is large once the event of admission to the nursing home occurs.[16] While only a small percentage of the elderly are admitted into a nursing home each year, the average length of stay (ALOS) ranges from one-half year to over a year, depending on age, and the variance is large. Around the ALOS are standard deviations of length of stay nearly twice the ALOS. For example, for persons aged eighty-five to eighty-nine years—an age range prominent in nursing home admissions—the ALOS is 1 year, and the COV is 1.6 years (584 days). We cannot compute the annual variance in spending from these data (to provide comparable figures to the spending variance from other risks), but it is clear that the risk is very large. To simplify the risk considerably, suppose that 2 percent of the Medicare population were admitted to a long-term care facility every year for the ALOS of one year. Then the average risk (at $50 per day) would be $365, and the variance in spending would exceed $125,000. If the probability of admission to a long-term care facility reaches 5 percent, the average risk would be $913, and the variance nearly $200,000. These estimates of risk understate the actual risk because of the large variance within the class of those who are admitted to long-term care facilities. Nevertheless, it is clear that the risk from long-term care approaches, if not exceeds, the risk imposed by the Part A or Part B structure alone.

Other uncovered services. Medicare does not cover certain medical services that create financial risk. The most obvious gaps, compared with private insurance coverage held by many under-sixty-five persons, occur for such services as dental care and vision care. Dental insurance has grown in popularity for the under-sixty-five, in great part because of the subsidy conveyed by the tax system (Phelps 1984, 1986). Although the risk is present for the elderly, we could find no data reliably describing the variability in expenses that the Medicare population confronts due to these services.

TABLE 5.8
Summary of Risk Confronting Medicare Participants (Standardized to 1987)

Medicare feature	Mean	Variance	Risk premium
Deductible Part A	$168	$183,500	$18
Coinsurance days[a] Part A	19	53,000	5
Lifetime reserve[b] Part A	18	Unknown	Unknown
Beyond coverage hospital days	Unknown	Unknown	Unknown
Part B (overall)	200	130,000	13
Uncovered services	—	Unknown	—

[a]This risk represents the 1983 distribution of copay days, evaluated at 1987 prices. The risk of incurring a copay day fell considerably subsequent to 1983, but no data exist yet on the distribution of the risk, and hence we cannot calculate the variance.

[b]This is the dollar value of an average of 0.063 LR days per enrollee in 1983, at $286 per day. In 1984 the average LR days fell to 0.037 per enrollee, or about $11 in average risk.

TABLE 5.9
Distribution of Large Expenses for Medicare (Total, Part A, and Part B, 1982)

Enrollee upper percentile	Percent of Expenses Attributed to Percentile Group		
	Part A	Part B	Total
8.8	80[a]	59	71
5.0	61	44	54
2.0	38[a]	26	32
1.0	24	17	20
0.5	15	11	13

[a]Approximation, interpolating from values in source.
Source: Riley et al. (1986) Table 1.

Summary of unresolved risks

We have summarized existing information on the financial risk arising under Medicare. Each of these discussions considered only the risk from each separate aspect of Medicare. Table 5.8 summarizes these separate studies.

We have found no data describing the overall financial risk generated by the structure of Medicare and the medical service use by the enrolled population.[17] In particular, although we know that Part A and Part B risk must be highly correlated, we do not know the extent of this correlation at the individual level. Thus, we can only conjecture about the overall risk confronting Medicare enrollees. Table 5.9 provides some indirect evidence on this issue: both expenditure distributions from Part A and Part B are similarly skewed, so that a small percentage of enrollees with large expenses accounts for large fractions of total expense. We cannot know from these data whether the same individuals are in both distributions, but it seems quite likely that in both distributions the hospitalized Medicare enrollees are those at largest risk in all cases.

Simulation of Part A Risks—the Upper Tail

Available data allow immediate calculation of the financial risk from the Part A deductible and from Part B overall. This leaves unanswered the extent of financial risk generated by the upper tail of the expenditure distribution from Part A, that is, expenditures for coinsurance days, LR days, and uninsured days. While some aggregate data show the average expense by individuals in this category, virtually nothing can show the financial variability. To resolve this, at least partly, we turn to a simulation of "deep risk" under Part A.

The overall simulation process is described in a heavily documented computer program available from the authors. We summarize the structure of the simulation here.[18]

1. An individual is "born" into the simulation at age sixty-five. Each person's probability of survival is taken from standard life tables, and a random number draw each year determines if the person lives or dies each year.

2. If the person lives, the number of hospitalizations encountered is generated according to a random distribution, with probabilities of number of admissions depending on age and sex.

3. On each hospitalization, the program generates a random probability that coinsurance days are incurred, using the observed probabilities from Medicare data. (The data reflect the use of coinsurance days for a single hospitalization, not a spell of illness. Thus, their use conditional upon a hospitalization is appropriate.) A Pareto distribution was fit to these data,[19] then this distribution was solved for the cumulative distribution function and inverted to find the number of days consistent with a random draw from the [0,1] range.

4. Aggregate data showed that in 1983, LR days were incurred at a rate of 0.063 per enrollee. Aggregate data show that 12.5 percent of persons using *any* LR days in a single year will run out during that year. Thus, we found a Pareto distribution with those characteristics. If 20 percent of the persons using any coinsurance days use some LR days, and if the conditional distribution of use of LR days is Pareto (alpha = 20, beta = 550), these aggregate phenomena are replicated.[20] This distribution has an average number of LR days—conditional upon there being any—of twenty-nine. This distribution forms the basis for our simulation of LR days and uninsured days.

5. If the drawing from the LR day Pareto distribution exceeds the remaining number of LR days for a person, uncovered days accumulate. Thus, the same process generates LR days and uncovered days. This model assumes that at these extreme lengths of stay, the length of stay is independent of insurance coverage, an assumption that cannot be supported or refuted by data in general. The actual distribution is unknown, so the simulation results depend heavily on the particular distribution of extended length of stay assumed in this process.

6. This process repeats until the person "dies."

7. The simulation is repeated over a sufficiently large sample. The estimates of risk remain stable as the number of lives in the simulation increases. Stability appears at about 10,000 lives. The results reported here represent 300,000 lives simulated.

Some results of the simulation appear in Table 5.10, showing the mean and variance first in days of care and then in dollars of risk. The average coinsurance days per enrollee per year closely replicates the Medicare data upon which the simulation was based. Our simulations show 0.135 coinsurance days per year,

TABLE 5.10
Variance in Spending from Medicare Part A (Results of Simulation)

	Days of care	
	Mean	Variance
Coinsurance days	0.135	2.60
Lifetime reserve days	0.0560	2.24
Uninsured days	0.011	0.68

	Financial risk (dollars)		
	Mean	Variance	Risk premium
Coinsurance days	19	53,000	5
Lifetime reserve days	16	184,000	18
Uninsured days	6	223,000	22

whereas Medicare shows 0.139 per enrollee per year. The financial risk from co-insurance days has a mean of $19 and a variance of $53,000. Our prototype risk-averse person would pay a premium to avoid this risk of about $5 on top of the $19 actuarial value of the risk.

The risk generated from LR days is much larger, primarily because the amount the individual must pay doubles from one-quarter to one-half of the average daily hospital cost. The simulation closely replicates the known average use of LR days in the Medicare population (0.063 per person per year, simulated as 0.056), and the variance is nearly $184,000. This occurs despite the average cost of such coverage being smaller ($16) than the average cost of the coinsurance day payments ($19). The annual risk premium our prototype Medicare enrollee would pay to avoid this risk is $18.

The risk created by uninsured days, beyond LR days for long hospitalizations, cannot be validated against Medicare data since by definition Medicare coverage has stopped, and no data exist to describe these occurrences. Our simulation employs the same probability distribution for generating uninsured days as we used for LR days. The estimated average annual use of uninsured days is 0.011 days per enrollee, or 11 per 1,000, with an average cost of $6. Even with this small average, the variance of risk is exceedingly large, estimated at $223,000. Our prototype risk-averse Medicare enrollee would pay a $22 risk premium on top of the actuarial average $6 expense in order to avoid this risk.

We have not simulated this process with perfect accuracy. Over Medicare's history, 1 in every 380 enrollees has run out of LR coverage. While our estimates of the aggregate use rate appear correct, we have simulated that approximately 1 in every 200 enrollees runs out of LR days. This may not be as inconsistent as it appears: the 1/380 ratio describes the entire lifetime of Medicare, and we know that both hospitalizations and life expectancy have increased for the elderly dur-

TABLE 5.11
Age-Sex Composition of Persons Running Out of Lifetime Reserve Coverage (Results of Simulation)

	Age						Total
	65–75	75–80	81–85	86–90	91–95	96+	
Male	6.4	11.5	7.0	12.1	6.4	2.5	46%
Female	3.2	8.3	12.8	15.9	8.9	5.1	54%

Note: All entries expressed as percent of the overall persons running out of LR coverage.

ing this period. Thus, our result, while biased, may not be as far from the recent occurrences as it might first appear. With this caveat, we discuss our results on this issue.

Running out of LR coverage, the most potentially devastating event imposed by Medicare's coverage structure is primarily a risk facing the very old, since the LR is a cumulative "bank account" of sixty days of coverage. Over half of the persons in our simulation who ran out of such coverage were eighty-six years old or more. Table 5.11 summarizes the age and sex characteristics of the persons in our simulation who ran out of LR coverage and confronted uninsured days.

The risks created by the LR feature of Medicare and the ultimate limitation of coverage create large financial risks (variance) with very small average costs. We have estimated that a premium of under $25 annually would cover these risks. This assumes—and we cannot test this—that there is no behavioral response to price in this range of hospitalization. But the events occur so infrequently (one person in every three thousand during any single year run-out of coverage) that there cannot be important price response. These are highly insurable events that Medicare does not cover.[21]

Finally, we note that the overall risk confronting individuals probably exceeds the sum of the individual components we have described in this chapter. This occurs because the risks are positively correlated. Because we cannot estimate this correlation factor from available data, we can only assert that the overall risks imposed by the partial coverage features of Medicare are larger than we can describe. However, since the large bulk of the Part A risks come from a few rare events (long hospitalizations), the correlations with the Part B risks are probably not as large as they might first seem.

Supplemental Coverage to Offset This Risk

Private health insurance

The financial liabilities incorporated into Medicare can be reduced or eliminated through the purchase of private supplemental insurance policies. Many Medicare beneficiaries choose to purchase private insurance to cover deductibles, co-payment amounts, and services not covered by Medicare. The benefit levels of private supplemental insurance policies vary considerably. Additionally, consumers' choices about the type and extent of coverage to purchase appear to vary with demographic factors such as age, income, and education. Thus, while private insurance may smooth the differences in the potential liabilities of various segments of the Medicare population, significant differences still exist due to the unevenness of private insurance coverage.

Some of this unevenness may have been ameliorated with the passage of the Baucus amendment to the 1980 Social Security Disability Act (PL 96-265). The Baucus amendment requires private supplemental insurance policies issued after July 1, 1982, to meet certain minimum standards if they are to be labeled or sold as "Medicare supplements." Policies issued before July 1982, group insurance offered by employers or labor organizations, and policies converted from group plans to individual policies are exempt.

The standards require coverage of all copayments for hospital days through the LR, coverage of 90 percent of hospital expenses past LR days for a lifetime minimum of 365 additional days, coverage of the 20 percent coinsurance for Part B expenses, a maximum deductible of $200, and a maximum benefit of no less than $5,000 (Cafferata 1984, p. 22). Since policies issued before July 1982 are not affected by the Baucus amendment, considerable variation in private supplemental coverage probably still exists. One major effect of this legislation that can be anticipated is an increase in premiums for these policies because the benefits may be substantially increased to meet the standards of the amendment. This can be expected to magnify any effect that income level has on the likelihood of purchasing supplemental insurance.

Detailed data on private supplemental insurance coverage is available from the National Medical Care Expenditures Study (NMCES) conducted in 1977, before the institution of the Baucus amendment. Since the data reflect choice made before the Baucus amendment became law, the characterization of private supplemental insurance coverage of the Medicare population drawn from this data can be taken as largely descriptive of freely selected policies.

As Table 5.12 shows, the Medicare population purchases private insurance for different types of medical care in accord with standard theories of insurance. They are more likely to buy more complete coverage for high-cost events with small probability of occurrence—hospital care—than for lower-cost, more predictable events—dental care, physician office visits, and so on. The likelihood of purchasing coverage is not constant across the Medicare population, however. The youngest of the old, those aged sixty-five through sixty-nine are more likely to purchase supplemental coverage for all of the services except hospital and in-

TABLE 5.12
Private Insurance Coverage of the Medicare Population: Percent of Medicare Beneficiaries Covered by Age, Education, Income, Health Status, 1977

	Any insurance	Hospital care	Inpatient physician care	Outpatient diagnosis	Physician office visit	Mental health care	Outpatient drugs	SNF care	Dental care
Total	14,518	97.6	88.4	64.5	61.6	58.0	40.6	60.8	4.1
Age									
65–69	5,244	97.9	88.6	68.4	65.7	63.1	48.0	58.3	5.2
70–74	4,131	97.9	90.8	65.0	62.3	57.2	41.0	62.0	5.5
75+	5,142	97.1	86.2	60.1	56.8	53.5	32.8	62.4	1.8[a]
Education									
<9 years	5,355	96.5	85.0	61.9	56.8	51.2	33.5	61.0	4.7
9–12 years	5,621	97.8	91.0	66.4	63.2	60.5	43.3	60.2	3.9[a]
13+ years	3,051	98.9	89.5	65.1	66.8	65.6	47.5	61.2	3.4[a]
Income									
Low	5,749	99.1	87.3	60.5	57.1	49.3	30.2	59.8	2.9[a]
Middle	5,197	95.7	88.7	68.0	63.1	63.5	46.6	62.0	4.8
High	3,572	97.9	89.7	65.8	66.5	64.1	48.6	60.8	5.0[a]
Health status									
Excellent	4,602	97.2	87.1	60.9	58.9	58.6	39.2	59.7	3.8[a]
Good	5,808	97.8	89.4	66.8	63.2	57.0	41.7	62.0	4.6
Fair	3,734	97.6	88.4	65.2	61.0	59.1	39.8	59.7	3.4

Note: Income adjusted for family size.
[a] Relative standard error > 30 percent.
Source: Cafferata (1984) Table 3.

patient physician care and skilled nursing facility care. The population with less than nine years of education is slightly less likely to have coverage for most of the services, and those with low income are less likely to have coverage for all services except hospital care. The final portion of Table 5.12 shows coverage for persons by health status. Interestingly, coverage does not vary in any consistent pattern with differences in self-reported health status.

Private supplemental insurance policies differ in the extent of coverage of each of these services. Consequently, consumer liabilities differ even among persons with private supplemental coverage for the same services. Table 5.13 shows the differences in private supplementation of Medicare Part A coverage for hospital care. Ninety-three percent of aged Medicare beneficiaries with private hospital coverage had full supplementary coverage for the Part A up-front deductible and copayments. Smaller percentages had coverage for copayments for days 61–90, for LR days, and for days beyond the exhaustion of LR days.

This pattern of coverage is inconsistent with the predictions of expected utility theory, which predicts that people will insure against low-probability, high-cost events like a long hospital stay.[22] Only 30 percent of aged Medicare beneficiaries with hospital coverage had full coverage for a long hospital stay; another 34 percent had partial coverage. Alternatively, 93 percent had coverage for the up-front deductible, a much more predictable and less costly event. If people behaved consistently with the theory, we would expect the largest number to insure for days beyond the LR, somewhat less against copayment days, and the smallest number for the deductible. As Table 5.13 shows, the pattern is just the opposite. Rice and McCall (1985) show similar patterns of purchases for data from 1982.

The extent of coverage for the Part A deductible and copayments varies with age and income. The oldest of the old, those aged over seventy-five, were less

TABLE 5.13
Private Supplementation of Medicare Part A: Distribution of Medicare Beneficiaries by Age and Income, 1977

Coverage	Deductible copayments	Copayments days 61–90	Copayments days 91–150	Partial days 151–365	Full days 151–365
Total	92.9	89.0	75.4	34.0	29.7
Age					
65–69	92.8	88.9	77.2	32.5	33.8
70–74	94.5	89.8	76.2	31.0	30.8
75+	91.7	88.4	73.0	38.0	24.3
Income					
Low	91.8	89.4	73.7	39.5	22.2
Middle	94.1	90.0	78.2	29.5	34.4
High	94.1	86.7	74.4	31.5	35.2

Note: Income adjusted for family size.
Source: Cafferata (1984) Table 4.

likely to have coverage for copayments for LR days and more likely to have partial rather than full coverage for days beyond the LR. Low-income beneficiaries had a similar coverage pattern for days beyond LR days.

Table 5.14 shows percentages of the aged Medicare population with private hospital insurance covered by different combinations of coverage levels for Part A liabilities. Twenty-seven percent had full coverage for the deductible, copayments, and some post-LR care. Another 45 percent had full coverage for only the first two liabilities and 21 percent had full coverage for only the deductible. Six percent had less than full coverage for each of these potential liabilities.

Private supplemental coverage of Medicare Part B insurance also varies within different segments of the Medicare population, as is shown in Table 5.15. Coverage of the deductible does not vary significantly with age, education, or income for either inpatient or outpatient physician care. Comprehensiveness of copayment coverage does vary with these characteristics, however. The most elderly, the least well educated, and the beneficiaries with the lowest incomes tend to have less comprehensive coverage, up to the Medicare allowable charge rather than to the usual, customary, and reasonable charge.

This review of data on private supplementary insurance coverage of Medicare beneficiaries suggests that a significant percentage of the Medicare population is uninsured for events that could cost them large amounts of money if they occurred. Furthermore, the oldest, poorest, and the least well educated of these beneficiaries are the most likely to be uninsured.

Medicaid coverage

Another possible source of coverage for risks not covered by Medicare is the Medicaid program. Medicaid coverage is available to low-income persons in every state and in thirty-eight states is also available for "medically needy" persons with high medical expenses relative to their incomes (Gordon 1986). Medicaid coverage differs by state, but it generally pays most of the Medicare deductibles and copayments (both Part A and Part B) and some services not paid for by Medicare.

TABLE 5.14
Medicare Part A Supplemental Coverage: Comprehensiveness of Coverage for Aged Beneficiaries, 1977

Part A deductible coverage	Copayments days 61–150	Benefits for days 151–365	Percent of beneficiaries
Full	Full	Full	26.8
Full	Full	Not full	45.2
Full	Not full	Not full	21.0
Not full	Not full	Not full	5.8

Source: Cafferata (1984) Table 10.

TABLE 5.15
Private Insurance Coverage for the Part B Deductible and Coinsurance: Distribution of Aged Beneficiaries, 1977

	Inpatient physician	Deductible	UCR[a]	Allow[a]	Physician office (thousands)	Deductible	UCR	Allow
Total	11,863	49.4	71.8	27.0	8,926	42.9	71.1	22.9
Age								
65–69	4,356	52.5	79.0	20.9	3,433	40.0	77.5	18.7
70–74	3,488	44.4	69.0	28.5	2,573	46.8	67.2	26.0
75+	4,018	50.2	66.3	32.3	2,920	42.8	67.0	25.1
Education (years)								
<9	4,150	51.4	64.6	34.4	3,039	43.8	65.2	28.3
9–12	4,726	49.4	75.0	23.0	3,539	45.7	74.8	19.7
13+	2,593	43.5	77.5	22.2	2,037	34.5	77.7	20.6
Income								
Low	4,546	48.8	65.7	32.1	3,286	48.6	66.0	27.1
Middle	4,294	52.2	72.3	26.9	3,266	37.8	71.5	20.3
High	3,023	46.2	80.2	19.5	2,374	42.1	77.7	20.6

Note: Income adjusted for family size.

[a] UCR = Usual customary-reasonable charge. Allow = fee above allowed.

Source: Cafferata (1984) Tables 6 and 7.

TABLE 5.16
Medicare Beneficiaries with Neither Private Supplemental Insurance nor Medicaid by Age and Income, 1984

	Beneficiaries (millions)	Percent with neither private insurance nor Medicaid
Total	25.6	20.1
Age		
65–69	8.6	17.3
70–74	7.2	19.1
75–79	4.9	20.1
80+	5.0	26.5
Family income (dollars)		
<5,000	3.1	28.5
5,000–8,999	5.6	29.9
9,000–14,999	6.2	20.8
15,000–24,999	5.9	13.7
25,000+	4.9	10.1

Source: Gordon (1986, 22).

The most prominent addition to the scope of benefits by Medicaid is for long-term care. Medicare's coverage of long-term care is substantially limited, both in law (a limited number of skilled nursing facility days of coverage) and in administrative practice (criteria for eligibility are administered very strictly). Medicaid provides long-term care coverage, mostly in intermediate-skill nursing homes, for large numbers of elderly, primarily female (because of differential survival rates of females over males).

In April 1984 approximately 2.5 million elderly persons were eligible for Medicaid benefits. The number varies somewhat but probably is not as sensitive to business cycle swings for the elderly as for other low-income Medicaid recipients.

Medicaid thus fills in some gaps in liability for those not covered by private supplemental insurance. Data from 1984 show, however, that 20 percent of the elderly Medicare enrollees were covered neither by private supplemental coverage nor by Medicaid. As Table 5.16 shows, Medicare beneficiaries with the lowest incomes, and the oldest portion of the Medicare population, are most likely to have no supplementation of Medicare, either through private plans or Medicaid.

The variability in Medicaid eligibility is in itself a form of risk borne by a part of the Medicare population. Since Medicaid is the mechanism to eliminate the risk imposed by Medicare for a significant number of persons, we can view Medicaid as a risk-reducing insurance plan only to the extent that coverage is stable and predictable for any enrolled individual. We have, unfortunately, found no information describing the transition into and off of Medicaid coverage for the Medicare population.

Recent Changes in Medicare—Consequences

Part A—the role of the DRG system

A recent change in the mechanism by which Medicare pays for hospitalization apparently has dramatically altered the risk confronting individuals—the DRG system. As is well understood, hospitals paid under a DRG system have strong incentives to reduce lengths of stay for every patient admitted under Medicare. These incentives blur once the patient stays in the hospital sufficiently long to become classified as an "outlier," but there are remarkable reductions in length of stay emerging from the changes in payment incentives. For the United States as a whole, Medicare enrollees had, respectively in 1984 and 1985, reductions of 8.9 percent and 8 percent for ALOS. To the extent that the changes in treatment cut off long lengths of stay (e.g., by discharging sooner to nursing homes), the chances of running out of Part A coverage can fall markedly for any individual.

Table 5.17 portrays these changes, which we have described briefly earlier, in aggregate data. The declines in numbers of persons ever using copayment days, ever using LR days, and running out of LR days have all fallen remarkably. From a strictly financial viewpoint, the DRG system has considerably reduced the risk confronting enrollees.

We must enter a note of caution here. By reducing length of stay, hospitals may have imposed a different sort of risk on Medicare patients—risk to their health status. We view this as a wholly open question, unanswered at present by any available data. While sporadic public hearings have provided examples of increased health risk due to early discharge, no systematic evidence is yet available on the consequences of earlier discharge. Conceptually, the risk may fall if, for example, the risks of iatrogenic illness increase rapidly with increased lengths of stay.

TABLE 5.17
Changes in Frequency of Long Stay-Related Risk to Medicare Enrollees (per 1000 enrollees)

	1982	1983	1984
Deductibles	285	285	271
Coinsurance days	148	139	96
Lifetime reserve days	67	63	37

Source: HCFA (undated).

Part B—assignment of benefits changes

A second change in Medicare's structure will affect the financial risk under Part B, relating particularly to the variability in prices confronting Medicare patients. Under previous Medicare law, physicians could choose on a patient-by-patient basis whether to accept assignment of benefits. (Recall that when the physician accepts assignment, he or she also agrees to accept the Medicare fee as the full fee. Thus, the patient is then responsible for the 20 percent copayment but no fees in excess of the Medicare fee level.)

Under provisions of the 1984 Deficit Reduction Act (DEFRA), Medicare again froze the allowed physician fees for July 1984 through September 1985. A second change established for the first time the concept of a "participating physician," who agrees to accept assignment on *all* patients. Participating physicians were allowed to increase charges to Medicare patients during the freeze period in order to establish a *higher* fee level for subsequent periods. Nonparticipating physicians could not raise fees during the freeze period. Thus, the decision to "participate" in this new plan amounted to a trade-off between accepting assignment now, in exchange for higher fees possible later, versus continuation of the old assignment system (patient by patient) but delays in ability to increase fees.

Apparently, a notable proportion of physicians decided to participate in this new plan. The proportion of Medicare claims for which assignment had been accepted had hovered steadily in the 51 to 53 percent range since 1975. In 1984 the proportion leaped to 59 percent and then again in 1985 to 68.5 percent (McMillan et al. 1985). This in turn implies a lower proportion of Medicare patients will confront risk from fees charged in excess of the allowed Medicare fee level and, eventually, reduced financial risk.

Medicare HMOs

Finally, we note that when Medicare allowed enrollment into health maintenance organizations (HMOs) as an alternative to the standard Medicare package, the opportunity arose for Medicare enrollees to eliminate great amounts of the risk they would otherwise confront. Since HMOs typically require few or no copayments (the Medicare HMO provisions severely restrict the level of such copayments allowed), virtually all of the Part B risk is eliminated. And since the Medicare HMO is obliged to extend hospitalization essentially without limit, the Part A risk from copayment days, LR days, and uninsured days is also essentially eliminated. (The same caveat applies as before: a health risk may also arise here if the HMOs discharge patients "too early." For the under-sixty-five population, results from the Rand Health Insurance Experiment showed no deleterious health effects for HMO enrollees unless they were lower-income participants (see Ware et al. 1986).

Conclusion: Potential Changes in Medicare

We have established a considerable financial risk confronting Medicare recipients, arising separately from (1) Part A deductibles; (2) Part A coinsurance days, LR days and, eventually, uncovered days; (3) Part B coinsurance; and (4) Part B excess physician fee payments. Uncovered services also create risks that we have not documented.

Private supplemental insurance greatly reduces these risks; indeed, the considerable popularity of these private plans is evidence of how intensively individuals wish to eliminate the risk confronting them from the original Medicare coverage.

As should come as no surprise, analysis shows that persons covered with supplemental insurance systematically use more health care than those without such coverage (Link, Long, and Settle 1980). Since much Medicare supplemental insurance is purchased individually,[23] this can either rise from self-selection (sicklier people buy better insurance) or from the usual effect of insurance lowering prices to consumers. At least on the basis of crude "self-perceived health status" measures, however, there appears to be no rampant self-selection in the choice of supplemental insurance plans (see Table 5.12).

Particularly if we view the increased spending of Medicare enrollees with supplemental insurance as a price effect, rather than a self-selection effect, it is clear that the presence of such plans increases Medicare's costs notably. As such, they create a fiscal burden not originally contemplated by the designers of Medicare, who obviously put some copayments in place to restrict overall health system use.

The Baucus amendment of 1980 is particularly puzzling in light of this issue: by *requiring* that Medicare supplemental plans cover first-dollar spending on both Part A and Part B (in addition to absorbing much of the outer-tail risk), these Baucus-type plans of necessity exacerbate the Medicare spending rate.[24] The effect of small copayments on overall use cannot be minimized: in the Rand Health Insurance Experiment (for an under-sixty-five population), imposition of a $150 annual deductible for out-of-hospital use reduced overall spending by 23 percent, compared with a full-coverage plan, with comparable reductions in inpatient utilization (Manning et al. 1987).

As a reasonable approximation, 80 percent of the Medicare population confronts very few, if any, copayments for first-dollar medical events. (This figure arises from the combination of persons with Medigap plans and Medicaid coverage.) These same plans have also greatly reduced the financial risk for low-probability events, the major source of risk confronting individuals under the original structure of Medicare.

As policy analysts, we are tempted to decry the mandatory front-end coverage generated by the Baucus amendment and, indeed, the front-heavy-but-tail-light coverage of the original Medicare law. The usual normative model of decision making under uncertainty (expected utility maximization) suggests that this structure is upside down. The obvious prescription arising from this model would have higher deductibles, at least under Part B, and better coverage at the tails of the expenditure distribution. Since its inception, the Part B deductible has eroded considerably in real terms. If the original $50 deductible had merely been adjusted for overall inflation, using the CPI, it would now be *twice* as high as the current level ($75). The increase in demand for medical services, both inpatient and outpatient, arising from this erosion of the Part B deductible is likely considerable, although we know of no direct estimates of the magnitude. Reinstating the original *real* Part B deductible seems an obvious move, particularly if traded for better extreme-risk protection (e.g., a stop-loss provision in Part B spending).

We must draw back with caution at this point, however. Such prescriptions flow naturally from the normative model of expected utility maximization, but all available evidence points to revealed preference of Medicare recipients in a different pattern. As we noted previously, even before the Baucus amendment requirements, consumers showed markedly higher preferences to insure away the more probable, less risky events—first, the Part A deductible, then coinsurance days, and last, LR day risk—in stark contrast to the predictions made from the standard model of behavior. While such choices appear "irrational" to the expected utility maximizer, they do in fact reflect the choices made by Medicare enrollees. Should policy choices force them into different paths?

In part, the most appropriate strategy for Medicare to follow depends heavily on consumers' motives for purchasing supplemental insurance. If the motives are primarily to avoid low-probability, high-risk events (i.e., the standard expected utility model), then the Baucus amendment obviously exacerbates Medicare's budget problems because of the induced medical care use arising from front-end coverage. Changing the law, perhaps even taxing such coverage, may be an appropriate choice.

In the same vein, if the most prominent concern of Medicare enrollees leading to purchase of Medigap policies is the high-risk event, then altering Medicare coverage to incorporate such events could possibly lead to major reductions in the amount of supplemental coverage purchased. The accompanying reductions in spending, as front-end coverage declined, would provide at least some funding to offset the increased costs of better back-end coverage. We know of no analyses allowing full consideration of this issue.

By contrast, if Medicare enrollees really make decisions according to alternative models such as Kahneman and Tversky's prospect theory approach or Kunreuther's analysis of consumer purchases of natural disaster insurance, then we would expect quite different responses to such changes in Medicare.[25] Instead of reducing the rate of supplementation, we might well find a higher rate of purchase of Medigap policies to cover front-end risk. (These models predict a strong demand for such coverage. In turn, if Medicare covered the high-end risks, the costs of the Medigap policy would naturally fall. Thus, the rate of purchase of supplemental policies would increase.)

In closing, we note with some pessimism that policy analyses of past behavior under Medicare have failed to provide what may prove to be crucial information—why do consumers actually choose supplemental policies under Medicare? Until we know which features of these policies are most wanted, we have little way to understand how consumers will eventually respond to any changes in Medicare itself. Thus, to predict Medicare and Medicaid spending or project demand for medical care resources overall, we may need to refocus Medicare analyses beyond the question of medical resource use and more on the prior question of choice of insurance. The consumer responses to the risk Medicare originally imposed, and the way such behavior would respond to any changes in Medicare, are still poorly understood.

We also note the inconsistent policy behavior of Medicare planners with regard to the Part A and Part B deductibles. By law the Part A deductible has increased through time, so this year it is ten times the original value (and over three times the original value in constant dollars due to increases in the relative price of hospital care). At the same time, Medicare planners have allowed the Part B deductible to erode greatly in real dollar terms, increasing it only nominally from $50 to $75. As a cost control device, the Part B deductible may be more important and could possibly achieve the same sorts of cost control as the Part A deductible, with much smaller financial risk generated. We urge attention of policymakers to this issue.

Our final attention, however, is drawn to the concept of the spell of illness. We do not know the original intentions of the persons framing Medicare's structure, but it appears likely that they intended the spell-of-illness concept to protect sickly individuals from financial double jeopardy. Whatever their purposes, it is now clear that one of the major sources of financial risk arising from the limited tail-end Part A coverage is due to the spell-of-illness concept. We have documented at least some of the risk this generates for coinsurance days and (partly) for LR days. The variability of risk confronting Medicare enrollees would drop considerably if the spell-of-illness concept were eliminated, with little added cost to the Medicare system. It appears that Medicare enrollees must pay for six times as many coinsurance days, for example, as would be true if the spell-of-illness concept did not exist. If no other single change in Medicare's structure were considered, this simple administrative change would serve the purposes of reducing risk considerably.

Notes

1. The importance of this tax subsidy is documented in Phelps (1986).

2. Due to limitations of data available, we can only make these calculations separately for various parts of Medicare's insurance structure, although new data files now becoming available from Medicare should allow a more complete calculation in the future.

3. Of course, if private insurance coverage is held, such insurance may cover some or all of the risks. Here, we merely portray the risk arising just from the structure of the Medicare program.

4. One story—perhaps apocryphal—suggests that this one-day deductible was instituted at the specific instruction of then-President Lyndon B. Johnson. According to the story, the initial proposed structure of Medicare that he reviewed contained no first-day payments, and he allegedly retorted, "Hell, my daddy will jump into the hospital every time he has a hangover. Make them pay for the first day."

5. In 1977, Medicare had 23.9 million enrollees, and 5.259 million had some hospital stay, representing 22 percent of the population at risk.

6. These are 1977 data, the most recent we could find. They reflect hospital admissions, not benefit periods. For example; in 1977, there were 6.577 million benefit periods and 7.768 million actual discharges. Thus 1.191 million discharges occurred as part of the same spell of illness, or some 15 percent of all discharges.

7. Thus, if a person has two admissions, the chances are 3/8 that only one benefit period occurs. If a person has three or more admissions, the chances are 3/8 that only one or two benefit periods occurred. We have had to make some arbitrary assumptions about the relationships between benefit periods and admissions to reach these numbers, but they are reasonably accurate, we believe. In particular, we had to exclude the possibility of a person with 3+ admissions having only one benefit period, and we had to assume that the chance of having two admissions collapse into a single benefit period was the same, no matter how many admissions occurred.

8. In particular, we use a utility function with a constant absolute risk aversion of 0.0002, equivalent to a relative risk aversion of 2 at an income of $10,000. This level of risk aversion is within the range employed by others and matches the risk aversion estimated in several studies. Other studies have used risk-aversion measures perhaps twice as large as this.

9. Pratt (1962) offers an approximate measure of the risk premium for distributions that are not "badly" skewed, proving that the risk premium is approximately $R = 0.5 * r * \text{Variance of risk}$, where r is the risk-aversion parameter. Since the variance here is $183,000, with a risk-aversion parameter of 0.0002, the approximation is $18. We have also made the exact expected utility calculation for a person with $10,000 income and a constant absolute risk-aversion utility function with a risk parameter of 0.0002. The results are very similar. Thus, we will use this approximation henceforth for calculating the risk premiums for various risks.

We should note that the risk premium concept measures the demand for risk removal only when there is no price effect on demand for the insured service (commonly described as "moral hazard"). When there is moral hazard, the willingness to pay for insurance is less.

10. Specifically, we are comparing actual distributions of coinsurance-incurring hospital days in 1983 with actual hospital length-of-stay data for 1977.

11. The chances of running out of LR days obviously increase with age, since the days accumulate through time. The persons who were quite old when Medicare began were unlikely to run out of LR days. For the youngest cohort entering Medicare in 1965, the full risk has not yet been realized.

According to life tables, for persons aged sixty-five in 1965, one-third would still be alive and accumulating days against their LR quota. Only when Medicare has "aged" through an entire cohort will the annual flow rate represent the steady state. We should be very near this state in another ten years.

12. The extent of subsidy has varied through time, but has increased considerably over the past decade. As Table 5.4 shows, the ratio of SMI premiums to benefit payments has fallen considerably since 1975.

At the conference where this chapter originally was presented, Wilbur Mills described how the original premium was set. It was intended to represent half of the actual cost of the program, with the intent to gain large rates of enrollment. At that time, nobody within the government was sure how many people would actually enroll in Part B, and they were concerned that a substantial underenrollment would discredit the program.

13. The choice of the 90th percentile probably does not reflect preferences of the providers. If physicians controlled the plans and voted for the level of payment they would most desire, then the median fee should emerge as the limit on payment (see Lynk 1981).

14. This requires assigning dollar values both to the closed intervals and the last open interval. The results are not very sensitive to alternatives we have used.

15. With a COV of 1.76 and an average risk of $200, the standard deviation will be approximately $360. Thus, the variance is approximately $130,000.

16. All data on length of stay in long-term care were drawn from the National Nursing Home Discharge Survey.

17. The very structure of Medicare prohibits this approach by segmenting Part A and Part B data. Different private insurance companies serve as "financial intermediaries" for Parts A and B, and they cannot combine their data. Only very recently, a new data retrieval system within the Social Security Administration allows the retrieval of information on all spending by the HCFA under Parts A and B. But even this data system cannot fully describe out-of-pocket expenses of individuals or families.

Household surveys provide an alternative approach for measuring risk. While such studies have been undertaken, they are very thin in sample, even for large national surveys, if one is concerned with the risks arising, for example, from the limitations on Part A coverage at the extreme tails of the expenditure distribution. This sample-sized problem requires adoption of highly specific functional forms for probability distributions of spending, and the results can depend heavily on such assumptions.

18. The program is written in BetterBasic, a structured language using the vocabulary of Basic. Thus, any person familiar with Basic should be able to understand the program's functions.

19. See Hogg and Tanis 1983, pp. 477–480. The distribution used in this study has parameters alpha = 20, beta = 255.

20. Notice that the distribution of coinsurance days (see Table 5.1) shows only 11 percent of persons using any coinsurance days in a single hospitalization actually using thirty coinsurance days. If this were the only path to use of LR days, only 11 percent of the coinsurance day users would eventually have LR day use. But we have assumed that 20 percent of all coinsurance day users require eventual use of LR days. This is consistent with Medicare reports that in 1985, 48,672 persons used at least one LR day. Scaled to 1983 levels of coinsurance day use, this creates the prediction that 20 percent of coinsurance day users required use of some LR days. This is another phenomenon of the spell-of-illness definition.

21. As we shall see in the next section, individuals purchasing private insurance often do not insure these same risks.

22. For example, Arrow (1971) proves that risk-averse, expected utility maximizing consumers will purchase full coverage above a deductible when confronted with a policy with a positive loading fee.

23. Readers should interpret past studies of group versus nongroup Medicare supplementation with caution. For example, the 1977 NMCES studies (Cafferata 1984) classify insurance purchased through the American Association of Retired Persons (AARP) as group insurance, which it is, but for purposes of understanding self-selection, it should be treated as individual insurance; individuals can

make the choice to enroll or not at will, just as with any nongroup plan (see AARP, undated for details of enrollment criteria).

24. The law specifies that advertising for the supplemental plans cannot use the word "Medicare" unless the plan conforms to the minimum amounts of coverage established by the legislation.

25. However, Hershey and Kunreuther (1984) report little of this phenomenon in their analysis of one group's purchases of health insurance.

References

American Association of Retired Persons, "Information on Medicare and Health Insurance for Older People," Washington, DC: AARP, 1986.

Arrow, K. J., "The Theory of Risk Aversion," *Essays in the Theory of Risk Bearing,* Chicago, IL: Markham Publishing Co., 1971.

Cafferata, G., "Private Health Insurance Coverage of the Medicare Population," Data Preview 18, National Center for Health Services Research, National Health Care Expenditure Study, Rockville, MD: Publication No. (PHS) 84-3362. September 1984.

Callahan, W., and T. Lawrence, "Medicare Prospective Payment System: Length of Stay for Selected DRGs," *Health Care Financing Review,* 7(4): 58–71, Summer 1986.

Gordon, N. M., Statement of Nancy M. Gordon, Assistant Director for Human Resources and Community Development, Congressional Budget Office, before the Subcommittee on Health and the Environment Committee on Energy and Commerce, U.S. House of Representatives, March 26, 1986.

Health Care Financing Administration, *Medicare Data,* HCFA, Office of Statistics and Data Management (undated).

Hershey, J., H. Kunreuther, J. S. Schwartz, and S. V. Williams, "Health Insurance Under Competition: Would People Choose What is Expected?" *Inquiry, The Journal of Health Care Organization, Provision, and Financing,* 21(4): 349–360, Winter 1984.

Hogg, R. V., and E. A. Tanis, *Probability and Statistical Inference,* New York, NY: Macmillan Publishing Co., 1983.

Kahneman, D., and Amos Tversky, "Prospect Theory: An Analysis of Decision Under Risk," *Econometrica,* 47(2): 263–291, March 1979.

Kunreuther, H., et al., *Disaster Insurance Protection: Public Policy Lessons,* New York, NY: John Wiley & Sons, 1978.

Link, C. R., S. H. Long, and R. F. Settle, "Cost Sharing, Supplementary Insurance, and Health Services Utilization Among the Medicare Elderly," *Health Care Financing Review,* 25–32, Fall 1980.

Lynk, W. J., "Regulatory Control of the Membership of Corporate Board of Directors: The Blue Shield Case," *Journal of Law and Economics,* 24:150–174, April 1981.

Manning, W. G. et al., "Health Insurance and the Demand for Medical Care," *American Economic Review,* 77(3): 251–277, June, 1987.

McMillan, A., J. Lubitz, and M. Newton, "Trends in Physician Assignment Rates for Medicare Services, 1968–85," *Health Care Financing Review,* 7(2): 59–75, Winter 1985.

Mitchell, J. B., K. A. Calore, J. Cromwell, et al., *Creating DRG-Based Physician Reim-*

bursement Schemes: A Conceptual and Empirical Analysis, Final Report, HCFA Grant No. 18-P98387/1-01, October 1984.

Phelps, C. E., "Taxing Health Insurance: How Much is Enough?" *Contemporary Policy Issues,* III(2): 47–54, Winter 1984–85.

———, "Large-Scale Tax Reform: The Example of Employer-Paid Health Insurance," Rochester Center for Economic Research, Working Paper No. 32, 1986.

Pratt, J. W., "Risk Aversion in the Small and in the Large," *Econometrica,* 32:122–136, 1964.

Rice, T., and N. McCall, "The Extent of Ownership and the Characteristics of Medicare Supplemental Policies," *Inquiry, The Journal of Health Care Organization, Provision, and Financing,* 22(2): 188–200, Summer 1985.

Riley, G., J. Lubitz, R. Prihoda, and M. A. Stevenson, "Changes in the Distribution of Medicare Expenditures Among Aged Enrollees, 1969–82," *Health Care Financing Review,* 7(3): 53–63, Spring 1986.

Ruther, M., and C. Helbing, "Medicare: Liability of Persons using Reimbursed Physicians' Services, 1980," *Health Care Financing Notes,* Number 3, U.S. Department of Health and Human Services, Health Care Financing Administration, December 1985.

Sadanand, A., and L. Wilde, "A Generalized Model of Pricing for Homogeneous Goods under Imperfect Information: A Theoretical Analysis with Policy Implications," *Review of Economic Studies,* 49:229–240, 1982.

Schwartz, A., and L. L. Wilde, "Intervening in Markets on the Basis of Imperfect Information: A Legal and Economic Analysis," *Pennsylvania Law Review,* 127: 630–682, 1979.

———, "Competitive Equilibria in Markets for Heterogeneous Goods Under Imperfect Information," *Bell Journal of Economics,* 13(1): 181–193, Spring 1982.

———, "Imperfect Information, Monopolistic Competition and Public Policy," *American Economic Review,* 72(2): 18–23, May 1982.

Tversky, A., and D. Kahneman, "The Framing of Decisions and the Psychology of Choice," *Science,* 211(3): 453–458, January 1981.

Ware, J., R. H. Brook, W. H. Rogers, et al., "Comparison of Health Outcomes at a Health Maintenance Organization with Those of Fee-for-Service Care," *The Lancet,* 1017–1022, May 3, 1986.

Wilde, L. L. and A. Schwartz, "Equilibrium Comparison Shopping," *Review of Economic Studies* 46(3): 543–553, 1979.

6. Should Medicare Provide Expanded Coverage for Long-term Care?

BERNARD S. FRIEDMAN

LARRY M. MANHEIM

Introduction

The question posed in the chapter title could be addressed from several different analytical, political, and ideological premises. This chapter adopts a relatively narrow approach, focusing on the net benefit of insurance to a citizen who must pay the full cost of insurance. Thus, we are asking whether the current "low-level equilibrium" in the private market for long-term care (LTC) insurance reflects inefficiencies that could be overcome with changes in Medicare together with changes in other government policies (e.g., Medicaid), leading to an increase in the expected well-being of individual consumers over their lifetime.

Our literature review and analysis emphasizes the following major influences on consumer demand (willingness to pay) for LTC insurance:

1. High loading charge (i.e., markup rates) associated with sales and screening costs to deal with selection bias in a nongroup market.
2. Accuracy of consumer information about existing coverage, as well as the risks and costs of LTC.
3. Replacement of family assistance to the person needing LTC and induced additional care by presence of financial benefits.
4. Availability of "backstop" Medicaid coverage after personal assets are exhausted or transferred.

Even with our narrowing of attention to efficiency in the provision of insurance, we do not expect to answer the title question definitively. A primary aim of this chapter is to demonstrate how the various factors affecting demand and equilibrium in a market for LTC insurance can be studied within a quantitative model that is tractable for simulating effects of policy changes. In order to formulate a useful model, we first review the history of Medicare limitations with regard to LTC and identify the rationales of past actions, and then we survey the progress of relevant research about the economics of insurance markets.

Our model is designed for simulating the maximization of expected utility by a representative consumer. We discuss the apparent importance and interaction of several underlying behavioral parameters (e.g., risk aversion, elasticity of benefit of LTC, share of income spent on LTC in the absence of insurance, probability estimates) that can, in principle, be estimated from market behavior and marketing research studies. This type of model helps to focus attention on areas where future research might be targeted, either because information is especially weak or especially important for effects for policy changes. For example, we find that the reduction of loading charges that could be obtained by large group sign-up could have relatively large effects, as could improved understanding about the limits of current public programs and the risk of needing LTC.

The model also indicates how variation in willingness to pay (across people) is likely to be great enough to warrant a system with optional choices by the retiree and with subsidies for people who would otherwise rely on the expectation of Medicaid coverage. This brokerage role for government would be capable of addressing several problems inhibiting the demand for LTC insurance. Our suggestions raise the issue of a general voucher system as a Medicare reform, about which we offer only a few points specific to LTC since other chapters in this text will treat that subject more intensively. The final section of this chapter offers a brief review of several other proposals involving more comprehensive public insurance of LTC.

Economic premises of Medicare

Our approach to the question of expanded public LTC coverage fits with certain basic premises about the rationale for the Medicare program as it stands, although these premises may not be shared by all supporters of Medicare. Most importantly, in 1965 one could say that the health insurance market for working people revealed a strong willingness to pay for hospital insurance—yet typically people had no opportunity to purchase equally extensive benefits for retirement years at the same loading charge rate. In addition, specific features of Medicare imply other economic premises.

The financing of hospital benefits out of a payroll tax fund reflects a general linkage of the value of coverage during retirement to the willingness to pay taxes during working years. The forced participation in hospital benefits could reflect the following premises: (1) that optimum coverage does not vary much from person to person and, therefore, a central decision based on pooled expertise is efficient in terms of cost of decision making; (2) the low screening and administrative costs associated with a large group plan has such a large cost advantage as to outweigh for nearly everyone the uniformity in the scope of benefits; and (3) government or charity payments for uninsured retirees are forced back on those individuals by requiring them to purchase health insurance.

The economic premises underlying Medicare hospital benefits may not carry over unchanged to LTC benefits. But before considering the logic of LTC coverage, we want to review and better understand the historical limitations of Medicare to "recuperative" LTC.

Medicare History

The history of Medicare reflects an almost total absence of debate about the appropriate coverage of LTC. LTC coverage was defined to allow substitution of nursing home care for the more expensive hospital care. The question of covering nonskilled care received little comment. In this context, it is interesting to examine the literature on national health insurance proposals in the early 1970s. Discussion was again devoid of any substantial discussion of appropriate LTC coverage. National health insurance coverage of LTC was generally modeled along the lines of Medicare's coverage at the time. In the one case where LTC was covered more significantly, the Kennedy-Mills bill, it was shifted to a voluntary Part C Medicare coverage (Davis 1975). This occurred despite the fact that many of these bills intended to fold Medicaid into their national health insurance programs.

This disinterest in the issue may have reflected in part an ignorance of the size of the LTC problem and its projected growth over the following decades. But in part it also reflected the distinction between custodial and medical needs. Vladek (1980) notes Wilbur Cohen was well aware that nursing home services tended to be more custodial than medical in nature, but it was for this very reason that they were not included in the Medicare bill. Cohen believed they belonged in an income maintenance program. Further, the cost of such custodial care was viewed as a "bottomless budgetary pit that would destroy the politically delicate budget for [Medicare] health insurance" (Vladek 1980, p. 49).

The federal view of what was to be covered under Medicare at the time of passage of these laws might therefore be stated as follows:

> The nursing home provides a measure of medical and nursing care to the long-term patient who, while not needing or perhaps not having access to the intensive and costly care of the hospital, does require more care than can be had in his home. Although precise lines of distinction may sometimes be hard to draw, nursing

homes are distinguished from the custodial or domiciliary care homes for the aged on the basis of the level of care provided. Thus skilled nursing homes provide not only residential and personal care, but more particularly services for the chronically ill, convalescent, infirm, or disabled, by professional or practical nurses who can administer treatment ordered by a physician. (Spiegelman 1960, p. 86)

Custodial care was more generally thought of as a concern of social welfare programs, whereas skilled nursing facilities (SNFs) involved medical care delivery. Income maintenance programs based partly on need might be expected to pay for domiciliary care, while the high medical expenses of skilled care would be an area of covered medical payments.

The Social Security Act of 1935 provided an income maintenance program for the aged, based on social insurance principles. Medicare provided medical insurance based on social insurance principles. However, the large extra expense of domiciliary care facilities or skilled facilities, either beyond the Medicare limit or needed for care not covered under Medicare, fell under neither of these plans. Rather, they came under needs entitlement programs (Kutza 1981). The crucial distinction here is between presumptive entitlement under the social insurance approach and needs-testing requirements. Thus, it was perhaps natural that the brunt of LTC coverage would be borne by the Medicaid program. A brief history of prior LTC coverage provides a backdrop to our discussion of current coverage under the Medicare and Medicaid programs.

Medicare and Medicaid and their antecedents

The form that nursing home coverage took under Medicare was, in part, the result of a thirty-year political debate. Although Roosevelt broached the subject of comprehensive national health insurance at the time Social Security legislation was introduced, vigorous opposition led to dropping this proposal. It was at this point that compulsory health insurance was divorced from Social Security, which had two important effects: (1) the definitions of medical care increasingly emphasized the medical aspects of health insurance and (2) it was an uphill battle to move care from a needs assessment (i.e. charity approach) to a social insurance approach (Marmor 1970).

Truman, however, introduced a comprehensive health care bill based on the social insurance model, which was defeated in 1949. From that point on, a strategy of incrementalism was adopted, and Ewing introduced a bill in 1951 that covered only hospitalization. It was not until 1960 that the Medical Assistance for the Aged bill (Kerr-Mills) was passed, which marginally expanded the role of the federal government in covering health care costs for the indigent. Prior to the passage of this bill, state welfare agencies could make direct payments to nursing homes for persons at or below the Old Age Assistance (OAA) eligibility level under provisions in amendments in the Social Security Act, which required the federal government to pay 50 percent of OAA program costs. Two significant aspects of the law that were retained, initially under Kerr-Mills and subsequently under Medicaid, was the states' ability to decide if they were going to have a spend-down provision, and the states' power to license nursing care facilities. Kerr-Mills expanded coverage to all the indigent (defined at the state level); the federal government was to assume from between 50 to 80 percent of the cost, and the ceiling of federal contributions was eliminated. Coverage included skilled nursing facilities, but the definition of such facilities was left to the states' discretion.

With the passage of Medicare in 1965, the social insurance approach was accepted into law for hospital and physician services. Nursing home and home care, however, were included only insofar as skilled care was to substitute for hospital care at the margins. The remainder of the federal coverage of nursing home care fell to Medicaid (a needs-based program), which replaced and extended the earlier Kerr-Mills Act. Medicaid also limited coverage of nursing homes to skilled care facilities, being less precise, however, as to what constituted a skilled care facility. However, previous coverage had provided states support for nursing homes under broader notions of service delivery, including domiciliary care. This potential reduction in the support of nursing home care resulting from the Medicaid replacement of Kerr-Mills resulted in the Miller amendment in 1967, which introduced payments for intermediate care facilities (ICFs) under the cash-assistance titles of the Social Security Act (SSA). This support of ICFs was shifted to Medicaid in 1971.

The definitional problems of what constituted ICFs and SNFs continued to plague lawmakers, and in what Vladek (1980) describes as the only serious consideration of nursing home issues in forty years, Congress passed the Moss amendment, which defined Medicare-covered nursing home facilities. ICFs were defined when their coverage was shifted to Medicaid. This amendment allowed the definitions of extended care facilities under Medicare and SNF coverage under Medicaid to both be defined as skilled nursing care services (Vladek 1980).

The definition of extended care under Medicare had already undergone tightening in response to its increased use. Revised instructions to intermediaries in 1968 listed services to be covered under Medicare, noting intermediaries should err on the side of denying claims, resulting in a 60 percent decrease in bills paid between 1968 and 1972 (Vladek 1980). The 1972 Social Security Act Amendments, which took effect in 1974, also provided payment to nursing homes under Medicare on a cost-related basis and guaranteed that the annual income of older or disabled persons would not fall below a minimum level. These Supplemental Security Income (SSI) features of the bill redirected responsibility from states to the federal government for the aged, blind, and disabled. Some states supplemented these payments, and some provided an additional amount for those receiving domiciliary care. The monthly cash benefits under SSI were limited to $25 per month for those in institutions covered under Medicaid (Waldman 1982).

Current coverage of LTC under Medicare. Coverage of medical care within the social insurance framework of Medicare has clearly been a slow incremental process, with substantial resistance to moving from a needs-assessment framework. Coverage of LTC under Medicare was included only to the extent that such coverage was seen as an extension of hospital care and, therefore, a lower-cost substitution of hospital care. Originally, nursing home care and home care services required a minimum of a three-day hospital stay to precede extended care coverage. This requirement was eliminated in July 1981, when the limit on the number of home care visits (100 per episode) was also removed. However, these extensions of coverage were justified as lower-cost replacements of hospital services and have been continued to be viewed as a response to acute care rather than LTC episodes. Skilled nursing home services were covered by Medicare up to 100 days per episode, with cost sharing (at one-eighth the rate for hospital care) introduced after 20 days of nursing home care. Most individuals use less than 100 days of care, due in part to the restrictions on coverage, with an average coverage by Medicare of 28 days, compared with a national average of 277 days for all patients in SNFs (Cohen 1983). Medicare accounted for just 2.1 percent of total nursing home payments in 1984, compared with 41.5 percent for Medicaid. Private payment accounts for almost all the rest, with LTC insurance covering only 1.1 percent of nursing home payments in 1984 (Table 6.1).

The question of social versus needs-assessment coverage cannot entirely be divorced from potential costs of the program. Given equal coverage, a social insurance program will clearly be more costly to the public budget; this is an important factor in defining future initiatives, given the government's budgetary problems, both with regard to general funds and Social Security trust funds. Thus, much of the recent discussion relating LTC and insurance has concerned

TABLE 6.1
Nursing Home Expenditures by Source of Payment (percentages)

Source	1977	1984
Medicare	3.3	2.1
Medicaid	41.6	41.5
Consumer	50.0	51.2
Out-of-pocket	49.2	50.1
Insurance	0.8	1.1

Source: Waldo and Lazenby (1984).

the expansion of private insurance to replace government payments for those who are ex ante able to pay. We, therefore, turn to the important question of the evidence on demand for LTC coverage, either privately or publicly provided. Of particular concern is integrating issues of private demand and availability of choice among LTC options with the fact of a need for some universal floor of coverage, whether provided on a needs-assessment or social insurance basis. Preliminary to such a discussion, we provide an indication of the extent of utilization of and expenditures for LTC services, emphasizing the trend in Medicare expenditures over time and its relationship to total LTC expenditures.

Nursing home expenditures

Expenditures on nursing home care have increased at a fast pace over the past two decades, faster than the growth of total health care expenditures. Nursing home expenditures grew from $2.1 billion in 1965 to $32.0 billion in 1984, with an increase in the percentage of all personal health care expenditures going to nursing home care increasing from 5.0 to 9.4 percent (Levit et al. 1985). These costs were not covered by Medicare. In 1967 nursing home care accounted for 4.6 percent of all Medicare expenditures; by 1975 nursing home expenditures were but 1.9 percent of all Medicare expenditures; by 1984 only 0.9 percent of Medicare expenditures went toward nursing home care. Table 6.1 shows the percentage of nursing home expenditures paid for by the individual, out-of-pocket, by Medicare and by Medicaid. Medicare's minuscule share has fallen to 2.2 percent in 1984, compared with 41.5 percent for Medicaid and 51.3 percent for consumer out-of-pocket expenditures.

These expenditures are incurred mainly by the oldest old (and their families). The use rate for SNF services increases sharply with age, with 2.7 users per 1,000 enrollees aged sixty-five and 31.2 users per 1,000 enrollees eighty-five or older (Davis & Rowland 1986). Compared with 1980, the population over eighty-five is projected to increase fivefold by 2040, from 2.6 to 13.3 million, of whom slightly more than 4 million would require some type of personal care assistance in the community and of whom 2.7 million may be in nursing homes (Manton and Soldo 1985).

Home care expenditures

It is frequently noted that nursing home expenditures characterize only a small percentage of the total population of potential users. Weissert (1982), using the 1979 Health Interview Survey, reported that 12.8 percent of the noninstitutionalized aged have some form of dependency—in personal care, household activities, or home-delivered health care services. In terms of most severe service need, the rate of personal care dependency (activities of daily living [ADL]) among the noninstitutionalized aged is 4.6 percent. Manton and Soldo (1985) estimate numbers of disabled in 1980 from the National Long Term Care Survey, conducted by the HCFA in 1982. They estimate that approximately 4.6 million individuals over age sixty-five and in the community (18.9 percent of this elderly population) have limitations in either instrumental activities of daily living (IADL) or ADL. Approximately 1.1 million of these individuals receive some level of formal care services; of these, 605,000 reported paying out-of-pocket for at least some portion of their formal care services. The estimated aggregate out-of-pocket expense is almost $1.2 billion a year. Over three-quarters of these elderly finance all of the service costs out-of-pocket. The probability of formal service receipt is found to decrease substantially if the individual lives with a spouse or other relative (Soldo and Manton 1985).

The average use of informal services also varies substantially by sex and type of residence. Estimates of excess hours of informal care and the cost of informal care are provided by Manton and Soldo (1985) and by Paringer (1985). For example, females over eighty-five with at least one ADL or IADL impairment receive an average of 9.85 hours of informal care per week. Paringer (1985) estimates the total cost of replacing informal care with aides at $9.6 billion, using 1978 aide wages, compared with $24 billion spent on nursing homes in 1981. These aggregate figures obscure the substantial variance in service use by age, household type, and severity of disability. For example, the monthly out-of-pocket expenditures on formal care in 1980 for disabled persons over sixty-five ranged from $82 for those with only one IADL limitation to $429 for those severely disabled with five to six ADL limitations (Manton and Soldo 1985).

The proportion of home care services funded under Medicare has been growing rapidly. While home care visits are no longer limited to 100 per episode, they must be tied to a need for skilled care related to an acute care episode. In 1980 Medicare paid an average of $760 per user of home health services, and there were a total of 888,200 users or 34.8 users per 1,000 enrollees. Total expenditures for home care services in 1980 were $675 million, up from $355 million in 1977. This rapid rise in home care expenditures has resulted in more stringent criteria being used to determine home care eligibility over the past few years.

Summary

Our overall interpretation of the policy history of LTC coverage is that influential leaders have viewed public payments for custodial LTC as an income supplementation program for retirees with the lowest asset levels. There was little preexisting insurance coverage for LTC, and correspondingly little evidence that people wanted to buy LTC coverage through the tax system. More recently, the risk of high expenses for LTC for the middle class appears large enough to argue for an insurance approach. Yet the number of private policies bought and sold for custodial LTC continues to be very small, despite initiatives over the last ten years. In reported discussions with potential insurers, the frequently mentioned obstacles to expanded offerings are concerns about weak demand due to under-estimation of needs by consumers, selection bias that requires counterbalancing screening and marketing costs, and "competitive" effects of Medicaid eligibility.

To clarify the current market situation, it becomes important to analyze with more quantitative rigor the determinants of demand and market equilibrium for LTC insurance. Purchasers in the marketplace may fail, for several reasons, to obtain the advantage of insurance for custodial LTC.

To begin with, now that Medicare and Medicaid are established, people may underestimate the risk of uncovered expenses for custodial LTC under Medicare. Also, people may not realize that the payment systems in Medicaid may increasingly constrain the quality of care offered by facilities and home care agencies. Finally, the high loading charges necessary in the nongroup Medigap market may greatly restrain demand from what would be observed in a group sign-up at age sixty-five, when people might be given a variety of retirement plan options, and the problem of adverse selection for LTC coverage would be less than in later years.

Progress of Relevant Research

While this section is targeted closely to issues of demand and market equilibrium for LTC insurance, we begin with a broader survey of major contributions to the economic analysis of health insurance during the past twenty years.

Economic analysis of health insurance
Within a short time after the enactment of Medicare, economists began to study carefully the effect of insurance coverage on demand for services. Pauly (1968) offered important clarifications of the concept of "moral hazard," extending the concept to the extra consumption of health care by each insured individual de-spite the welfare loss to the group of insureds. Ehrlich and Becker (1972) ana-lyzed the effect of insurance on reduced investment in self-protection. Zeckhauser (1970) and Feldstein (1973) addressed "optimum" coverage in quantitative models that included risk aversion and inefficient demand induced by insurance. It is not that all additional health care utilized as a result of insurance coverage is useless, but since it is worth less than its full cost, and since the full cost is built into the premium that is charged, the consumer may prefer to have less insurance coverage than if there were no induced utilization through moral hazard.

Optimal insurance in economic models is usually discussed within the frame-work of expected utility maximization (EUM) by a representative citizen who must pay the full cost of insurance. Some questions of distributional equity have also been addressed in the context of public programs, where the financing and benefit levels may take into account the income of the covered person. "Market failure" is a situation in which willing buyers and sellers of a particular service must settle on some inferior contract or perhaps no transactions are achieved. In the case of externalities, not all of the affected parties can be easily brought into the contract. In the case of differences in information affecting the likely outcomes of a contract, each party must take into account how hidden information will affect the behavior of the other party. In various writings, Arrow and others have clarified the situation of market failure as one in which higher than normal "transaction costs" are embodied into the final price of a product, reducing demand or preventing transactions altogether.

The problem of information differences has been analyzed in the context of insurance by Arrow (1963, 1970, 1976), Spence and Zeckhauser (1971), Pauly (1974), and Rothschild and Stiglitz (1976). The problem is sometimes referred to as "adverse selection" or self-selection bias, but those terms are prone to be used loosely in public debates. For example, if it is easy to classify people into different risk classes, price differences can be used efficiently to sort people into a variety of policies and there is no market failure and, therefore, selection bias is not a problem.

When selection bias is a problem, potential buyers of insurance policies have information about their expected losses that insurers cannot obtain, except perhaps at high cost. Sellers might like to offer policies to different people at different premiums, reflecting different risks of loss. However, if they do not have information about the individual's risk, they have to be prepared for the eventuality that the individual may self-select into a policy that was priced on the basis of lower risks. In the case where the seller cannot obtain accurate information about the individual's risk class, Rothschild and Stiglitz show that a "high-benefit" plan pooling all people may not survive because of the incentive for a competing insurer to try to attract away the lower risks with a "low-benefit" plan, until even the people with higher risks would prefer to join the low-benefit plan. Pauly analyzes how the public offering of a minimum coverage plan would provide useful information to private insurers about the potential demanders of supplementary coverage. Pauly also argues that an efficient role for government is to reduce the cost of information to insurers by various means that would permit more accurate individual pricing of contracts.

The high loading charge of health insurance sold to individuals rather than groups reflects costs of screening and marketing efforts to obtain a normal or favorable pool of buyers, relative to the actuarial cost embodied in the premiums.

If insurers are not permitted by public regulations to vary prices to reflect information that they obtain about individual risks, they will refuse to offer any policy to the higher risks. The market outcome in this case is a partial failure in the sense that high-benefit plans may survive, although the price will be so high as to discourage some buyers, and high-risk individuals may be given no opportunity to buy policies. The outcome for high-risk buyers may be viewed by some policy analysts as a market failure—in the sense of a lifetime insurance market in which forecasted risks of health care needs are much more equal at younger ages than after environmental exposures.

The attention given to analyses of selection bias has increased in view of the options offered to individuals within employer groups. Such studies are currently at the forefront of empirical research about demand for health insurance, for example, Price et al. (1983) and Schuttinga et al. (1985). These studies and the other conceptual treatments of the problems of market failure do not supply much quantitative information bearing on the issue of the demand for LTC insurance and the contributing role of selection bias, operating in part via high loading charges, to explaining the very small volume of private coverage sold and bought.

Medicare consumer issues
In the remainder of this section, we would like to contrast the evidence of latent demand from marketing survey research with the small amount of market activity and proceed to discuss problems of consumer information and decision making that have lately received careful empirical attention.

LaTour, Friedman, and Hughes (1986) asked Medicare eligibles to consider a variety of choices in the context of a Medicare voucher system. Prices for each option were developed from actuarial data and a random increment was added. A prominent finding was significant demand for expanded LTC coverage that would include services at home if the monthly extra cost were $15. In addition, price sensitivity was statistically significant but not high. Meiners and Tave (1985), in another national survey of willingness to pay for LTC insurance, found a wide distribution in the demand for hypothetical LTC insurance and explored reasons for buying or not buying such insurance. Nearly 40 percent of their respondents thought they could afford $30 per month or more for LTC insurance. Reliance upon potential Medicaid eligibility was not expressed by respondents as a major factor in reasons for not buying private insurance. Other findings from their study are discussed in the next section.

The quality of consumer information about Medicare and about existing supplementary insurance may affect demand for LTC insurance, although this type of question has not been previously studied with regard to insurance markets in general. Cafferata (1984b) found that knowledge about Medicare coverage of LTC was much poorer than knowledge about coverage of hospital and physician services. Lambert (1980) found that Medicare beneficiaries tended to overestimate the percentage of medical expenses typically paid by Medicare. McCall et al. (1986) found that only 25 to 47 percent of samples of beneficiaries in six states knew that Medicare does not cover all costs for a six-month stay in a nursing home. In addition, they found that about the same proportions of holders of Medigap insurance knew if their policy covered custodial care or SNFs. These results explain why the market for LTC insurance is not universal, but they do not explain why even the sizable minority who knows the limits to Medicare coverage fail to insure privately.

Marquis, Kanouse, and Brodsley (1985) reviewed research findings about elasticity of demand with respect to insurance prices and found that the price elasticity was not higher for presumably better-informed groups of consumers. Because of this and the evidence that when purchasing supplementary coverage, people seem to prefer plans that fill in Medicare copayments but do not extend catastrophic coverage. Marquis et al. suggest that more attention be given to psychological aspects of health insurance choice than has previously been done. Hershey et al. (1984) cite evidence of low demand for catastrophic coverage in earlier studies of flood and auto insurance, but in a new hypothetical choice study they find a substantial latent preference for increased catastrophic coverage in health insurance and about half of their population willing to give up first-dollar coverage for actuarially fair reductions of premium.

The question of whether EUM is a useful conceptual framework for predicting behavior is examined at some length by Schoemaker (1982), who argues that whenever empirical tests conflict with EUM, modeling changes of an ad hoc nature tend to be proposed. One way to view this literature is that EUM itself is accepted as an almost tautological and normative framework, within which some particular parameters can be estimated. Alternatively, if one seeks primarily behavioral predictions, a set of tested propositions about choice under uncertainty are emerging from the psychological literature, featuring authors such as Tversky, who deserve to be recognized. In the present context, for a multiattribute good such as health insurance, actual choices may reflect "elimination by aspects" and other phenomena. It is unclear to us if these behavioral models have something to offer in understanding the virtual absence of a market in LTC insurance despite survey evidence of latent demand. The EUM models continue to have appeal as normative and heuristic methodologies for "expert" decisions made on behalf of others—in that situation, it is argued that axioms of rational choice are more appropriate than "shortcuts" that would otherwise be used by consumers on their own.

Simulation Model and Tentative Findings

This section develops a quantitative model of demand for LTC insurance within the framework of EUM but with some extensions for inaccurate information. The model isolates key behavioral parameters and how they interact. Although we adopt simplifying assumptions, the quantitative solutions are not simple and direct. We do not have a data base suitable for jointly estimating all the underlying parameters. Therefore, we can only roughly "calibrate" the model by determining ranges of parameter values that are consistent with independent but fragmentary sources of empirical data and reasonable a priori assumptions. The model can be used to explore the importance of several contributing explanations for "market failure" in private LTC insurance. Simulations indicate possible changes in optimal LTC coverage that would result from policy changes, and a sensitivity analysis explores how much the outcomes vary with changes in each underlying assumption. Finally, the entire exercise helps to target issues for better empirical research.

We assume that a typical retired person may either live out a normal lifespan and die suddenly or may acquire serious illness and disability that persists until death. Such long-term disabilities result in the high expenses not covered under current Medicare policies. The assumed time pattern of expenses for medical care and related personal care is depicted in Fig. 6.1.

Point H is the level of expense per unit of time for routine housing and personal care in the absence of the major illness. Areas indicated by M represent expense for acute hospital and medical care covered by existing Medicare and supplementary insurance. Area S represents skilled nursing care of a short-term "recuperative" nature that is also covered by Medicare and supplementary insur-

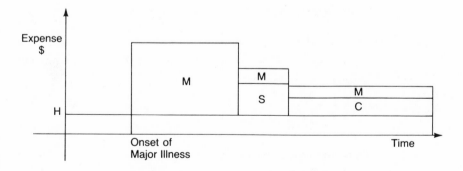

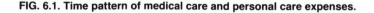

FIG. 6.1. Time pattern of medical care and personal care expenses.

ance and may be provided in an institution or at home. Area C represents the long-term nursing and custodial care for which most people currently have no third-party coverage, except Medicaid after their assets are exhausted.

The person has income and annuitized wealth of an amount A and can draw on time and resources of other family members up to an amount R per unit of time. A hypothetical insurance policy offers a benefit of B per unit of time after onset of illness. This type of indemnity, based only on the occurrence of severe functional dependence, would give the least bias on the types of services purchased. A simpler operational program might involve only candidacy for nursing home placement, but the consumer research reveals stronger interest for coverage that includes services at home.

We adopt a simplifying assumption that illness may occur with probability p, but we do not consider variation in the age of the retiree when the illness occurs. A more sophisticated model with more attention to the timing of occurrence of disability and the purchase of insurance and the effects of mortality risk is under development, but it is not yet suitable for quantitative applications.

If illness does not occur, the payment for insurance per unit of time is

$$\pi = (1 + L)\frac{p}{1 - p}B$$

where L is the "load" factor. We now proceed to determine an optimal level of B given the load factor, the probability p, resources A and R, and underlying preference parameters for risk aversion and benefits of care. The general technique is to solve first for the optimal consumption of care C in the event of illness conditional upon benefit level B. Then, the expected utility (EU) with insurance is condensed to a function of B and maximized.

In the event of illness, we specify the utility model to be maximized as

$$U_i = C^a (A + R - C + B)^{1-r}$$

where a is the elasticity of utility benefit with respect to LTC expense, and $r < 1$ is the proportional risk aversion for monetary gains and losses. The condition for a maximum of U_i leads to a solution

$$C^* = \frac{a(A + R + B)}{1 - r + a}$$

Notice that insurance benefits cause an increase in expenses by $a/(1 - r + a)$ for each dollar of benefit. This increase represents an "income effect" of insurance indemnities on demand for covered care. This type of indemnity insurance, based on occurrence of disability, does not have the substitution effects that would be present if benefit payments were contingent on consumption of particular services. If LTC services are completely elastic in supply, then the extra consumption by each individual induced by the indemnity insurance does not result in higher prices that could limit demand for insurance. In practice, some feedback from changes in market prices could become important in limiting demand for insurance. Note that a problem of moral hazard for this type of insurance is that some people may wish to misrepresent their disability in order to receive indemnity payments.

Another important refinement to this model would be to allow the use of an individual's "own" resources and the use of family resources to have different effects on the utility outcome. Thus, replacement of services bought with insurance benefits for services contributed by family members could be explicitly analyzed. In that type of model, an inverse relationship of demand for coverage with respect to availability of family resources might be expected (insurance would make a bigger difference in the amount of care people could afford for those with less family support), while the net effect of total resources available might still be positive (more wealth to protect).

When the formula for optimal C is replaced in the utility function for the illness state, the result is

$$U_i(B) = k(A + R + B)^s$$

where

$$s = 1 - r + a \quad \text{and} \quad k = \left(\frac{a}{s}\right)^a \left(\frac{1 - r}{s}\right)^{1-r} < 1$$

Utility when well is characterized by $C = 0$ and $B = 0$, or $U_w = (A + R - \pi)^{1-r}$. In order for there to be any demand for insurance, the marginal utility of a dollar of resources in the illness state, μ_i, must be greater than the marginal utility when well, μ_w, at the origin $B = 0$. In the present case

$$\frac{\mu_i}{\mu_w} = \frac{ks}{1 - r} (A + R)^a$$

which is greater than unity for all levels of income if $ks > (1 - r)$, and that occurs if r is relatively high and larger than a.

EU to be maximized with respect to B is

$$EU = pU_i(B) + (1 - p)U_w(B)$$

In the more elaborate model, recognizing that the age at which the disabling illness occurs is a random variable, the EU would be obtained by summing the utility for periods of premium payment before illness with the sum of utility for benefit periods after onset of illness and then averaging the result, using the probability of the illness beginning at each specific age.

The condition for a maximum EU in the simplified model equates the expected marginal utility of a dollar in the sick and well states and can be expressed as follows, after substituting $b = B/(A + R)$:

$$\frac{ks}{1 - r} (1 + b)^{a-r} = (1 + L)\left(1 - \frac{b(1 + L)p}{1 - p}\right)^{-r}$$

As b increases from zero, the left side of the equation falls, while the right side rises leading to a solution.

Baseline solutions

We first attempt to calculate solutions of the optimal b for the "well-informed" consumer (who has accurate knowledge about p and costs of care) under conditions similar to the current Medigap market of individual insurance policies, using fragments of evidence from which starting values of the underlying parameters can be estimated.

Currently, individual policies in the Medigap market carry a loading charge of about 100 percent, compared with about 11 percent for group policies (Cafferata 1984). The higher load for individual policies covers costs of screening and marketing aimed at enrolling a population with health status no worse than the assumptions embodied in the premiums charged.

The probability of needing LTC is estimated for the baseline simulations as follows. Using data for 1976, Liu and Palesch (1981) estimated that 6 percent of the elderly population used nursing home services for more than three months. In the 1982 National Long-Term Care Survey of the noninstitutionalized elderly, it was found that about 4 percent of this population required formal LTC services that they had to pay something for. By combining these two prevalence rates, we begin with an estimate of p to be about .10.

Estimation of the benefit elasticity, a, and the risk aversion, r, can be attempted by both indirect methods and direct methods. An ideal direct method of calibration would be to fit the model to statistical data about insurance purchases and derive separate parameter estimates by maximum likelihood methods. This is not possible in the present case. An indirect method uses evidence about expenses on LTC in the absence of insurance and also some a priori assumptions about risk aversion. A more direct method uses survey evidence on willingness to pay for specific insurance policies.

Previous studies and commentaries about health insurance markets infer a relatively high degree of risk aversion (Friedman 1974; Marquis and Phelps 1985). Another theme of the general literature about insurance is that demand appears to be more evident for "shallow" coverage (i.e., filling in deductibles and coinsurance) than for catastrophic coverage (Hershey et al. 1984). But the problem of relatively low demand for catastrophic coverage is often viewed as a problem of subjective probability distortions or psychological aspects of decision making that depart from EUM. Alternatively, the low demand for catastrophic health insurance, especially by people with low wealth, has been linked to the presence of all-or-nothing subsidized care, as in Medicaid (see, e.g., Friedman 1979).

To clarify the effects of assumptions about the risk-aversion parameter in the present context, consider a person with wealth of $10,000, facing a risk of losing $3,000, with a probability of 10 percent. (The dollar values are chosen with some relevance to the problem of LTC, as shown later.) The highest premium that a person with constant relative risk aversion would offer varies with r as follows: at $r = 0.3$, a premium of $315; at $r = 0.5$, a premium of $324; at $r = 0.7$, a premium of $334; and at $r = 0.9$, a premium of $345. Although the "pure premium" in excess of $300 does vary noticeably with r, the percentage variation in the total premium is not large.

Given a value of r, only particular values of the benefit elasticity, a, will be consistent with observed evidence about the fraction of family resources spent on LTC in the absence of insurance. Data from a 1982 survey of noninstitutionalized elderly (Manton and Soldo 1985) reveal that for the people who paid for all their formal home care, the monthly cost was about $141, on average, and $429 for the most disabled. The figure for the most disabled is more appropriate than the average for this simulation exercise, since these people are presumably more similar to the institutional residents who would also be included in the broad LTC insurance. This expense amounts to about 45 percent of average household income for the elderly. But since the appropriate measure of financial resources of the elderly would allow for the consumption of assets, a lower ratio of perhaps about 33 percent will also be considered (see e.g., ICF 1985 for data on asset holdings of the elderly). Further refinement to this assumption would require estimation of the value of informal care—adding the value used (particularly the time of family members) to expenses and adding the availability to financial resources. A more complete model would allow for the resources of the elderly and their families to be "taxed" at different rates, as noted above.

We learned immediately that for any plausible values of r and a, at the loading factor of 100 percent, the optimal b is 0. Therefore, all the remaining discussion posits a group load charge of 11 percent. At this lower load rate, and with an

TABLE 6.2
Baseline Results (Load Factor = 11%, *p* = 10%)

r	*b*	Premium (median household)	Induced Care
0.7	0.02	$2/month	+1% of income
0.9	0.23	$26/month	+8% of income

expense ratio of one-third in the absence of insurance, there is demand for insurance only if *r* is about 0.7 or higher. Two examples are given in Table 6.2.

In Table 6.2, the premium is calculated on the basis of household income of $11,000 per year (Waldo and Lazenby 1984), since that income level was also used in estimating the proportional expense on LTC in the absence of insurance. Obviously, the premium could be quite different for single households with lower average income and for households with higher income. But this variation in demand cannot be assessed without better information about how the expenses in the absence of insurance vary with household resources. The rightmost column shows the increase in proportion of income expended on covered services as a result of insurance. Note that the increase results not from lower consumer prices for care but rather from the increased income in the insured disability state.

At the higher level of risk aversion, we found that demand was choked off by loading rates exceeding 30 percent.

Calibration with marketing survey results
It is clear that the initial results are quite sensitive to the assumption about the degree of risk aversion. While one has the impression from actual choices that *r* is high, the question of exactly how high is quite important to policy debates. For some improvement in calibration of the model, we can refer to marketing research surveys that ask people how much they are willing to pay for improved coverage. In LaTour, Friedman, and Hughes (1986), there was a significant preference for Medicare options with increased coverage of "custodial" LTC in institutions or at home that raised the cost of all such options by $15 per month. A doubling of this implicit cost did not remove the significant preference for plans with expanded LTC. In another national survey, Meiners and Tave (1985) report a median willingness to spend about $20 per month on LTC, with considerable variance in what people said they could afford and in their expectations about the cost of LTC services per day when needed.

We suppose that respondents envisioned extensions of Medicare with implicitly low load factors. Using the load factor for group coverage of 11 percent, the premium of $20 per month implies an optimum *b* of about 0.177, which, under the assumption of the one-third *ex ante* expense ratio, implies a risk-aversion parameter value of 0.84, within the range of the two lines of Table 6.2. The marketing evidence is thus roughly consistent with a demand for coverage that would offset between one-half and two-thirds of preexisting home care expenses of those in the most severe class of dependence.

The demand for insurance would be much greater than shown in the above table if the *ex ante* expense ratio were one-half rather than one-third. The higher ratio would be more appropriate when thinking about nursing home care. However, if insurance were for institutional care only, other elements of the model would have to be changed, and one should recognize that survey respondents are less interested in buying insurance for institutional care than for more general policies that include services in the home. At the one-half expense ratio in the absence of insurance, if the risk parameter were 0.7, the optimal benefit would be 41 percent of income, and the monthly premium paid would be $46. The premium at $r = 0.9$ would be $68. The latter premium, however, seems significantly larger than survey evidence on what median elderly respondents would be willing to pay. The indicated discrepancy might be traceable with more research to particular assumptions, especially the accuracy and completeness of information provided to survey participants, the risk-aversion assumption, and/or the assumption about expense rates of the median uninsured person in the event of dependence.

Sensitivity to accuracy of information
The average findings from the marketing surveys are consistent with the lower end of the range of plausible demands for well-informed utility maximizers. Rather than infer that typical respondents are not very risk averse, we should also consider that (1) the typical respondent may seriously underestimate the cost of care if needed and (2) the probability of needing care may be underestimated, perhaps because the coverage of Medicare and Medicaid is overestimated, as suggested by the literature reviewed in the previous section.

To show the sensitivity of demand to inaccurate estimates about the needs for care (and scope of current public coverage), we reestimated demand, assuming lower estimated probabilities but with the premium still determined by a probability of 10 percent. One finds that at an estimated risk of 9 percent, only a relatively small underestimation, the demand of insurance falls greatly, from $b = 0.23$ to only $b = 0.03$ at an average premium of $3 per month. This high sensitivity to the accuracy of probability estimates has a major influence on our view of policy options, as explained later. This issue is already being taken more seriously by federal officials in their guide booklets for people contemplating purchase of supplementary policies—restrictions on the definitions of covered LTC are now highlighted. However, there is still a seriously misleading summary table saying that "home health care" is covered in full. In fact, all this means is that someone needing periodic visits by professional nurses for an approved skilled nursing procedure will have no limit on the number of days of coverage. This does not mean in practice that all nursing necessary to keep the person at home will be covered.

Effects of Medicaid coverage

If people with relatively low financial resources anticipate that they will be eligible for Medicaid after some time of spending their own assets on LTC, they may rationally prefer not to buy insurance to cover LTC expenses. This would be particularly attractive to people who do not wish to avoid institutional nursing home care, which is the bulk of Medicaid coverage. There appears to us to be little to be gained in a formal quantitative extension of the simulation model to address this issue, as it probably plays a small role in the demands of the average citizen. On this point, the survey evidence reported by Meiners and Tave report that only 19 percent of respondents said that the availability of welfare benefits was an important reason for not buying LTC insurance. There is already recognition about the limitations of type and quality of service availability in public programs—23 percent of respondents said the most important factor in buying LTC insurance was to have a choice of services, and 8.4 percent said avoiding welfare was most important. The remainder were primarily concerned with protecting family resources and assuring access to care as posited in the basic model.

It is plausible to assume that because of altruistic concern for people who have few resources going into retirement, or who make unwise choices regarding insurance, there will always be a need for some backstop free services or subsidies. These cannot be too generous if they are not to discourage purchase of private insurance. For many of the group, who might be tempted to rely on the availability of public coverage, this might be overcome by instituting a partial subsidy geared to income and assets toward the purchase of optional coverage that is available to other elderly people at full cost. The efficiency advantage of this type of partial subsidy, rather than relying on the all-or-nothing Medicaid program, was previously argued in Friedman (1979). If there were a political consensus that the minimum acceptable LTC benefit had to be "reasonable" for even an average citizen, then such a minimum benefit could have substantial depressing effect on demand for supplementary insurance.

Implications for Government Policies

The simulation exercise has impressed upon us several considerations for economic efficiency in the expansion of insurance for LTC. We cannot answer quantitative questions about the "best" approach to the problem at this time. But we do tentatively infer that there is a considerable latent demand and willingness to pay by the typical elderly citizen if (1) load charges can be brought down to group coverage rates, (2) people can be better informed about costs of care if needed, and (3) tendencies to distort probabilities and to overestimate existing public programs can be overcome.

It is not necessary that the government manage a long-term insurance program in order to satisfy the latent demand that appears to exist. But it seems desirable to have the government act as a broker for participating plans and regulate the terms of competition among the plans, as well as oversee the marketing of insurance. By offering an optional "sign-up" for LTC coverage to all Medicare beneficiaries, the government addresses problem (3) above by offering clear signals to consumers that they must take action to attain coverage for LTC.

The inclusion of optional and contributory LTC plans within Medicare should eventually reduce utilization of Medicaid and thereby save money for federal and state governments. However, people with low income may prefer to rely on the continuance of Medicaid eligibility, rather than contribute to LTC insurance. This behavior could be counteracted by partial government subsidies for enrolling in LTC insurance for people with low incomes, coupled with reductions in coverage by the existing Medicaid programs.

In a brokerage or "market simulation" role, the government also addresses problem (1) above by offering to each insurer a large group of beneficiaries at the time they retire and in return demanding that all applicants be accepted and screening/marketing costs be minimized. It might be helpful to allow age-related premiums and restrictions (waiting periods and/or surcharges) for enrollment after the first time of eligibility, in order to deal with biased self-selection by people switching between plans. A practical system for optional enrollment in a variety of LTC plans would require much careful analysis beyond the basic outline herein suggested. Actuarial studies, as well as advice from political officials and possibly further consumer survey research, would serve to refine such practical issues as price variation with age or previous plan choices, exclusions, degree of subsidy, reserve requirements for participating plans, minimum standards in benefit packages, regulation of marketing activities, and so forth.

The brokerage approach, rather than a centrally defined program, has efficiency advantages that depend largely on how much variation there is in consumer demand, other than variation due to poor information or poorly conceived choices. Our model emphasized the sensitivity of demand to information about how much expense might be needed if one became disabled. Even for the same disability, the average expenses would probably vary a great deal by geographic area and in relation to household composition and other highly particular factors.

(The same could be said for other Medicare benefits, and yet for basic hospital and medical care the variation is not due primarily to equally effective substitute inputs.) Research is not yet sufficient for a centrally defined program to be based on variation in underlying demands—but if on the basis of such research, contributions or payments under such a program were graduated by household composition, location, or other such factors, far-reaching alterations in those aspects of family life may have greater consequences than the induced utilization when people purchase their own indemnity policies.

It should be noticed that the brokerage approach suggested above would fit neatly with a more general voucher approach to Medicare benefits. The full range of issues about a voucher system is discussed by other chapters in this text. One special point emerges from the work of LaTour et al. (1986), namely that the inclusion of LTC benefits in a voucher system could reduce overall problems of biased selection in the current experience of health maintenance organization (HMO) options for Medicare beneficiaries. As LTC is a major new type of benefit, and one that may be very salient to people with poorer health status, options with LTC would tend to reverse the current pattern of people with lower expected utilization opting into the alternative plans.

Brief Review of Alternative Proposals

Several proposals for major government initiatives in the financing of LTC services have been published. While a presumption of market failure underlies these proposals, the authors go beyond the potential welfare gain of the individual insured who would be willing to pay for the expected benefits. It will not be possible in this brief review to explain the broader policy frameworks and social values with which these proposals were developed. We will consider their specific operating designs and their possible effects, compared with the more modest public brokerage approach to LTC insurance.

In general, with a comprehensive public program to pay for health services, some major issues are (1) the distribution of costs and benefits, (2) the management of eligibility and benefit payments to restrain induced demand, (3) the effects on overall supply and cost of LTC services via exertion of monopsony power, (4) the effects on the program from lobbying by supplier groups, and (5) the flexibility of the program to evolve over time to reflect consumer and taxpayer preferences. These issues are not peculiar to LTC coverage, and it may be helpful to indicate briefly how some of the issues relate to Medicare coverage of hospital and physician services.

The enrollee "premiums" for hospital benefits are reminiscent of a "whole life" insurance policy (accumulated during working years to cover larger losses later), except that payments are proportional to taxable earnings up to the maximum applicable earnings, and there is no strict policy that each cohort's future expenses are fully covered by its earlier contributions into the fund. The distribution of benefit payments, controlling for incidence of illness, appears to favor particular geographic regions, races, and other population categories associated with differential utilization rates (see, e.g., Davis 1975). Whether the distribution of benefits by income class closely approximates the distribution of contributions is unknown.

Management of benefit payments to restrain induced demand has been a major preoccupation of government officials. Prior approval for capital construction, scrutiny of new technologies prior to approval, retrospective review of charts to penalize unwarranted admissions, peer group limits on reimbursable cost per diem, and, finally, prospective pricing using diagnosis-related groups (DRGs) have been employed to restrain payments. The prospective pricing, with ad hoc annual adjustments to reflect general inflation and other policies, is now a tool for monopsonistic advantage, given that hospitals cannot charge patients for "reasonable" costs not covered by Medicare. This type of policy will eventually constrain the supply of care—the volume, average quality, and variety—since consumers can't voice demands for higher-cost varieties in the marketplace.

The central determination of the scope of current Medicare benefits is subject to the influence of concentrated lobbying. For example, hospitals until very recently preserved reimbursement on the basis of individual circumstances, while other providers were subject to "prevailing rate" screens. The issue of flexibility over time is important—when one recognizes that for more than ten years catastrophic protection has been common in employment-based plans but not in Medicare. More recently, coverage of prescription drugs, which has been expanded in employer group contracts, is another case in point. These are all concerns that have potential analogies in a direct government program to finance LTC services. Yet several knowledgeable policymakers and analysts are convinced that a direct program would have the scale to define and solve problems of LTC that no private insurer would be large enough to overcome.

Davis and Rowland (1986)

Davis and Rowland propose an optional program within Medicare that would charge enrollees 4 percent of income at age sixty, with a minimum of $200 per year and with rising premiums at later ages. Given the income-related premium, Medicaid supplementation of benefits would receive reduced federal contribution. Prospective payment methodologies would be established for nursing homes, based on patient functional impairment. Preadmission assessment would be required for nursing homes, and utilization review would be applied to all claims falling outside established profiles of appropriate utilization.

Davis and Rowland would include some limited LTC services other than institutional residence. Day hospital services would be an alternative to nursing homes in some cases, and respite care could assist family members to maintain a person at home. Grants would be offered to community agencies for home services that help to keep people at home.

The income-related premium does reflect an increasing value of coverage with income in the current environment (i.e., those with higher income have more to "spend-down" before becoming eligible for Medicaid). Until private insurance at lower loading charges is available to higher-income people, many of them would be attracted to the optional coverage, even at premiums greater than expected benefit. The premium charge in relation to family composition raises some questions. In the case of a married couple, would each pay 4 percent of the household income? This would result in much higher total payment than if they were living separately with divided income. And since couples have more self-help capability, this might encourage them to insure only the spouse expected to outlive the other and "self-insure" the spouse expected to die sooner.

The Davis-Rowland proposal gives serious attention to control of induced demand for purchased care, and the mechanisms for claims review and prospective payment are likely to show economies of scale. Essentially, benefits are approved when institutional care is deemed necessary, but for the subset of approved persons with a preference for staying at home, supplementary financing will be available to families and community agencies to support home care. By controlling the pricing of nursing home stays and the preadmission assessment, the government can control the overall supply of institutional care and thereby exert pressure for local expansion of alternative services. (This is already true to some extent as a result of state controls and Medicaid payment policies.) The proposal does not attempt to provide an expensive home care option for which some people might be willing to pay the full premium.

Davis and Rowland also provide some critical views of other policy approaches. Home equity conversions might be encouraged as a source of funds for the elderly to purchase LTC insurance or enrollment in a social/HMO or other managed care system. Obstacles include the legal and tax issues that may discourage lenders, the unwillingness of the elderly to view their home equity as a spendable asset, and the high cost of enrollment in private insurance plans that are subject to adverse self-selection (the latter issue being a prime concern of this chapter).

Tax incentives could be used to foster saving toward costs of LTC in retirement and to reward families who provide more home care and save expenses to the Medicaid program for institutional care. Davis and Rowland do not strongly criticize this type of policy, except to question the volume of new funds and services that would actually flow into LTC. The present authors are more critical of the tax incentive approach. It is questionable why the government should subsidize modest amounts of saving for LTC for everyone, when the risk of needing care is small but can exhaust a great deal of assets—arguing for insurance rather than savings as a solution—and why the subsidy should increase with income, despite the value of protection rising with income. Moreover, if the government is going to commit substantial tax revenue to LTC, it would be reasonable to insist on the cost control impact that could be attained with a direct program.

Bishop (1980)

Bishop proposes a system of benefit payment options to be chosen by a disabled person, contingent on the assessment of disability level by a "gatekeeper." The options would include cash indemnities, vouchers toward enrollment in a capitated delivery system, and reimbursement with coinsurance for a wide range of covered services. This system would provide a significant adaptation to consumer preferences beyond the Davis-Rowland proposal. The Bishop proposal could include a wide variety of regulatory and review mechanisms, as in the Davis-Rowland proposal.

The financing of the Bishop proposal does not include premiums, as it is a compulsory program. Regardless of how the tax financing of the program is related to income, Bishop proposes income-related deductibles before benefits are paid. With such deductibles and with coinsurance, the program could have a somewhat wider scope of services and providers covered, as well as more generous definitions of certifiable disabilities. The deductibles and coinsurance would encourage people with higher incomes to shop around among competing suppliers and thereby exert some market pressure beneficial to all consumers.

The Bishop proposal could potentially mean a much larger federal expense than the Davis-Rowland proposal, which is more restricted to people approved for institutional care. Bishop proposes that deductibles and coinsurance for home care be larger for people with more family resources (i.e., imputed values for family time available or available housing could be added to financial resources). This approach is essentially a refinement of Medicaid spend-down regulations, with the same incentives to misrepresent or revise family arrangements. Bishop admits that this way of addressing cost containment for noninstitutional care is "speculative."

Somers (1982)

The American Public Health Association has officially adopted a position calling for a national program to provide comprehensive LTC services. Somers has developed a proposal of this type, which has been debated in bodies such as the White House Conference on Aging. She proposes a wide scope of eligible LTC services covered within Medicare and the replacement of all applicable Medicaid programs. Cost sharing would be retained, although the issue of income-related coinsurance or deductibles is considered secondary. She proposes that cost sharing might be formulated to increase at higher levels of expense, although the explicit argument for that is not stated. She envisions a role for private supplementary insurance, on the grounds that the coverage of the deductibles and coinsurance amounts dictated by the public program is a type of insurance that private carriers can efficiently undertake.

The critical element of the Somers proposal is a local agency charged with coordination among suppliers of service, comprehensive patient assessment, and "cost-effective case management." Unlike most proposals dealing with LTC, the case management agencies would also include acute care services in their purview. Somers contrasts her proposal with alternative case management approaches, in which an agency receives a capitation contract and is thereby held at risk for the cost of care.

The argument for this program appears to rely on the scale economies of having a single local agency determining cost-effective patterns of care. But this kind of local authority goes beyond any previous mechanism to delegate authority in Medicare and could be subject to "capture" by providers. If the management agency is not at risk, it would appear that there would be unbalanced pressures from expensive service providers to buy influence over decisions. Criticisms raised against strict health-planning programs should also be weighed in this context, particularly the restriction of entry from new suppliers who may be more adaptive to consumer locations and tastes. One virtue of the capitated agency, or risk-sharing approach, is that this could be made an option for consumers who would otherwise have simple indemnity coverage, and, therefore, the capitated agency would have to justify to consumers that restriction on use of costly treatments was not injurious.

Concluding Observations

We doubt that there is sufficient quantitative understanding of the welfare effects and hazards of a comprehensive Medicare expansion into LTC to justify that approach at this time. However, there is evidence of latent demand for insurance protection by people who would pay the full cost of such coverage if it were available at the lower loading charges that we think would be achievable with a government brokerage approach. In addition, the government brokerage approach, or a more general voucher system, would work to supply better information to consumers and tend to increase demand for coverage on that account.

There are already a variety of models of LTC coverage under development that might be suitable alternatives to indemnity plans for inclusion in a set of approved offerings to Medicare enrollees. These alternatives are packaged in various ways with housing and nonmedical services, including programs of managed care at home, social/HMOs, and continuing care retirement communities. If there are substantial efficiencies in the operation of case management agencies in LTC, then with some start-up public funds to demonstrate their value, such agencies might undertake joint ventures with insurers to provide an increasingly desirable variety of available plans.

References

Arrow, K. J., "Uncertainty and the Welfare Economics of Medical Care," *American Economic Review,* 53(5): 941–973, December 1963.

———, "Political and Economic Evaluation of Social Effects and Externalities," in J. Margolis, ed., *The Analysis of Public Output,* New York, NY: Columbia University Press, 1970, p. 11.

———, "Welfare Analysis of Changes in Health Coinsurance Rates," in R. Rosett, ed., *The Role of Health Insurance in the Health Services Sector,* New York, NY: NBER, 1976, pp. 3–23.

Bishop, C. E. "A Compulsory National Long Term Care Insurance Program," in J. J. Callahan, Jr. and S. S. Wallack, eds., *Reforming the Long Term Care System,* Lexington, MA: Lexington Books, 1980, pp. 61–94.

Cafferata, G. L., "Private Health Insurance Coverage of the Medicare Population," Data Preview 18, National Center for Health Services Research, National Health Care Expenditure Study, Rockville, MD: U.S. Department of Health and Human Services, Publication No. (PHS) 84-3362, September 1984a.

———, "Knowledge of Their Health Insurance Coverage by the Elderly," *Medical Care,* 22:835, September 1984b.

Callahan, J., et al., "Responsibilities of Families for Their Severely Disabled Elderly," *Health Care Financing Review,* 1(3): 29–49, Winter 1980.

Cohen, J., "Public Programs Financing Long Term Care," Urban Institute Working Paper, January 1983.

Davis, K., *National Health Insurance: Benefits, Costs and Consequences,* Washington, DC: The Brookings Institution, 1975.

Davis, K., and D. Rowland, *Medicare Policy: New Directions for Health and Long-Term Care,* Baltimore, MD: Johns Hopkins University Press, 1986.

Ehrlich, I., and G. Becker, "Market Insurance, Self-Insurance, and Self-Protection," *Journal of Political Economy,* 80: 639, July/August 1972.

Feldstein, M. S., "The Welfare Loss of Excess Health Insurance," *Journal of Political Economy,* 81(2): 377–434, March/April 1973.

Freeland, M., and C. Schendler, "Health Spending in the 1980's: Integration of Clinical Practice Patterns with Management," *Health Care Financing Review,* 1–68, March 1984.

Friedman, B., "Risk Aversion and the Consumer Choice of Health Insurance Option," *Review of Economics and Statistics,* 7: 209–213, May 1974.

————, "Rationale for Government Initiative in Catastrophic Health Insurance," in M. Pauly, ed., *National Health Insurance: What Now, What Later, What Never?* Washington, DC: American Enterprise Institute, 1979.

Hershey, J. C., et al., "Health Insurance Under Competition: Would People Choose What is Expected?" *Inquiry,* 21:349–360, Winter 1984.

Holmer, M., "Tax Policy and Demand for Health Insurance," *Journal of Health Economics* 3:203–221, December 1984.

Hughes, S. L., *Long Term Care Options in an Expanding Market,* Homewood, IL: Dow Jones Irwin, 1986.

ICF Inc., "Private Financing of Long Term Care: Current Methods and Resources," final report submitted to Office of Assistant Secretary for Planning and Evaluation, U.S. DHHS, January 1985.

Kutza, E. A., *The Benefits of Old Age: Social-Welfare Policy for the Elderly,* Chicago, IL: University of Chicago Press, 1981.

Lambert, Z. V., "Elderly Consumers' Knowledge Related to Medigap Protection Needs," *Journal of Consumer Affairs,* 14:434–451, 1980.

LaTour, S. A., B. Friedman, and E. F. X. Hughes, "Medicare Beneficiary Decision Making About Health Insurance: Implications for a Voucher System," *Medical Care,* 24(7): 601–614, July 1986.

Levit, K. R., et al., "National Health Expenditures, 1984," *Health Care Financing Review,* 7(1): 1–35, Fall 1985.

Liu, K., and Y. Palesch, "The Nursing Home Population: Different Perspectives and Implications for Policy," *Health Care Financing Review,* 3: December 1981.

Manton, K., and B. Soldo, "Dynamics of Health Changes in the Oldest Old: New Perspectives and Evidence," *Milbank Memorial Fund Quarterly,* 63:206–285, Spring 1985.

Marmor, T. R., *The Politics of Medicare,* Chicago, IL: Aldine, 1973.

Marquis, M. S., D. E. Kanouse, and L. Brodsley, "Informing Consumers about Health Care Costs: A Review and Research Agenda," Rand/UCLA Center for Health Care Financing Policy Research, Santa Monica, CA: The Rand Corporation, September 1985.

Marquis, M. S., and C. E. Phelps, "Demand for Supplementary Health Insurance," Rand Corporation R-3285-HHS, July 1985.

McCall, N., T. Rice, and J. Sangl, "Consumer Knowledge of Medicare and Supplemental Health Insurance Benefits," *Health Services Research,* 20(6): 633–658, February 1986.

Meiners, M., and A. Tave, "Consumer Interest in Long-Term Care Insurance: A Survey of the Elderly in Six States," unpublished, February 1985.

Meiners, M. R., and G. R. Trapnell, "Long-Term Care Insurance: Premium Estimates for Prototype Policies," National Center for Health Services Research Working Paper, Baltimore, MD: NCHSR, 1983.

Merritt, R. E., and D. B. Potemken, eds., *Medigap: Issues and Update,* Washington, DC: Intergovernmental Health Policy Project, 1982.

National Association of Insurance Commissioners and Health Care Financing Administration, *Guide to Health Insurance for People with Medicare,* Baltimore, MD: U.S. Department of Health and Human Services/Health Care Financing Administration, April 1983.

Paringer, L., "Forgotten Costs of Informal Long-Term Care," *Generations* 9(4): 55–58, Summer 1985.

Pauly, M. V., "The Economics of Moral Hazard: Comment," *American Economic Review* 58(3): 531–537, June 1968.

———, "Overinsurance and Public Provision of Insurance: The Roles of Moral Hazard and Adverse Selection," *Quarterly Journal of Economics,* 88(1): 44–62, February 1974.

———, "Taxation, Health Insurance, and Market Failure in the Medical Economy," *Journal of Economic Literature,* 24(2): 629–675, June 1986.

Price, J. R., J. W. Mays, and G. R. Trapnell, "Stability in the Federal Employees Health Benefits Program," *Journal of Health Economics,* 2(3): 207–223, December 1983.

Rothschild, M., and J. Stiglitz, "Equilibrium in Competitive Insurance Markets: An Essay on the Economics of Imperfect Information," *Quarterly Journal of Economics* 90(4): 629–649, 1976.

Schoemaker, P. J., "The Expected Utility Model: Its Variants, Purposes, Evidence and Limitations," *Journal of Economic Literature,* 20, June 1982.

Schuttinga, J. A., M. Falik, and B. Steinwald, "Health Plan Selection in the Federal Employees Health Benefits Program," *Journal of Health Politics, Policy and Law,* 10:119–140, Spring 1985.

Somers, A., "Long-Term Care for the Elderly and Disabled: A New Health Priority," *New England Journal of Medicine* 307 (22): 221–226, July 1982.

Spence, M., and R. Zeckhauser, "Insurance, Information, and Individual Action," *American Economic Review, Papers and Proceedings,* 61:380–387, May 1971.

Spiegelman, M., *Ensuring Medical Care for the Aged,* Homewood, IL: Richard Durwin, 1960.

Storfer, M., "Medicaid Data Report July–September 1980," Working Paper #ER-MED-3-80, City of New York, Human Resources Administration, January 1981.

U.S. Congressional Budget Office, *Changing the Structure of Medicare Benefits: Issues and Options,* The Congress of the United States, March 1983.

U.S. General Accounting Office, *Entering a Nursing Home: Costly Implications for Medicaid and the Elderly,* Washington, DC: U.S. Government Printing Office, 1979.

Vladek, B. C., *Unloving Care: The Nursing Home Tragedy,* New York, NY: Basic Books, 1980.

Waldman, S., "A Legislative History of Nursing Home Care," in J. R. Vogel and H. C. Palmer, eds., *Long-Term Care: Perspectives from Research Demonstrations,* Health Care Financing Administration, U.S. Department of Health and Human Services, 1982 (undated), pp. 507–535.

Waldo, D. R., and H. C. Lazenby, "Demographic Characteristics and Health Care Use and Expenditures by the Aged in the United States: 1977–1984," *Health Care Financing Review,* 6(1): 1–29, Fall 1984.

Weissert, W., "Size and Characteristics of the Non-Institutionalized Long Term Care Population," Urban Institute Working Paper No. 1466-20, Washington, DC: Urban Institute, September 1982.

Zeckhauser, R., "Medical Insurance: A Case Study of the Tradeoff Between Risk Spreading and Appropriate Incentives," *Journal of Economic Theory,* 2(1): 10–26, March 1970.

7. An Analysis of "Medigap" Enrollment: Assessment of Current Status and Policy Initiatives

□ □ □

RICHARD M. SCHEFFLER

Introduction

Medicare was enacted in 1965 to ensure access to medical treatment for Americans over sixty-five years old. Even when it was passed, Medicare was never intended to provide total coverage of medical care. Although coverage of services has expanded and program expenditures continue to increase, the elderly are still responsible for a significant portion of their total medical expenses. Coverage not provided either under Medicare Part A (hospitalization) or Part B (physician services and other medical services) leaves an individual at considerable risk, particularly at an age when sources of income to pay for these items are diminishing (see the chapter by Phelps and Reisinger in this text for estimates of that risk).

A market has been created in the private sector to sell Medicare supplementary insurance, more commonly referred to as "Medigap." Medigap insurance basically supplements the coverage provided by Medicare. Individual policies vary considerably in coverage provided. Regulation ensures coverage of the Medicare copayment and coinsurance provisions, but many policies also cover deductibles and other items either not covered or partially covered by Medicare. However, larger "gaps" remain—coverage of routine, preventive, and long-term care—which are covered neither by Medicare nor by supplemental policies.

The amount of private insurance acquired to supplement Medicare has grown steadily. The percentage of Medicare beneficiaries estimated to have private supplemental coverage has grown from 45.5 percent in 1967 (Mueller 1972) to approximately 67 percent in 1980, while an additional 13 percent were covered by Medicaid (Garfinkel and Corder 1985). Another analysis estimated Medigap ownership to range between 69 percent and 82 percent in the six states surveyed (Rice and McCall 1985). Traditionally, the insurer with the largest market share has been the aggregate of Blue Cross and Blue Shield Plans. Garfinkel and Corder (1985) estimated that in 1980 approximately 54 percent of Medicare beneficiaries with private supplemental insurance had Blue Cross and Blue Shield policies. In the Health Insurance Association of America's (1986) estimates of coverage of persons with private insurance over sixty-five years of age for both 1983 and 1984, the Blue Cross and Blue Shield Plans held 59 percent of the private insurance market for hospital coverage and 69 percent of the private insurance market for medical coverage (other than hospital).

Given the prevalence of Medigap policies (which developed in response to specific provisions in the Medicare legislation), it is important to be aware of the provisions of current Medigap policies and how those policies might change due to legislative action to respond to a new market situation. In addition, the assessment of the impact of potential legislation requires a knowledge of who is buying Medigap policies, the type of policy they are buying, and how purchase affects utilization (and, therefore, Medicare costs). As an initial step in such an effort, this chapter first describes the nature of Medicare and Medigap coverage and speculates about the impact proposed changes would have on the Medigap market. It then reviews existing research on supplementary insurance and presents an analysis that utilizes enrollment data of sixty-three Blue Cross Plans to describe group and nongroup beneficiaries over sixty-five years of age. This study analyzes the demand for Blue Cross nongroup supplementary coverage, using an econometric model. Further, this model attempts to associate the purchase of Blue Cross Medigap supplementary coverage with Medicare expenditures.

Overview of Medicare and Medigap

Medicare coverage

Medicare provides coverage under two categories. Part A covers inpatient hospitalizations, skilled nursing facilities, and qualified home health care. Coverage is effective for any U.S. citizen aged sixty-five and over, who is eligible for Social Security. Those persons aged sixty-five years and over and ineligible for Social Security or resident noncitizens can purchase Part A coverage through payment of a monthly premium. Part B, or Supplementary Medical Insurance (SMI), covers physician services, home health, and other qualified medical services. Coverage is voluntary and a monthly premium must be paid for these additional services. It serves as a public supplementary insurance to Part A.

Despite the coverage provided by Medicare, the elderly are still at financial risk for the deductibles, copayments, and coinsurance for services covered by Medicare, as well as for those services that remain uncovered. Medicare accounted for less than 49 percent of the payments for health care provided to the elderly in 1984 (Waldo and Lazenby 1984). The deductible for Part A is approximately equal to the cost of the initial day of hospitalization. It has grown from $40 in 1966, when Medicare was implemented, to $492 in 1986. Medicare pays for the initial 60 days of a hospital stay after the deductible is paid for the benefit period. A copayment equal to one-fourth of the deductible is then charged for the 61st through 90th days; a copayment of half of the deductible is assessed for the next 60 lifetime reserve days of stay. If a patient is discharged to a Medicare-qualified skilled nursing facility, the first twenty days are covered, but a copayment of one-eighth the deductible must be made for additional days up to 100 as long as the services are rehabilitative. After that time, the patient is responsible for the entire cost. The recent (1987) legislative proposals provide stop-loss coverage without deductibles or copayments. There is usually a "spend-down" period, whereby the individual makes out-of-pocket payments until reaching the level of impoverishment for Medicaid eligibility. Then, Medicaid is relied on for the balance of long-term care support.

Part B, which operates nominally as a voluntary insurance plan, requires the payment of a monthly premium ($15.50 in 1986), an annual deductible ($75.00 in 1986), and 20 percent coinsurance of allowable charges for covered services used. In addition, the patient could be liable for the difference between the actual and allowable costs of services. Approximately 75 percent of the cost of Part B is covered by a subsidy from general revenue taxation, so that very few elderly decline coverage.

Medical reimbursements for the elderly covered by Medicare totaled $41.7 billion in 1980, according to Garfinkel and Corder (1985). Of this amount, the federal government paid 56 percent ($23.4 billion) through Medicare expenditures, 18 percent ($7.6 billion) was paid by the beneficiaries or their relatives, 15 percent ($6.3 billion) was paid by private insurance, Medicaid paid 7 percent ($3.1 billion), and the remaining 3 percent ($1.2 billion) was paid by other sources. Thus, for those items covered by Medicare, individuals were still liable for a larger portion than private insurers, and Medicaid, as the public supplement, covered nearly half of what the private insurers reimbursed.

Medigap coverage
The approximately 67 percent of the Medicare-aged population who buy Medigap policies are offered basically three categories of private insurance to supplement the public coverage provided under Medicare: major medical, indemnity,

and limited policies. The major medical policies cover the copayment provisions and, depending on the extent of coverage of the policy, may include the deductibles, coinsurance, and other items, such as prescribed drugs, not covered by Medicare. Payment for covered services is usually coordinated between government and the private insurer for payment to the provider of the service. Indemnity policies usually provide a sum of money to the beneficiary in the case of hospitalization or a stay in a nursing home. The individual is then liable for payments to the providers. Limited policies, or what have become known as "dread disease" policies, usually insure against a single disease, such as cancer.

For these elderly who have both Medicare and private insurance, Medicare paid 54 percent of expenditures for this subgroup, 21 percent was paid by private supplemental insurance, 20 percent was paid by the individual or relatives, and the balance (5 percent) was paid by other sources, such as prepaid organizations and Medicaid. Although Medicare paid a slightly lower percentage overall for this group, their total expenditures were higher. On a per capita basis, an individual with private supplemental coverage in addition to Medicare incurred approximately $1,818 in expenses, of which $363 would have been paid out-of-pocket, $988 paid by Medicare, with private insurance responsible for most of the balance. In contrast, the individual with Medicare only (no private or public supplement) incurred approximately $1,087 in per capita expenditures and was responsible for $318 out-of-pocket, while Medicare reimburses $729 for each individual in this subgroup (Garfinkel and Corder 1985). These data suggest that those with Medigap coverage have per capita medical expenditures nearly 70 percent higher than those with Medicare coverage only, and the per capita cost to Medicare is approximately one-third higher for those beneficiaries with private supplemental coverage, which has important implications when considering changes in legislation regulating Medigap policies and/or Medicare coverage. Increasingly, state and federal regulations have defined the more traditional major medical coverage as "qualified Medicare supplement" insurance.

Regulation and Assessment of Private Medicare Supplementary Insurance

Private insurance sold as a supplement to Medicare has existed nearly as long as the Medicare program itself. In the late 1970s the issue of Medicare supplementary insurance coverage was brought to the attention of the public through a series of congressional hearings and reports (DeNovo and Shearer 1978). Concern was raised about product misrepresentation, inefficacy, and the advantage being taken of the vulnerable elder segment of the population.

The National Association of Insurance Commissioners (NAIC) appointed a special task force in 1978 to examine the issue of marketing private supplementary insurance to the elderly. Despite increased state monitoring, as a result of the NAIC study and recommendations, there was a consensus that federal government involvement was needed to strengthen the state efforts. Subsequently, in 1980 Congress passed a voluntary certification program as an amendment to PL 96-265, Section 507, which has become known as the Baucus amendment (named after its sponsor, Senator Max Baucus of Montana). The law basically adopted the NAIC minimum standards and set July 1, 1982 as the implementation date. The law further required subsequent evaluations of each participating state's effectiveness in regulating Medicare supplemental policies.

The Baucus legislation required minimum benefit standards, including but not limited to the following:

☐ Standardization of coverage terms used in policies
☐ Loss ratios (ratios of total benefits to total premiums paid) of 75 percent for group and 60 percent for nongroup policies
☐ Linking of the policies' cost-sharing provisions to changes in Medicare
☐ Ability of purchasers to review a policy prior to purchase agreement
☐ Outline of coverage and replacement stipulations
☐ Buyers' guide and written receipt upon application

Specific to Medicare supplementation, the Baucus legislation further stipulated that a policy's coverage include the following:

Part A
☐ Required coverage of copayments for days 61–90 of a hospital stay
☐ Required coverage of copayment for lifetime reserve days (91–150)
☐ Required coverage of 90 percent of hospitalization expenses to a lifetime minimum of 365 additional days
☐ Six-month or less "preexisting condition" clause

Part B
☐ Maximum $200 deductible for eligible charges
☐ Required coverage of 20 percent copayment
☐ Maximum of $5,000 out-of-pocket costs per calendar year

Many private policies cover much more than the minimal requirements stipulated by this legislation. A description of Blue Cross and Blue Shield nongroup, Medicare complementary policies from their recent survey is included as Table 7.1 to indicate the diversity of options available through one insurer that meet and exceed Baucus standards.

TABLE 7.1
Blue Cross and Blue Shield Nongroup Medicare Complementary Products
(N = 119)

	Included	Not included	Data not provided in survey
Part A			
Copay, days 61–90[a]	102	2	17
Copay, lifetime reserve days[a]	101	2	16
90%[a] or 100% of additional 365 days	83	14[b]	22
Hospital deductible	88	17	14
Skilled nursing facility copay, days 21–100	88	14	17
Extension of skilled nursing facility days	37	67	15
Prescription drugs	42	61	16
Part B			
$75 Deductible	63	36	20
20% Copay above $200 and less than $5,000	c	c	28

[a]Baucus minimum benefit standard.

[b]12 of these 14 products are offered by plans that also offer a Medicare complementary policy, which does not cover 90–100% of an additional 365 days, as required by Baucus. The other two are in non-Baucus states.

[c]Two plans cover the Part B copayment, as specified by Baucus, 20% copay above $200 and less than $5,000; 11 require a $200 deductible but do not limit payments to $5,000; 10 products use a $5,000 maximum but require only a $75 or $0 deductible; 68 products pay the 20% copay, with a deductible of only $75 and no $5,000 maximum.

Sources: Medicare Complementary Survey Report, Blue Cross and Blue Shield Association, Product Development, July 1986.

Policy Issues: the Gaps Remain

Issues: demography, coverage, and the role of insurance

As the population ages, a demographic imperative for medical care coverage looms as the age cohort of those sixty-five years and over expands. A larger percentage of the population will live longer as the twenty-first century is reached. The first issue that must be addressed is whether existing "catastrophic" coverage can be expanded just to meet the anticipated needs of the growing elderly population.

Another issue is whether or not the elderly should have comprehensive coverage for medical care. As stated earlier in this chapter, there are many items that Medicare does not cover. If it is agreed that medical care coverage for the elderly should be comprehensive, how is medical care to be defined? At present, items that are categorized as health promotion and disease prevention, as well as other actions to assess health status, such as routine physical examinations, remain uncovered. Should all of these be included in a comprehensive plan for the elderly?

The role of public versus private insurance is important, particularly with respect to coverage and enrollment concerns. The incorporation of deductibles, copayments, and coinsurance in Medicare (Parts A and B) was intended to serve as a utilization control by maintaining an individual's involvement in the cost of obtaining medical care. Buyers and sellers in the private market chose to cover these cost-sharing provisions instead of services not covered by Medicare, such as long-term care. The Baucus legislation and subsequent state mandates required such coverage in policies offered. In doing so, both the direct cost of medical care and the premium cost of Medicare facing an individual elder are made less than the true cost of either to society. While the Medicare Prospective Payment Systems (PPS) may control inpatient hospital utilization (quantity of care), medical care expenditures for this segment of the population continue to increase.

What impact will a change in Medicare have on the private insurance market, and what role will private supplemental insurance play in the future?

Alternative recommendations
If, in fact, medical care coverage is to be defined more comprehensively, a number of alternatives have been proposed to cover long-term care, ranging from cash accumulation instruments to the addition of a "Part C" to Medicare (Davis and Rowland 1986; Knickman et al. 1986; Blumenthal et al. 1986). The effect on private Medicare supplementary policies of instituting an alternative coverage plan is difficult to assess, given that empirical evidence is unavailable. The degree to which the public and the private sectors will continue to play important roles insuring the elderly against the cost of illness varies, depending on the characteristics of the alternative and the degree to which the existing system would be changed by its possible implementation. Proceeding with conjecture, the effects upon the viability of continued and/or expanded private supplemental Medicare coverage would most likely be produced through at least two avenues of change: (1) through modifications in the financing of care and (2) through changes in health care delivery.

Under the scenario of more comprehensive coverage, as proposed by Davis and Rowland (1986), a stipulated ceiling on annual out-of-pocket expenses of $1,500 for acute care and $3,000 for long-term care would set a maximum personal liability of 44 percent of average annual income for elderly individuals ($10,150). Currently, that liability is limitless, and the uncertainty regarding expenses for medical care, combined with the Medicare "subsidy" to private coverage, has induced the elderly to purchase private plans to supplement Medicare. The question then arises whether the elderly would continue to purchase private supplemental insurance policies if Medicare is revised to provide greater comprehensive coverage for both acute and long-term care, while continuing to charge the same premium, regardless of whether or not private coverage is bought. Assuming the elderly to be risk averse, our best guess is that they would continue to be interested in such supplementary insurance.

From the standpoint of financing, implementation of strict Medicare cost-containment policies would be needed to avoid escalating costs brought on by the extension of coverage. Private third-party payers would probably react favorably by continuing to offer supplemental policies since public cost-containment measures would help to lessen variability in costs. As a result, the level of financial risk borne by insurers would be reduced and premiums would be easier to determine.

A similar design has been recommended by the Harvard Medicare Project (Blumenthal et al. 1986). This proposal suggests that Medicare be simplified by combining the two existing parts and extending coverage to include long-term care and chronic illness. Premiums would be increased and based on an elderly person's ability to pay. Copayments would be decreased and, in some cases, eliminated, such as for long hospital stays. Further recommendations are made to restructure the physician reimbursement policy, including expansion of prepaid or managed care arrangements, prospective budgeting, and mandatory acceptance of assignment. Private supplemental policies would have to extend their range of coverage and modify the premium structure concomitant with the alternative proposals for the cost-sharing provisions of the public programs. The elderly would still be likely to purchase such policies, assuming risk aversion, unless total individual liability for copayments was so limited that an individual need not insure against these occurrences of illness. However, proposing a reduction in each beneficiary's maximum liability would foretell large increases in public expenditures to fund the program and thus would make this alternative unlikely in the present era of containment and deficit reduction.

Thus, in both of the scenarios described above, the market for private supplemental Medigap insurance could be expected to grow if Medicare coverage provisions are changed by the government. Standardization and increased public sector coverage of long-term care will open the market for private long-term care insurance paralleling the one currently available for acute care. With such changes, premiums could be set at a level compatible with the budgets of the elderly, and the level of risk borne by the private insurers would be decreased substantially, giving them an incentive to expand coverage of the over-sixty-five market.

If, on the other hand, publicly funded coverage is scaled to ensure adequate access to health care and protection against catastrophic costs, the Medigap market would still grow, although the incentives would be different. Under this scenario, Medicare would remain basically the same as it is now but with an expansion of the scope of coverage to include more long-term care. A ceiling would be proposed limiting individual liability, although it would be higher than the other two proposals. Due to a broadening of coverage provided, both government and private insurers would have increasingly important roles in the development and implementation of utilization and cost-containment measures. Alternative forms of delivery, for example, private health plans, health maintenance organizations (HMOs), and social HMOs, could be utilized more extensively since they are better able to monitor costs and limit access to unnecessary care. Because coverage would establish a relative ceiling on personal liability, private insurers would expand the Medigap market because their liability would be better defined, even though it may be greater than at present. In other words, the risk of providing private supplemental insurance would be lessened, even though the scope of both publicly and privately supported coverage may be increased. Recently (1987) proposed legislation that is likely to pass includes stop-loss coverage against catastrophic costs but does not cover long-term care.

Support for these two options or other proposals (such as no change or further regulation of Medigap) depends, in part, on an understanding of the current Medigap market and consumer behavior. A number of studies address these issues.

Previous Research

Definitions and assessments of private Medicare supplementary insurance could be grouped by data sources utilized for analysis. Most of the prior research has been performed on an individual level of analysis from national sample surveys, with estimates made for the general population.

The Survey of Income and Education, a national sample of 150,000 households, was used to assess the cost-sharing impacts of 30,000 elderly households in regard to private insurance as a supplement to Medicare. In estimating demand for supplementation, Long and Settle (1982) found that the probability of acquiring private supplemental insurance rises sharply as income increases from the lowest reported levels, but that income made relatively little difference after it reached a level of $10,000. Further, they found that changes in Medicare cost-sharing provisions do affect demand for private insurance supplements and, apart from income, that age and race had significant influence on supplementation rates. The aged elderly and black Medicare beneficiaries were less likely to have private supplements. The difference in racial supplementation rates is significant (approximately 80 percent for whites and 65 percent for blacks), even when income is above the $9,000 to $10,000 income level. Long and Settle propose possible explanations for this racial disparity in supplementation rates as due to factors of demand (differences in risk aversion correlated with race) and supply (discriminatory marketing practices). Long, Settle, and Link (1982) conclude that cost sharing has a different impact, depending on whether or not one has a private supplement, uses Medicaid as a supplement, or has no supplement.

The National Medical Care Expenditure Survey (NMCES) is a nationally representative survey of 14,000 households, performed during 1977 and 1978. It has been used with respect to the Medicare private supplementary insurance issue to describe the characteristics of the elder population at the time and to predict possible effects of the Baucus legislation (Cafferata 1985a). Part of the analysis in this study includes a breakdown of group and nongroup insurance by coverage of health services. Although both group and nongroup insurance cover nearly all hospital and inpatient physician care, there are notable differences in other service areas, particularly outpatient diagnostic services, outpatient prescribed medicines, dental care, and mental health. Cafferata and Meiners (1984) also assessed the impact of Medigap on out-of-pocket expenses of the elderly. More recently, Cafferata (1985a) used this data to determine coverage characteristics and distribution of policies meeting Baucus minimum standards. Her analysis evaluated whether perceived health status (excellent, good, fair, or poor), source of insurance (group or nongroup; Blue Cross and Blue Shield, commercial, or other), geographic census region of the country and place of residence (Standard Metropolitan Statistical Area [SMSA] or not) increased the likelihood of one having had private insurance in 1977 that would have met the Baucus standards established in 1980. For example, an individual self-perceived to be in excellent health, not living in an SMSA, with a group Blue Cross and Blue Shield policy in 1977 would be most likely to have had coverage meeting Baucus- like standards. The same data base was used to assess the elderly population's coverage of nursing home care (Cafferata 1985b).

The National Medical Care Utilization and Expenditure Survey (NMCUES) was undertaken in 1980 to compile detailed national estimates of the utilization and expenditures for various types of medical care. Part of the rationale for doing this extensive survey was to compile more detailed information on the Medicare and Medicaid population. Garfinkel and Corder (1985) use this database to describe supplemental health insurance among Medicare enrollees over sixty-five years of age. Their work indicates that in 1980 approximately 80 percent of Medicare beneficiaries reported having some kind of supplemental insurance. Approximately 67 percent reported having private, or commercial, supplements, while an additional 13 percent reported having Medicaid. Further analysis showed that 54 percent of the 67 percent with private supplements had Blue Cross and Blue Shield Plans.

NMCUES was used in conjunction with the National Nursing Home Survey (NNHS 1977) by Rice and Gabel (1986) to construct a data source representative of the entire elderly population that would include both their noninstitutional and institutional health care costs. Their analysis indicates that the elderly have increased protection through private supplemental coverage until health care costs reach a level of about $7,500. After costs reach that critical level, supplementation through private insurers declines as a percentage of total expenditures for health care. Rice and Gabel (1986) show that for those who experienced catastrophic costs (defined as over $2,000 annually), over 80 percent were due to nursing home care.

As part of the legislated requirements, subsequent evaluations were to be done to assess the effectiveness of the Baucus regulations on private supplementary insurance. The Stanford Research Institute (SRI) was awarded a contract to assist the Department of Health and Human Services (DHHS) in performing the initial studies to survey consumers and determine the state regulatory impact. In 1982 six states identified by the Health Care Financing Administration (HCFA) and NAIC were surveyed: California, Florida, Mississippi, New Jersey, Washington, and Wisconsin. The initial survey results suggest that specific state regulations expand the Medicare supplemental health insurance market in the individual states studied (McCall and Rice 1983). Further review of individual policies was done by Rice and McCall (1985) to describe and analyze policy ownership characteristics of supplementary policies for a broader assessment of the effectiveness of this legislation. Other actions such as labeling, standardization, dissemination of buyers' guides, and referral services serve not only to increase consumer knowledge but also aid in protecting the elderly against potential sales abuse practices (McCall, Rice, and Sangl 1986).

These studies are largely descriptive but do establish the following facts:

☐ Demand for insurance is influenced by income up to a threshold of $10,000 (in 1982), when the vast majority of white beneficiaries purchased some kind of supplementary coverage. Blacks, however, were less likely to buy Medigap policies, even at upper income levels.
☐ Demand apparently is also influenced by the nature of state regulation, with states that require a certain minimum benefit level having higher Medigap enrollment.
☐ Medigap policies tend to reduce out-of-pocket expenditures up to a ceiling of about $7,500. Most catastrophic care payments are paid by the elderly or their families, with 80 percent of personal expenditures going to nursing home care.
☐ There is some evidence that use of Medicare-covered services tends to be higher among holders of Medigap policies, thereby increasing the payments made by Medicare.

The intent of this research is to analyze purchase of Blue Cross Medicare supplemental policies by providing more descriptive information about policy and purchaser characteristics and, further, to explore how the purchase of supplementary coverage affects Medicare expenditures. This is particularly important because an understanding of demand and utilization behavior is essential for predicting the impact of various policy options. The Blue Cross Plans were selected because they offer a wide range of policies, operate nationwide, and account for over 50 percent of Medigap purchases.

The Blue Cross Experience—Medicare Complementary Coverage: Determinants of Blue Cross Medigap Enrollment

Description

The Blue Cross and Blue Shield Plans were early entrants in the Medicare supplementary insurance market. In a recent survey of the individual Blue Cross and Blue Shield Plans conducted by the national Blue Cross and Blue Shield Association, it was reported that all of the Plans offer some type of "Medicare complementary" coverage and are also subject to state regulatory review of premiums for nongroup Medicare supplementary insurance. Even in states without enacted Baucus legislation, the policies marketed by the Blue Cross and Blue Shield Plans meet or exceed the NAIC minimums of these amendments. For example, in six states the Blue Cross and Blue Shield Plans are required to provide benefits, such as chiropractic services, which are in excess of the Baucus minimums but mandated by the states (Blue Cross and Blue Shield Assoc. 1986).

The wide range of premiums charged is dependent on policy benefits for Blue Cross and Blue Shield Medicare supplementary insurance, which vary from coverage approximating the Baucus minimum to comprehensive coverage far exceeding the minimal standards. A national survey of Blue Cross Medigap products found that the lowest premium charged by a Blue Cross Plan for basic coverage (comparable to the Baucus minimums) was $18.13 per month or $217.56 per year. On the other hand, the highest premium charged for the most comprehensive coverage was $130 per month ($1,560 per annum), which included deductibles, drugs, home and office visits, complete psychiatric coverage, and so forth. Because these premiums differ across both Plans and types of coverage, the prices reflect regional medical care cost differences, as well as varying degrees of insurance coverage. Among the Plans reporting in the recent survey, 75 percent of nongroup enrollees pay a premium less than $43 per month ($516 per annum), and approximately 80 percent pay less than $50 per month ($600 per annum) (Blue Cross and Blue Shield Assoc. 1986).

Blue Cross regular enrollment data are reported for Medicare complementary categories broken down by group and nongroup policies. A separate tally records regular Medicare "carve-out" enrollment. Since 1984 plans have subdivided their HMO and preferred provider organization (PPO) enrollment totals into the

three Medicare components as well. The group and nongroup Medigap enrollment analyzed in this chapter necessarily excludes Medicare HMO members
prior to 1984. Based on evidence from subsequent years, this omission is of
minor concern. In 1984 only 0.09 percent of Medicare-aged Blue Cross policyholders were enrolled in HMO options. The unique Blue Cross "carve-out" category includes retirees whose medical insurance benefits after retirement remain
the same as those actively employed. There is a coordination of Medicare and
employer-sponsored benefits that usually includes services additional to those
usually provided as Medicare complementary. Many Plans offering carve-out
coverage are unable to report it separately from the group covered, making analysis of this category impossible.

For descriptive purposes, Blue Cross group and nongroup (individual) enrollment of those over sixty-five years of age for 1981 through 1985 is analyzed by
the four large census regions of the country. The regional distribution of Blue
Cross Medicare complementary enrollment (sixty-five years of age and over) in
1985 indicates that 42 percent of Blue Cross nongroup Medigap enrollees lived
in the Northeast, 30 percent in the north central region, 22 percent in the South,
and 6 percent in the West. This distribution has been relatively stable over the
past five years. By contrast, in 1983 the regional distribution of all Medicare
enrollees shows that the highest percentage of beneficiaries lived in the South
(approximately 33 percent), with 26 percent in the north central region, 24 percent in the Northeast, and 17 percent in the western region. The West has the
lowest number of both Medicare and Blue Cross enrollees. These distributions
are similar to those found in the analysis of the NMCES data (Cafferata 1984),
which indicate that there is a higher percentage of private supplemental insurance coverage in the northeastern and north central regions than in the South and
the West.

Over the past five years, Blue Cross Medicare supplemental insurance enrollment has shown a small decline. Blue Cross under-sixty-five enrollment has
shown a similar decline over these years. However, the data indicate that group
Medigap enrollment has remained relatively steady, while the decrease has been
in the nongroup, or individual, Medigap enrollment (Table 7.2). Regionally, as
seen in Table 7.2, the largest declines have been in the West, although the north
central and southern regions have also decreased more rapidly than the Northeast, which is Blue Cross' strongest area in under-sixty-five enrollment as well.

The Blue Cross share of the private insurance market for the population aged
sixty-five years and over seems to be remaining relatively stable. It is difficult to
compute actual market share as information on all of the other private insurers is
not readily available, and Medicare supplementary policies have not traditionally
been reported separately. However, in the 1986 Update to the *Source Book of*

TABLE 7.2
Blue Cross Medicare Complementary Enrollment Annual Percent Changes
1981–85 (percents)

| | By category | | |
	Group	Nongroup	Total
1981–82	−0.7	−0.9	−0.9
1982–83	−1.3	−1.8	−1.6
1983–84	0.3	−3.3	−2.4
1984–85	1.0	−3.0	−2.0
Average annual percent change	−0.2	−2.2	−1.7

| | By region | | | | |
	Northeast	North central	South	West	Total
1981–82	0.3	−2.1	−1.3	−1.5	−0.9
1982–83	−1.4	−2.6	−1.3	0.3	−1.6
1983–84	−0.8	−3.2	−3.4	−6.1	−2.4
1984–85	−1.0	−2.3	−2.2	−6.3	−2.0
Average annual percent change	−0.7	−2.5	−2.0	−3.3	−1.7

Source: Blue Cross and Blue Shield Association Enrollment Reports.

TABLE 7.3
Blue Cross Regional Market Penetration by Census Region

	Northeast	North central	South	West	Total
Blue Cross >65 enrollment as percent of Medicare >65 enrollment					
1981	58.8	39.0	23.6	12.9	34.3
1982	58.1	37.6	22.7	12.4	33.3
1983	56.4	36.1	21.9	12.0	32.1
Blue Cross Medicare complementary insurance annual percent change in regional market penetration					
1981–82	−1.2	−3.6	−3.5	−4.2	−2.9
1982–83	−3.0	−4.2	−3.7	−2.7	−3.7
Average annual percent change	−2.1	−3.8	−3.6	−3.4	−3.2

Sources: Blue Cross and Blue Shield Association Enrollment Reports, 1981–83, HCFA Annual Medicare Program Statistics, 1981–83.

Health Insurance Data, statistics are published separating out the population aged sixty-five and over for 1983 and 1984. Blue Cross and Blue Shield Plans, as a percentage of all insurers for the category aged sixty-five and over, held 59 percent of the private market for hospital insurance and 69 percent of the private "medical other than hospital expense protection" market for both years, respectively (HIAA 1986). It should be noted that some of the data in these calculations are based on estimates. Using Blue Cross enrollment data and HCFA Medicare program statistics, regional market penetration was calculated as the percentage of the Medicare enrollees over sixty-five years old that held Blue Cross nongroup Medigap policies. HCFA data were available at the county level for the years 1981 through 1983. Table 7.3 shows these calculations by region. As with the enrollment figures, a slight decline is evident with a total penetration of 34.3 percent in 1981, dropping to 32.1 percent in 1983. The regional changes shown in Table 7.3 indicate that the north central region, and the South and West are losing more of their respective markets than the Northeast.

Methodology and empirical results

This section of the chapter provides an empirical examination of Blue Cross nongroup Medigap enrollment. As noted earlier, Blue Cross holds more than half of the market for Medigap policies sold in the United States. Our empirical work focuses on nongroup Blue Cross policies, which represent over six million of the eight million Medigap policies sold to the Blue Cross population aged sixty-five years and older. The unit of analysis is the Blue Cross Plan area. Plan areas vary in size, according to the geographic coverage of the sixty-five Blue Cross Plans. Only sixty-three of the sixty-five Blue Cross Plans are included in our analysis: two plans were excluded because of incomplete enrollment data. These Plans represented less than 1 percent of total Blue Cross enrollment in 1985.

Our empirical model analyzes a number of variables that have previously been associated with Medigap policy demand (Long and Settle 1982; Long, Settle, and Link 1982; Rice and McCall 1985). Theoretically, we assumed the demand for Blue Cross supplemental insurance coverage to depend on the relative price of Blue Cross Medigap policies, income, race, regulatory factors, and the strength of Blue Cross in the under-sixty-five market for insurance in the Plan area. Because our analysis is conducted at the Plan rather than the individual level, we used the percentage of Medicare enrollees over age sixty-five with Blue Cross nongroup Medigap policies to represent quantity of policies demanded in each Plan area. The variables analyzed are listed and defined in Table 7.4. Table 7.5 reports simple descriptive statistics for the variables included in the analysis, and Table 7.6 summarizes our ordinary least-squares results. Data sources are reported in Appendix 7.1.

As depicted in Table 7.6, we estimated separate regressions on the sample of sixty-three Blue Cross Plans in 1981 and 1984, with and without regional dummy variables. Based on the results of statistical testing described in Appendix 7.2, we concluded that the two cross-sections could also be pooled. Results from the pooled runs, with and without regional dummy variables, also appear in Table 7.6. In each case, the regional dummy variables add little to the predictive power of the model but, in most cases, are statistically significant at the 5 percent level.

TABLE 7.4
Variable Definitions: Medigap Regressions

Variable	Definition
Dependent variable	
N	Blue Cross nongroup Medigap enrollment as a percent of Medicare enrollees over age 65 in relevant Blue Cross Plan area; in 1984 non-group Medigap enrollment includes elderly with HMO and PPO arrangements, as well as those enrolled in traditional Medigap plans
Independent variables	
DEDUCT	Medicare Part A hospital deductible deflated by estimated consumer price index for medical care expenditures for an intermediate budget of a retired couple living within Blue Cross Plan area; deflated deductible is measured in 1981 dollars
RACE	Percent of elderly population reported as nonwhite in 1980
BAUCUS	Dummy variable indicating state legislative approval of Baucus amendment; for the 1984 model, BAUCUS equals 1 if the state(s) corresponding to Blue Cross Plan area had passed Baucus legislation by January 1, 1983, and equals 0 otherwise; for 1981 BAUCUS equals 0 for all Plans
BCMS	Total group and nongroup Blue Cross members under 65 years of age as a percent of under-65 population within the Blue Cross Plan area; because only total HMO enrollment was reported in 1981, HMO enrollment is excluded from total under-65 Blue Cross enrollment in that year; during 1981 HMO members comprised only 0.9% of total Blue Cross enrollment; in 1984 BCMS includes both HMO and PPO members under 65 years of age
NE	Regional dummy variable equals 1 if Blue Cross Plan is located in the northeastern census region and equals 0 otherwise
NC	Regional dummy variable equals 1 if Blue Cross Plan is located in north central census region and equals 0 otherwise
S	Regional dummy variable equals 1 if Blue Cross Plan is located in southern census region and equals 0 otherwise
T	Time dummy variable for pooled cross-sectional analysis equals 1 in 1984 and 0 in 1981

Source: See Appendix 7.1.

Because we used cross-sectional data, we also tested for heteroscedastic errors. Results from the heteroscedasticity tests also appear in Appendix 7.2 and indicate that heteroscedasticity does not appreciably affect the results reported in Table 7.6.

Prices. Because we were unable to include actual data on Blue Cross or its competitors' Medigap policy prices in our regression analysis, we included an estimated price faced by the elderly not owning Medigap supplemental coverage.[1] As discussed earlier, most Blue Cross nongroup Medigap policies cover some combination of Medicare deductibles and copayments. Although these Medicare coverage gaps are set nationally, the impact of the Medicare deductible and the related copayments on the individual will vary, depending on the cost of

TABLE 7.5
Summary Statistics for Variables Used in Blue Cross Medigap
Ordinary Least-Squares Model

Variable	Mean (standard deviations in parentheses)		
	1981 ($n = 63$)	1984 ($n = 63$)	Pooled ($n = 126$)
N	27.44	25.09	26.27
	(13.48)	(12.79)	(13.14)
DEDUCT	206.63	287.56	247.09
	(4.36)	(8.93)	(41.22)
RACE	8.76	8.76	8.76
	(8.86)	(8.86)	(8.83)
BAUCUS		0.86	0.43
BCMS	36.04	29.30	32.67
	(20.38)	(21.12)	(20.95)
NE	0.27	0.27	0.27
NC	0.25	0.25	0.25
S	0.32	0.32	0.32

Source: See Appendix 7.1.

TABLE 7.6
Blue Cross Nongroup Medigap Market Penetration

Independent variables	Coefficient estimates (t-statistics in parentheses)					
	1981		1984		Pooled	
CONSTANT	−168.63[b]	−46.45	−12.55	10.73	−20.31	18.33
	(2.303)	(0.473)	(0.298)	(0.229)	(0.745)	(0.639)
DEDUCT	0.8990[c]	0.2860	0.0672	−0.0221	0.1652[a]	−0.0343
	(2.504)	(0.586)	(0.471)	(0.138)	(1.262)	(0.244)
RACE	−0.1303	−0.1833	−0.2220[a]	−0.2463[a]	−0.2016[b]	−0.2335[b]
	(0.879)	(0.940)	(1.479)	(1.362)	(1.907)	(1.814)
BAUCUS			7.968[b]	7.529[b]	6.959[b]	6.249[b]
			(1.954)	(1.835)	(1.860)	(1.734)
BCMS	0.3178[c]	0.2340[c]	0.4588[c]	0.2381[c]	0.4266[c]	0.2385[c]
	(4.347)	(2.545)	(6.676)	(2.446)	(9.212)	(3.661)
NE		13.208[b]		17.506[c]		16.572[c]
		(1.854)		(3.142)		(4.195)
NC		9.519[b]		9.382[b]		10.782[c]
		(1.708)		(2.137)		(3.441)
S		6.245[a]		7.376[b]		7.632[c]
		(1.239)		(1.763)		(2.503)
T					−18.806[b]	−3.324
					(1.695)	(0.277)
$\bar{R}^2$	0.5053	0.5099	0.4788	0.5352	0.4833	0.5415

[a]Significant at the 10% level.
[b]Significant at the 5% level.
[c]Significant at the 1% level.

medical care in each Plan area. In effect, the fixed national deductible will appear to be a lower relative price in an area where medical care costs are higher in general. To adjust the standard, nationally set Medicare deductibles for health care price differences across Plan areas, we constructed a medical care price index for each Blue Cross Plan area, based on the 1981 Bureau of Labor Statistics (BLS) intermediate budgets for retired couples living in certain SMSAs. Details of the price index estimation are available from the author. The 1981 Medicare Part A deductible of $204 was adjusted for price differences across areas in 1981. Then, the 1984 deductible of $356 was deflated to 1981 dollars, using the same medical care indices, which were adjusted for changes in Blue Cross area prices over time by region and size class.

Although the estimated coefficient for the adjusted deductible was highly significant in 1981, before controlling for regional specific effects, its impact could not be interpreted as statistically different from zero in the 1984 cross-section. One possible explanation for this could be the introduction of the Baucus regulations—in many states requiring private insurers to cover Medicare copayments, which are based on the deductible. Prior to the Baucus legislation, higher real deductibles might have encouraged the elderly to purchase Blue Cross policies that typically covered such gaps (Cafferata 1985a). Since the legislation required more universal coverage of some gaps related to the deductible, real deductible prices may have become less of a choice consideration for the elderly by 1984. In any event, these results suggest a possible change in the significance of deductible price effects over time. Introduction of the regional dummy variables diminish the independent effect of the price variable and may be related to the method used to construct the price index.

Income and race. Nearly every empirical analysis of Medigap policy demand has found income and race to be important explanatory variables. Even controlling for income (Long and Settle 1982; Rice and McCall 1985; Rice 1986; Rice and Gabel 1986), race has had an independent effect on the purchase of private supplementary policies. Because our analysis involved aggregate data, we were unable to isolate a precise measure of elderly income within each Plan area. Instead, we hypothesized that higher overall per capita income in an area might be positively correlated with the share of elderly owning Blue Cross nongroup Medigap policies, while the percentage of nonwhite elderly would be negatively correlated with Blue Cross Medigap market share. Because of its statistical insignificance and lack of measurement precision, we omitted area-wide per capita income from our current analysis.

As in the earlier studies, our results generally support the hypothesis that nonwhite elderly purchase fewer Medigap policies. In particular, we tested whether areas with higher percentages of nonwhite elderly also tended to be areas with lower Blue Cross nongroup Medigap market shares. However, because of our income measurement error problem, we were unable to isolate the independent effects of race after controlling for income variation. Part of the racial variation in our model might capture the tendency for nonwhites to be among the lower-income Medicare recipients and, thus, more likely to be eligible for Medicaid supplementation. The racial variable also reflects other possible explanatory factors, such as unique cultural preferences among the nonwhite elderly or selective insurance marketing.

The results reported in Table 7.6 suggest a negative correlation between the percentage of nonwhite elderly and the percentage of elderly Medicare beneficiaries with Blue Cross nongroup Medigap coverage in 1981, but it is not statistically significant at conventional levels. However, the estimated coefficient is statistically different from zero in the 1984 and pooled runs. On average, controlling for the variables in our equations, we find that a 1 percent increase in the percentage of the elderly population that is nonwhite in plan areas reduces the market share of Blue Cross Medicare supplemental policies in the 1984 and pooled runs by less than one-tenth of 1 percent. The small size of this elasticity may be due to the higher price of Blue Cross Medigap policies relative to competing Medigap policies or may be related to the tendency for lower-income and nonwhite elderly to be eligible for Medicaid. The negative relationship between race and the purchase of Medigap policies is, however, consistent with previous research in this area (Long and Settle 1982; Rice and McCall 1985; Rice and Gabel 1986).

Regulation. In addition to independent price and race variables, we included a dummy variable to measure the possible impact of the Baucus legislation passed in 1980 on the market share of Medigap held by Blue Cross. Because the Baucus regulations were not implemented by the respective states until 1982 and 1983, we assumed any effect caused by the Baucus legislation would not appear in the 1981 cross-sectional results.[2] The regression results reported in Table 7.6 suggest that the adoption of Baucus standards was positively correlated with the market share of Blue Cross nongroup Medigap policies (N) for Plans in covered jurisdictions, holding constant all other explanatory factors indicated.[3] The relationship is highly significant in 1984 and in the pooled (1981 and 1984) regressions. This variable was not included in the 1981 regressions because voluntary compliance with the Baucus legislation was not fully implemented until later. One explanation for the significance of the regulatory variable could be that the Baucus legislation made other insurers provide more comprehensive and expensive policies, hence increasing the relative attractiveness of the high-coverage policies already offered by well-established Blue Cross Plans. Of course, quality assurance through the establishment of minimal standards for compliance may have helped to increase the enrollment of other insurers as well, but we cannot assess that possibility with our data, which is limited to Blue Cross nongroup enrollment.

Blue Cross under-sixty-five market penetration. As expected, the percentage of the population under age sixty-five enrolled in a Blue Cross medical insurance plan is positively related to Medigap (over-sixty-five) market penetration. A 1 percent increase in the under-sixty-five market share, or BCMS, increases the market share of Blue Cross over sixty-five (N) by an average of 0.5 percent in the regression runs, without the regional variables. This result suggests that in areas where the elderly population was more likely to have had Blue Cross coverage before retirement, Blue Cross continued to exhibit strong Medigap market penetration.

In summary, our ordinary least-squares regressions explain approximately half of the variation in Blue Cross nongroup Medigap market share. While the real price of the Medicare deductible and copayments might have been more important in 1981 than in 1984 (see further discussion in Appendix 7.2), the model appears to be relatively stable over time, especially with respect to the influence of the existing under-sixty-five market share on Medigap market share. Both the regression results and earlier descriptive tables indicate that Blue Cross nongroup Medigap market share has declined slightly since 1981. As with its under-sixty-five health insurance market penetration, Blue Cross maintains its strongest presence in the northeastern and north central states, with lower market shares in the southern and western states.

Further analysis

In addition to further refining the Blue Cross Medigap models presented in the last section, we have also begun to investigate the possible relationship between Medigap policy ownership and rising Medicare expenditures. Table 7.7 outlines

TABLE 7.7
Annualized Percent Changes in Medicare Expenditures and Blue Cross Non-group Medigap Policies by Census Region, 1981–83

Region	Annual percent change in Medicare expenditures[a]			Annual percent change in Blue Cross nongroup Medigap enrollment
	Total	Part A	Part B	
Northeast	10.9	9.7	13.5	−0.8
North central	7.9	6.5	11.6	−2.4
South	14.3	13.7	15.6	−1.5
West	11.0	9.5	13.9	0.2

[a]Expenditures are in real terms (1981 dollars) and are deflated by the regional consumer price index for all urban consumers (all items).

Sources: HCFA, Blue Cross and Blue Shield Enrollment Reports, Bureau of Labor Statistics.

TABLE 7.8
Variable Definitions: Medicare Regressions

Variable	Definition
Dependent variable	
MDCR	Medicare expenditures per enrollee deflated to 1981 dollars, using estimated consumer price index for medical care expenses of an intermediate-budget for a retired couple; expenditure and enrollment data exclude disability and end-stage renal disease beneficiaries under 65 years of age
Independent variables	
NHAT	Predicted Blue Cross nongroup Medigap enrollment as a percent of Medicare enrollees over age 65 from Medigap regression (see Table 7.6)
HSTAT	Health status measured as total deaths in Blue Cross Plan area per thousand population
HBEDS	Total hospital beds in Blue Cross Plan area per thousand population
NE	Regional dummy variable equals 1 if Blue Cross Plan is located in northeastern census region and equals 0 otherwise
NC	Regional dummy variable equals 1 if Blue Cross Plan is located in north central census region and equals 0 otherwise
S	Regional dummy variable equals 1 if Blue Cross Plan is located in southern census region and equals 0 otherwise
T	Time dummy variable for pooled cross-sectional analysis equals 1 in 1984 and 0 in 1981

Source: See Appendix 7.1.

the annualized increase in Part A, Part B, and total Medicare expenditures, adjusted for regional price increases between 1981 and 1983 for each census region. Except for the north central region, the annualized percentage changes in real Medicare expenditures for the three other census regions were over 10 percent between 1981 and 1983, the latest year complete county-level expenditure data are available from HCFA. The north central states experienced a slightly lower rate of inflation-adjusted Medicare expenditure growth (7.9 percent annually) than states in the other census regions between 1981 and 1983.

Theoretically, Medicare copayments and deductibles are intended to serve as cost-containment measures. By requiring the elderly to pay for some out-of-pocket health care costs, Medicare beneficiaries face an incentive to avoid obviously unnecessary or unreasonable medical procedures, thus moderating their consumption of medical care and tempering Medicare expenditures. Because ownership of Medigap policies tends to diminish this cost-containment incentive, we are interested in whether or to what extent Medigap policy ownership contributes to rising Medicare expenditures.

In preliminary analysis we regressed deflated Medicare expenditures in 1981 and 1983 on a selection of control variables listed and defined in Table 7.8. Results of the estimation appear in Table 7.9. Of particular interest are the results

TABLE 7.9
Medicare Expenditure: Two-Stage Least-Squares Regression Results

Independent variables	Coefficient estimates (t-statistics in parentheses)					
	1981		1983		Pooled	
CONSTANT	985.76[c] (4.666)	946.80[c] (3.520)	1118.66[c] (5.218)	928.67[c] (3.502)	999.20[c] (6.747)	818.32[c] (4.403)
NHAT	6.097[b] (1.978)	5.378 (0.754)	6.200[b] (1.948)	14.400[b] (1.772)	6.690[c] (3.084)	12.690[c] (2.478)
HSTAT	17.478 (0.564)	30.301 (0.901)	10.163 (0.300)	18.693 (0.531)	11.520 (0.515)	27.522 (1.185)
HBEDS	−6.595 (0.257)	−10.269 (0.378)	2.777 (0.103)	14.512 (0.457)	−2.891 (0.159)	−1.018 (0.052)
NE		−48.556 (0.215)		−305.168[a] (1.240)		−254.108[a] (1.598)
NC		32.212 (0.204)		−136.158 (0.858)		−99.378 (0.928)
S		−85.158 (0.771)		−143.225[a] (1.255)		−137.214[b] (1.800)
T					129.18[c] (3.690)	143.40[c] (3.932)
$\bar{R}^2$	0.0727	0.0790	0.0704	0.0640	0.1653	0.1893

[a]Significant at the 10% level.
[b]Significant at the 5% level.
[c]Significant at the 1% level.

pertaining to the predicted market share variable, or NHAT. The market share of Blue Cross Medigap policies was predicted using the regression results shown in Table 7.6 to produce Table 7.9. Although this equation performs poorly overall, the predicted Blue Cross market share of the over-sixty-five policies does relate positively to real Medicare expenditures. It does have at least one suggestive result; on average, a 1 percent increase in the Blue Cross Medigap market share raises real Medicare expenditures by less than 0.2 percent. Assuming that Blue Cross Medigap market penetration is correlated with overall Medigap market penetration, this result could suggest that Medigap ownership contributes to higher Medicare expenditures. Care should, however, be taken in interpreting this result because more work is needed in the specification of this model. With Blue Cross enrollment data, we are constrained to test only the possible simultaneous impact of increased Blue Cross Medigap market share on Medicare expenditures and not the impact of all Medigap ownership on rising Medicare outlays. Nevertheless, our analysis of the Blue Cross experience may allow us to speculate on the overall impact of Medigap policy ownership on Medicare expenditures and on the implications that changes in the existing Medicare structure might have on the private Medigap market.

Conclusion

The analysis of Blue Cross nongroup market penetration for the population over sixty-five does suggest that, especially before the Baucus standardization, Medigap purchases were sensitive to the price proxy. Although the elderly surely desire financial protection, that desire is not unlimited.

The major result of interest is the effect of the Baucus program. It apparently did what it was intended to do. Additionally, it increased the market share of policies that provide a generous minimal, standard coverage of the Medicare cost-sharing features, while protecting the elderly in acquiring this insurance. While our results are somewhat tentative, they do suggest that this expansion of coverage came at a cost—an increase in total Medicare expenses. In any event, this effect would not necessarily mean that the presumably greater access that the expansion of coverage represents is not worth this cost: the fact that especially nonwhites currently lack Medigap coverage and are, therefore, presumably deterred from care is significant. The result does, however, suggest concern for the cost-increasing consequences of the removal of Medicare cost sharing unless it is accompanied by other control mechanisms that have the potential to contain costs, such as HMOs or PPOs.

Appendix 7.1: Data Sources

Data	Year(s)	Source
Blue Cross nongroup Medigap enrollment	1981, 1984	Blue Cross Plan Enrollment Reports
Blue Cross under-65 enrollment	1981, 1984	Blue Cross Plan Enrollment Reports
Medicare enrollments and reimbursements	1981	Office of Data Analysis and Management (ODAM) Area Resource File, Bureau of Health Professions (February 1986)
	1983	HCFA, *Medicare Reimbursement by State and County, 1983* Table 8. Enrollment and Reimbursement for Hospital and Medical Insurance by State and County of Residence: Persons Aged 65 and Over (unpublished) We used Medicare enrollment in 1981 and 1983 to approximate over-65 population in 1981 and 1984, respectively
Medicare deductible	1981	HCFA, *The Medicare and Medicaid Data Book, 1981*
	1984	Health Insurance Association of America (HIAA), *Source Book of Health Insurance Data, 1984–85*

Data Sources Continued

Data	Year(s)	Source
Percent nonwhite elderly	1980	ODAM Area Resource File, Bureau of Health Professions (Feb. 1986), 1980 Census of Population and Housing: Summary Tape File 1A
Total population	1980, 1982, 1984	U.S. Bureau of the Census Tape, 1985, Population (1984) and Per Capita Income (1983) Estimates: Governmental Units 1981 population is a simple average of 1980 and 1982 1983 population is a simple average of 1982 and 1984
Total deaths	1980	ODAM Area Resource File, Bureau of Health Professions (Feb. 1986) Mortality Data Tapes NCHS: Scientific and Technical Information Branch
Total hospital beds	1981 and 1984	ODAM Area Resource File, Bureau of Health Professions (Feb. 1986) American Hospital Association (AHA) Annual Survey of Hospitals
Baucus legislation	1983	McCall, Rice and Hall, *Final Report* (1983)

Appendix 7.2: Statistical Testing

In order to test the stability of the ordinary least-squares estimates reported in Table 7.6 of the text, we subjected the Blue Cross nongroup Medigap market share regressions to a series of hypothesis tests. This appendix briefly discusses each statistical test and reports our findings.

Pooling 1981 and 1984 cross-sections

In order to test our null hypothesis that the 1981 and 1984 nongroup Blue Cross Medigap cross-sections could be described by a single regression equation, we calculated appropriate F-statistics using the error sums of squares from the separate 1981 and 1984 regressions reported in Table 7.6 and the same regression on the two years of pooled data (Pindyck and Rubinfeld 1981). In doing so, we implicitly assumed that the Baucus legislation had no effect on the Blue Cross Medigap market shares in 1981. The pooled regressions used for these tests are nearly the same pooled specifications reported in Table 7.6, except that we omitted the time dummy in the F-test runs. The resulting F-statistics are reported in Table 7.2.1 and indicate that the null hypothesis cannot be rejected at the 5 percent level.

Using a time dummy variable to test whether each of the intercept and parameter estimates remained stable over time, the following pooled results were

TABLE 7.2.1
Joint F-test on the Null Hypothesis of the Equality of Coefficients in 1981 and 1984 Nongroup Medigap Market Penetration Cross-Sections

Model	F-Statistic	Critical F
Without regional dummies	1.61	2.29
With regional dummies	0.15	2.02

estimated with t-statistics reported below each coefficient in parentheses. Notice that the null hypotheses of no change in the intercept and the deductible slope coefficient can be rejected at the 5 percent level but only in the case where the regional dummy variables are excluded.

$$N = - 168.63 + 0.90 \text{ DEDUCT} - 0.13 \text{ RACE} + 7.97 \text{ BAUCUS}$$
$$(2.33) \quad (2.54) \quad\quad (0.89) \quad\quad (1.93)$$

$$+ 0.32 \text{ BCMS} + 156.08 \text{ T} - 0.83 \text{ T} * \text{DEDUCT} - 0.09 \text{ T}$$
$$(4.40) \quad\quad (1.86) \quad\quad (2.17) \quad\quad\quad (0.44)$$

$$* \text{RACE} + 0.14 \text{ T} * \text{BCMS}$$
$$(1.41)$$

$$\bar{R}^2 = 0.4926$$

$$N = - 46.45 + 0.29 \text{ DEDUCT} - 0.18 \text{ RACE} + 7.53 \text{ BAUCUS}$$
$$(0.49) \quad (0.61) \quad\quad (0.98) \quad\quad (1.76)$$

$$+ 0.23 \text{ BCMS} + 13.21 \text{ NE} + 9.52 \text{ NC} + 6.25 \text{ S} + 57.18 \text{ T}$$
$$(2.64) \quad\quad (1.93) \quad\quad (1.77) \quad\quad (1.29) \quad (0.54)$$

$$- 0.31 \text{ T} * \text{DEDUCT} - 0.06 \text{ T} * \text{RACE} + 0.004 \text{ T} * \text{BCMS}$$
$$(0.62) \quad\quad\quad (0.24) \quad\quad\quad (0.03)$$

$$+ 4.30 \text{ T} * \text{NE} - 0.14 \text{ T} * \text{NC} + 1.13 \text{ T} * \text{S}$$
$$(0.48) \quad\quad (0.02) \quad\quad (0.17)$$

$$\bar{R}^2 = 0.5216$$

Heteroscedasticity
Because the nongroup Medigap market penetration models analyze cross-sectional data, we tested the error structure for heteroscedasticity. Following the methodology of Park and Glejser (Pindyck and Rubinfeld 1981), we suspected that our error variances might be correlated with either of three possible factors: Blue Cross plan under-sixty-five market share, Blue Cross Plan under-sixty-five total enrollment, or the entire population of the geographic area within which particular Blue Cross plans operate. For each of these three possible correlates, we tested two different functional forms, as suggested by Pindyck and Rubinfeld

(1981). We regressed transformations of the predicted error on the three possible correlates as follows.

$$\log(\hat{e}_i^2) = \cancel{c} + \pounds \log X_i + u_i \tag{1}$$

$$|\hat{e}| = \cancel{c} + \pounds X_i + u_i \tag{2}$$

These two equations were estimated for all three hypothesized variance relationships for each of the six equations reported in Table 7.6.

Of the six heteroscedasticity tests run on the 1981 sample data without regional dummy variables, the null hypothesis of homoscedasticity could not be rejected with 90 percent confidence in all cases except one. Similar results were noted for the model specification, including regional dummy variables. In both 1981 models, the absolute value of the residual appeared to be negatively correlated with population in the Blue Cross Plan area. Weighted least-squares regressions run on the 1981 data confirmed that the heteroscedasticity correction did not substantially alter the results reported in Table 7.6. Of the twelve heteroscedasticity tests run on the 1984 subsample, the null hypothesis of homoscedasticity could only be rejected with just less than 90 percent confidence, assuming functional form 1, with X equal to the under-sixty-five Blue Cross Plan market penetration rate and omitting the three regional dummy variables.

Stronger evidence suggested that the pooled error variances might be correlated with the Blue Cross plan's under-sixty-five market penetration. For the specifications reported in Table 7.6, the null hypothesis of homoscedasticity could be rejected with 95 percent confidence for both market penetration functional forms when the regional dummies were excluded. Including the regional dummies, only one pooled error variance test suggested possible correlation between the errors and the market penetration rate. The null hypothesis of homoscedasticity could be rejected with approximately 90 percent confidence for functional form 2. As with the 1981 cross-section, weighted least-squares results did not substantially alter the pooled results, as reported in Table 7.6.

Notes

The author thanks Barbara Holland, Mark Pauly, and Thomas Rice for helpful comments. I am grateful to Dolores Gurnick, Denise Jarvinen, and Eric Nauenberg for their research assistance.

1. The author thanks Mark Pauly for suggesting that plan-specific Medigap loss ratios be used to measure the price facing Blue Cross Medigap policyholders. Because the loss ratios could not be obtained before the publication of this chapter, we were unable to incorporate the suggestion at this stage of the analysis.

2. We recently ran the 1981 model with the Baucus legislation dummy variable and observed a positive, significant (at the 5 percent level) coefficient. This is consistent with the hypothesis that

conditions affecting Medigap policy ownership may have "caused" the Baucus legislation to be enacted. The author again acknowledges Mark Pauly for suggesting this result.

3. It should be noted that Massachusetts and New York, which are included among the non-Baucus states, are among the most highly regulated states for mandated insurance benefits. Their regulations are more stringent than the minimums established by the Baucus legislation. Blue Cross lost penetration in both its under- and over-sixty-five product markets between 1981 and 1984. While the decline in under-sixty-five Blue Cross enrollment was more pronounced in the non-Baucus states, nongroup Medigap enrollment declined less rapidly than under-sixty-five coverage in both the Baucus and non-Baucus states. The regulatory nature of the two predominant states without Baucus legislation perhaps accounts for the similar, less rapid rates of decline in the over-sixty-five markets.

References

American Association of Retired Persons, "Long-Term Care Research Study," Washington, DC: Towers, Perrin, Forster & Crosby, January 1984.

American Health Care Association, Summary of Proceedings, "Policy Forum: Private Insurance for Long Term Care," Washington, DC, May 15, 1984.

Blue Cross and Blue Shield Association, "Medicare Complementary Survey Report," Product Development, July 1986.

Blumenthal, D., M. Schlesinger, P. B. Drumheller, and The Harvard Medicare Project, "The Future of Medicare," *New England Journal of Medicine,* 314(II):722–728, 1986.

Cafferata, G. L., "Private Health Insurance of the Medicare Population and the Baucus Legislation," *Medical Care,* 23:1086–1096, 1985a.

———, "The Elderly's Private Insurance Coverage of Nursing Home Care," *American Journal of Public Health,* 75(6):655–656, 1985b.

———, "Private Health Insurance Coverage of the Medicare Population," Data Preview 18, National Center for Health Services Research, National Health Care Expenditures Study, Rockville, MD: U.S. Department of Health and Human Services, Publication No. (PHS) 84-3362, September 1984.

Cafferata, G. L., and M. R. Meiners, "Public and Private Insurance and the Medicare Population's Out-of-Pocket Expenditures: Does Medigap Make a Difference?" paper presented at Anaheim, CA: American Public Health Association Annual Meeting, 1984.

Davis, K., and D. Rowland, *Medicare Policy: New Directions for Health and Long-Term Care,* Baltimore, MD: Johns Hopkins University Press, 1986.

DeNovo, A., and G. Shearer, *Private Health Insurance to Supplement Medicare,* Washington, DC: Federal Trade Commission, 1978.

Garfinkel, S. A., and L. S. Corder, "Supplemental Health Insurance Coverage among Aged Medicare Beneficiaries," NMCUES Descriptive Report No. 5, DHHS Publication No. 85-20205, Office of Research and Demonstrations, HCFA, Washington, DC: U.S. Government Printing Office, August 1985.

Health Insurance Association of America, *Source Book of Health Insurance Data,* Washington, DC: Public Relations Division, 1984–85 and 1986 Update.

Knickman, J., N. McCall, J. Gollub, and D. Henton, "Increasing Private Financing of Long-Term Care: Opportunities for Collaborative Action," Conference Report, Menlo Park, CA: SRI International, March 1986.

208   Scheffler

Long, S. H., and R. F. Settle, "Medicare Cost Sharing and Private Supplementary Health Insurance: Selected Research Findings," paper presented at the Medical Care Section, American Public Health Association Annual Meeting, Montreal, November 15, 1982.

Long, S. H., R. F. Settle, and C. R. Link, "Who Bears the Burden of Medicare Cost Sharing?" *Inquiry,* 19:222–234, Fall 1982.

McCall, N., "Health Insurance," *Generations,* 36–39, Summer 1985.

McCall, N., and T. Rice, "Medigap—Study of Comparative Effectiveness of Various State Regulations: Executive Summary," Menlo Park, CA: SRI International, September 1983.

McCall, N., T. Rice, and A. Hall, "Medigap—Study of Comparative Effectiveness of Various State Regulations," *Journal of Health Policy, Politics and Law* 12(1):56–76, Spring 1987.

———, "The Effect of State Regulations on the Quality and Sale of Insurance Policies to Medicare Beneficiaries," (unpublished), 1985.

McCall, N., T. Rice, and J. Sangl, "Consumer Knowledge of Medicare and Supplemental Health Insurance Benefits," *Health Services Research,* 20(6):633–657, February 1986.

"Medicare Supplement Insurance," *Consumer Reports,* 347–355, June 1984.

Merritt, R. E., and D. B. Potemken, eds., *Medigap: Issues and Update,* Washington, DC: The Intergovernmental Health Policy Project, June 1982.

Mueller, M. S., "Private Health Insurance in 1970," Social Security Bulletin no. 35, Washington, DC: U.S. Government Printing Office, February 1972.

Pindyck, R. S., and D. L. Rubinfeld, *Econometric Models and Economic Forecasts,* New York, NY: McGraw-Hill Book Co., 1981.

Rice, T., "Ownership and Characteristics of Medigap Policies," *Health Policy Research Series,* Menlo Park, CA: SRI International, January 1985.

———, Prepared Statement to the Subcommittee on Health and the Environment, Committee of Energy and Commerce, U.S. House of Representatives, March 26, 1986 (unpublished).

Rice, T., and J. Gabel, "Do 'Medigap' Policies Cover High Health Care Costs?" revision "Protecting the Elderly Against High Health Care Costs" submitted to *Health Affairs* for publication in Fall 1986.

Rice, T., and N. McCall, "The Extent of Ownership and the Characteristics of Medicare Supplemental Policies," *Inquiry,* 22:188–200, Summer 1985.

Taylor, A. K., P. J. Farley, and C. M. Horgan, "Medigap Insurance: Friend or Foe in Reducing Medicare Deficits?" forthcoming in H. E. Frech III, ed., *Health Care in America: The Political Economy of Hospitals and Health Insurance,* San Francisco: Pacific Institute for Public Policy Research.

Waldo, D. R., and H. C. Lazenby, "Demographic Characteristics and Health Care Use and Expenditures by the Aged in the United States: 1977–1984," *Health Care Financing Review,* 6(1):1–29, Fall 1984.

III
Medicare Payment and Provider Behavior

8. The Impact of Medicare's Prospective Payment System on the Use of Hospital Inpatient Services

□ [□] □

GERALD F. KOMINSKI, DENA S. PUSKIN,
MERYL F. BLOOMROSEN, AND JOLENE A. HALL

Introduction

The Medicare Prospective Payment System (PPS) was enacted by the Congress in April 1983 to control the growth in expenditures for hospital inpatient services. To accomplish this objective, PPS pays hospitals a fixed payment amount for 475 different categories of patient illness that are defined using diagnosis-related groups (DRGs). This system of fixed payment amounts is designed to provide strong financial incentives for hospitals to reduce the cost of hospital inpatient care.

The Prospective Payment Assessment Commisson (ProPAC) was created by Congress to advise the legislative and executive branches on changes needed to maintain and update the payment system. The commission's primary responsibilities are to make annual recommendations to the secretary of Health and Human Services concerning the annual percentage change in Medicare payments (i.e., the update factor) and necessary changes in the DRGs. In addition, the commission provides an annual report to Congress on the overall impact of PPS on the delivery and financing of health care.

This chapter presents the conceptual framework used by the commission to support its recommendation for fiscal year 1987 regarding the update factor for Medicare inpatient payments. It presents some of the empirical evidence considered by the commission in arriving at its recommendation and discusses the strengths and the weaknesses of the information that was available for evaluating the impact of PPS.

Background

The commission's annual recommendations become part of the policy-making process in the following way. The commission issues its annual recommendations in April. The secretary of Health and Human Services then issues a notice of proposed rule making (NPRM), outlining proposed changes in PPS, in June. In this document, the secretary is required to respond to ProPAC's recommendations and to explain why each recommendation has been accepted or rejected. ProPAC then has thirty days to respond to the secretary's proposed rule.

The secretary issues a final rule in September that usually becomes effective with the beginning of the federal fiscal year on October 1. In November ProPAC issues its final comment on the secretary's final rule. The process begins again in April. Beginning in 1988 ProPAC's recommendations will be issued in March and the secretary's NPRM will be issued in May to permit a longer comment period.

The commission is required to recommend an annual percentage change to update hospital payment amounts under PPS. Table 8.1 compares ProPAC's recommended update factor for fiscal year 1987 with the secretary's recommended

TABLE 8.1
ProPAC and HCFA Recommendations for Increases in Medicare Payment Amounts for Fiscal Year 1987

	Recommendation	
Update factor component	ProPAC	HCFA
FY 87 market basket forecast	4.0%	3.7%
FY 86 market basket forecast correction	0.0	0.0
Discretionary adjustment factor	0.6	−1.7
Scientific and technological advancement	0.7	0.7
Productivity	−1.5	−1.0
Site-of-care substitution	−0.6	−2.0
Real case-mix change	2.0	0.6
Across DRGs (DRG case-mix index)	1.3	0.6
Within DRGs (case complexity)	0.7	0.0
Subtotal	4.6	2.0
Adjustment for total change in DRG case-mix index (real case-mix change and upcoding)	−2.7	−2.6
Total	1.9%	−0.6%

Note: Recommendations assume that capital expenses remain excluded from PPS.

update factor, which was issued by the Health Care Financing Administration (HCFA). The update factor consists of the following four components:

- [ ] Market basket forecast
- [ ] Correction for errors in the previous market basket forecast
- [ ] Discretionary adjustment factor
- [ ] Case-mix change

The market basket forecast measures expected changes during the upcoming year in the input prices of a fixed basket of goods and services purchased by the typical hospital. ProPAC and HCFA use the same index for determining the market basket forecast.[1] The discrepancy between ProPAC's recommendation and the secretary's recommendation occurred only because the secretary had access to a later forecast.

The second component of the update factor corrects for errors in the market basket forecast from the previous year. For fiscal year 1986 the market basket forecast correction was −0.3 percent. The commission, however, chose to recommend a zero percent correction. This partially reflects the commission's belief that the actual update factor for fiscal year 1986 was originally too low.

In arriving at its recommendation for the update factor, the commission is required by law to consider changes in hospital productivity, scientific and technological advancement, and the quality and long-term cost-effectiveness of services provided. These factors are combined into a discretionary adjustment factor (DAF). As Table 8.1 shows, ProPAC and the secretary differed substantially concerning the level of the DAF for fiscal year 1987. The reasons for these differences are explained in detail elsewhere.[2]

The commission regards the annual update factor as the minimum increase in Medicare payments consistent with maintaining access to high-quality hospital services. For fiscal year 1987 the commission's DAF recommendation considered the following four areas affecting the use of hospital inpatient services:

- [ ] Scientific and technological advancement
- [ ] Hospital productivity
- [ ] Site-of-care substitution
- [ ] Real case-mix change

The commission's final recommendation for these DAF components was 0.6 percent, while the secretary's recommendation for these components was −1.7 percent. The DAF components reflect actual changes in the use of hospital inpatient resources. The next section discusses the DAF components and summarizes some of the empirical evidence that was available to the commission in arriving at its recommendation for fiscal year 1987.

The final component of the update factor is an adjustment for changes in the DRG case-mix index. Changes in case-mix index are automatically reflected in hospital payments and are, therefore, subtracted from the update factor. However, case-mix change can increase the average cost of treating Medicare patients. The commission believes, therefore, that the DAF should include a case-mix adjustment.

Changes in the distribution of patients across DRGs (i.e., the DRG case-mix index) may result from true changes in the patient population or from incentives to improve coding. The commission has adopted the position that an allowance for true changes in the patient population should be incorporated into the DAF. In addition, the commission recognizes that real changes in case complexity may occur within DRGs. These within-DRG changes are not reflected in the DRG case-mix index. The commission's allowance for real case-mix change contains both an across-DRG and a within-DRG component.

The commission's policy is to subtract the total change in the DRG case-mix index from the update factor but to add back the components of across- and within-DRG change attributable to real case-mix change as part of the DAF. The final update factor is then applied to the average standardized payment amounts for the upcoming year. The commission's policy, therefore, provides an allowance only for annual increases in the average cost per case associated with changes in the type of patients treated.

ProPAC depends upon HCFA for its estimate of the change in the DRG case-mix index. This estimate is based on actual Medicare claims data. The difference between ProPAC's adjustment and the secretary's adjustment for case-mix change occurred because the secretary had access to later data.

The secretary's final recommendation for the update factor was +0.5 percent, rather than the −0.6 percent shown in Table 8.1. The secretary explained that this increase in the update factor was necessary to avoid the possible adverse effects of a negative update factor.[3] ProPAC's final recommendation was for an update factor of 1.9 percent. Each percentage point in the update factor represents almost $600 million in additional Medicare payments.

Empirical Evidence

Scientific and technological advancement

The allowance for scientific and technological advancement is a future-oriented policy target to provide hospitals with the additional funds for acquiring new technologies that are both quality enhancing and cost increasing. Under current policy, new technologies that require capital expenditures are financed as a pass-through because capital costs are excluded from the prospective payment amounts.

These new technologies, however, may also have a considerable impact on operating costs. Furthermore, many scientific and technological advances may not require any capital expenditures.

A broader definition of scientific and technological advancement includes changes in practice patterns. These changes may have a more substantial impact on total operating costs than high-cost technologies.

The allowance for scientific and technological advancement also reflects the commission's belief that most expenditures are for diffusing technologies, rather than for newly introduced technologies. This component of the DAF is currently based primarily on the collective judgment of the commission, rather than firm empirical evidence. Therefore, it represents a policy target more than an adjustment for recent changes in the use of hospital resources.

Hospital productivity

The allowance for productivity is a future-oriented policy target that translates expected productivity gains into reductions in the Medicare payment amounts. The commission has adopted the principle that productivity gains should be shared equally between the hospital industry on the one hand and the Medicare program and Medicare beneficiaries on the other. The commission has considered three primary indicators when evaluating productivity gains. These indicators are changes in length of stay, ancillary services, and staffing patterns.

Length of stay. The rates of growth in admissions and admission rates during the period 1971 to 1982 were much lower for patients under age sixty-five than for patients aged sixty-five and above (Table 8.2). Admission rates have declined steadily since 1981 for patients under age sixty-five. Admission rates for patients aged sixty-five and above, however, did not begin to decline until 1984, the first year of PPS. Furthermore, in 1985, admissions and admissions rates fell more for patients aged sixty-five and above than for patients under age sixty-five, for the first time in fifteen years.

TABLE 8.2
Annual Percent Change in Hospital Admissions and Admission Rates, 1971–85

Year	Admissions		Admission rates	
	Under 65	65+	Under 65	65+
Annual average 1971–82	1.4	4.9	0.5	2.4
1983	−2.8	4.7	−3.6	2.6
1984	−4.2	−2.6	−5.0	−4.7
1985[a]	−5.9	−6.1	−6.6	−8.1
Annual average 1983–85	−4.3	−1.3	−5.1	−3.4

[a]1985 estimate based on first eight months of data compared with the first eight months of 1984.
Source: Admission data from the AHA National Panel Survey. Population data from the Bureau of the Census.

TABLE 8.3
Ancillary Service Utilization by Medicare Patients, 1980–84

A. Laboratory tests

Year	Proportion with laboratory tests	Average number of lab tests	Percent change
1980	0.990	15.43	—
1981	0.990	15.58	1.0
1982	0.990	15.82	1.6
1983	0.989	15.63	−1.3
1984	0.986	10.30	−34.1

B. Diagnostic tests

Year	Proportion with diagnostic tests	Average number of tests	Percent change
1980	0.776	1.124	—
1981	0.787	1.154	2.7
1982	0.794	1.183	2.5
1983	0.790	1.176	−1.3
1984	0.746	1.003	−14.7

C. Drugs

Year	Proportion with drugs	Average number of drugs	Percent change
1980	0.834	1.975	—
1981	0.836	2.013	1.9
1982	0.848	2.073	3.0
1983	0.849	2.092	0.9
1984	0.863	2.172	3.8

Source: Analysis conducted by CPHA under contract with ProPAC.

TABLE 8.4
Annual Percent Change in Hospital Employment and Employment-Related Expenses, 1971–85

	Percent change in full time equivalent employees			
	Total	Inpatient only		
Year	Number	Number	Per admission	Per day
Annual average 1971–82	4.3	3.9	2.6	3.0
1983	1.4	0.8	1.4	3.4
1984	−2.3	−3.5	0.2	5.6
1985[a]	−3.0	−5.0	1.0	3.2
Annual average 1983–85	−1.3	−2.6	0.8	4.1

[a]1985 estimate based on first eight months of data compared with the first eight months of 1984.
Source: AHA National Panel Survey.

Using American Hospital Association (AHA) Panel Survey data, the change in average length of stay for all patients aged sixty-five and above between 1984 and 1985 was −2.9 percent. Adjusting this reduction in length of stay for site-of-care substitution and real case-mix change, and applying a 60 percent marginal cost assumption, yields an estimated 2.2 percent reduction in costs. Sharing half of this productivity gain with the hospital industry results in a 1.1 percent reduction in the payment amounts.

Ancillary services. The utilization of some ancillary services changed dramatically during the first year of PPS. The use of laboratory and diagnostic tests decreased rapidly in 1984 among Medicare patients, while the use of drugs continued to increase slightly (Table 8.3). The proportion of Medicare patients receiving laboratory and diagnostic tests did not change significantly during the period from 1980 to 1984. The decreased use of these tests resulted from a decline in the number of tests administered.[4]

Staffing patterns. During the first year of PPS, the number of full-time equivalent employees declined for the first time during the fifteen-year period from 1971 to 1985 (Table 8.4). Because this decline was less than the decline in admissions and length of stay, staffing patterns continued to increase when measured per admission or per day. This pattern continued during the second year of PPS (i.e., 1985).

Site-of-care substitution

This DAF component reflects changes resulting from the substitution of services provided outside of the hospital for services formerly provided during the inpatient stay. Using discharge destination as an indicator of shifts in the site of care, Medicare patients during the first year of PPS were discharged more often to other short-term hospitals, skilled nursing facilities (SNFs), intermediate care facilities (ICFs), and home health care, when compared with the period from 1980 to 1983 (Table 8.5). The trends for non-Medicare patients, on the other hand, remained relatively constant during the period from 1980 to 1984.

TABLE 8.5
Percent of Medicare and Non-Medicare Discharges, by Discharge Disposition Status, 1980–84

Discharge disposition	1980	1981	1982	1983	1984
Medicare					
Home	80.6	80.5	80.6	80.0	77.2
Short-term hospital	1.7	1.7	1.7	1.8	2.0
SNF or ICF	8.9	8.9	8.8	9.0	9.9
Home health	2.3	2.6	2.7	3.3	5.0
Deceased	6.5	6.3	6.2	5.9	5.9
Non-Medicare					
Home	97.4	97.4	97.3	97.1	96.8
Short-term hospital	1.1	1.1	1.2	1.3	1.4
SNF or ICF	0.2	0.2	0.2	0.2	0.2
Home health	0.4	0.4	0.4	0.5	0.6
Deceased	0.9	0.9	0.9	0.8	0.9

Source: Analysis conducted by the CPHA under contract with ProPAC.

TABLE 8.6
Annual Percent Change in the DRG Case-Mix Index (CMI) and in Case Complexity, 1981−85

Year	Medicare		Non-Medicare	
	DRG	Complexity	DRG	Complexity
1981	0.1	0.7	1.3	0.5
1982	0.3	0.9	1.4	0.5
1983	1.1	2.8	1.9	1.1
1984	2.9	2.4	2.8	1.1
1985	3.8	0.7	2.6	0.1
Annual average 1981−83	0.5	1.5	1.5	0.7
Annual average 1984−85	3.4	1.6	2.7	0.6

Source: Analysis conducted by CPHA under contract with ProPAC.

Real case-mix change

The DRG case-mix index changed dramatically during the first two years of PPS for both Medicare and non-Medicare patients (Table 8.6). Changes in case complexity (i.e., within DRGs), however, returned to pre-PPS levels in 1985 after substantial increases during the previous two years.

Case complexity was defined using the body-systems-count approach developed by the Commission on Professional and Hospital Activities (CPHA). This approach assigns a score of from one to five for each patient, depending on the number of the patient's diagnoses that fall into unique major diagnostic categories under the DRG patient classification system. The CPHA developed empirical weights, based on average length of stay, for each level of body system counts within DRGs. Then, controlling for changes in the distribution of cases across DRGs, the CPHA measured the impact on average length of stay of changes in the proportion of cases within DRGs having one, two, three, four, and five or more body system counts.

Discussion

Changes in case mix and in case complexity can occur because of three factors: improved coding practices (i.e., more complete and accurate coding), strategic coding practices (i.e., DRG creep), or actual changes in the distribution of hospitalized patients. Recent studies by the Rand Corporation[5] have attempted to disaggregate case-mix change into changes in patient distributions and changes in coding. These studies, however, do not provide an estimate of changes in case complexity.

The commission's findings regarding changes in case complexity are relevant to Medicare policy for several reasons. Under PPS, changes in case mix result directly in higher (or lower) hospital payments. When setting the annual update factor, therefore, the secretary recommends an adjustment to remove price increases that are related to case-mix change. Changes in case complexity, however, are difficult to measure directly and thus represent an unobserved component of case-mix change. If case-complexity change represents a true change in the type of patients hospitalized, PPS will underpay hospitals. These underpayments will continue unless a specific adjustment is made in the annual update factor or in the patient categories.

Changes in productivity result in lower or higher hospital costs, holding all other factors constant. Changes in the hospital product, however, represent a shift in the site of service from the hospital inpatient setting to other settings, rather than a true productivity gain. The commission's estimates of changes in productivity include an adjustment for changes in the hospital product. This adjustment is necessary to prevent overpayment for services that were formerly provided during the inpatient stay. The estimates of site-of-care substitution indicate that the hospital product has changed considerably since the beginning of PPS.

One important consideration in evaluating the impact of PPS and the adequacy of the annual update factor is the level of Medicare payments. If payment levels are too low, some Medicare beneficiaries may no longer have access to hospital care. During the first two years of PPS, Medicare payments per day and per admission have increased considerably, while Medicare charges per day have increased only slightly (Table 8.7). Revenue per day for non-Medicare patients, however, has declined slightly during the same period.

TABLE 8.7
Average Annual Percent Real Change[a] in Medicare and Non-Medicare Payments, 1979–85

	Medicare			Non-Medicare
Period	Payment[b] per day	Payment per stay	Charge per day	Revenue[c] per day
Annual average 1979–83	5.1	3.2	7.2	5.5
Annual average 1984–85	15.8	6.4	8.4	2.9

[a]Real percent change, adjusting for price inflation.

[b]Medicare payments include program benefit payments and beneficiary liabilities.

[c]Non-Medicare revenue represents the difference between AHA inpatient revenue and Medicare payments.

Source: HCFA, "Final Rule," *Federal Register,* 51(170):31512, September 3, 1986. Medicare payment data from HCFA, Office of the Actuary. Medicare charge data from the Medicare statistical system. Non-Medicare revenue data for AHA Panel Survey for Community Hospitals.

Conclusions

The data presented in this chapter represent some of the best indicators that are currently available to assess the impact of PPS on the use of hospital inpatient services. The indicators substantiate that PPS has had a considerable impact on hospital resource use. Trends in the use of hospital services and in hospital staffing showed dramatic changes beginning in 1984, the first year of PPS. These indicators play an important role in determining the amount of the annual update factor, which in turn affects the annual rate of growth for Medicare inpatient expenditures.

The following conclusions can be drawn concerning the relationship between research and the policymaking process related to the annual update factor. First, in the short run, wide discrepancies will continue to occur between the secretary's recommended update factor and ProPAC's unless better indicators are developed to assess annual changes in hospital resource use. The two indicators most in need of improvement are those dealing with site-of-care substitution and real case-mix change.

A second conclusion is that the research community can make a substantial contribution to the policy-making process by helping to develop better indicators of the impact of PPS, both inside and outside of the hospital setting.

The final conclusion is that the shorter lengths of stay under PPS are calling attention to the lack of adequate coverage by Medicare for services provided outside of the hospital, especially subacute and long-term care services. The challenge for researchers and policymakers in the future will be to reduce these gaps in the coverage of Medicare beneficiaries, while maintaining incentives for cost-effective and high-quality care.

Notes

Primary data analysis for this study was performed by the Commission on Professional and Hospital Activities under ProPAC Contract #T33726021. Any conclusions are solely those of the authors and do not necessarily represent the views of the Prospective Payment Assessment Commission or its contractor.

1. The market basket was first published in the article by Mark S. Freeland, Gerard Anderson, and Carol Ellen Schendler, "National Hospital Input Price Index," *Health Care Financing Review,* 1(1):37–61, Summer 1979. Revisions in the categories and the weights of the market basket appear in the *Federal Register,* 51(170):31461–31468, September 3, 1986.

2. See the Health Care Financing Administration, "Medicare Program; Changes to the Inpatient Hospital Prospective Payment System and Fiscal Year 1987 Rates; Proposed Rule," *Federal Register,* 51(106):19970–20034, June 3, 1986. See also Prospective Payment Assessment Commission, *1987 Adjustments to the Medicare Prospective Payment System: Report to the Congress,* November 1986.

3. Health Care Financing Administration, "Medicare Program; Changes to the Inpatient Hospital Prospective Payment System and Fiscal Year 1987 Rates; Final Rule," *Federal Register,* 51(170): 31519, September 3, 1986.

4. In Table 8.3, the number of tests indicates the number of different *types* of tests administered, rather than the total number of each type of test.

5. Paul B. Ginsburg and Grace M. Carter, "Medicare Case-Mix Index Increase," *Health Care Financing Review,* 7(4):51–65, Summer 1986.

9. Prospective Payment and Hospital–Medical Staff Relationships

□ [□] □

WILLIAM S. CUSTER, JAMES W. MOSER,
ROBERT A. MUSACCHIO, RICHARD D. WILLKE

Introduction

The impact on hospitals and patients resulting from Medicare's Prospective Payment System (PPS) of hospital reimbursement is the subject of considerable interest. Preliminary evidence suggests the introduction of PPS has been followed by a decline in the average length of a hospital stay. Public policy analysts are concerned with the effect PPS will have on the access to and quality of care, as well as its effect on the out-of-pocket costs for Medicare beneficiaries.

In addition, concern has been expressed regarding Medicare's transition from cost-based reimbursement for hospitals to PPS and its likely impact on the relationship between hospitals and their medical staff. A literal cost-based reimbursement system minimized the potential for conflict between hospitals and their medical staff, since hospitals were assured of reimbursement for the inputs ordered by the physician. PPS changed the hospital's incentives. As Glandon and Morrisey (1986, p. 166) have stated, "PPS fundamentally changed the financial incentives facing hospitals but left physician . . . incentives unaffected. A conflict of incentives resulted." Since physicians allocate hospital resources in the treatment of patients, they have a direct impact on the hospital's financial well-being.

The traditional organization of the hospital makes the relationship between the hospital and its medical staff symbiotic. A change in hospital reimbursement is likely to affect physician behavior by changing the environment in which they practice medicine. Consequently, the effects on physician revenues and practice expenses, as well as on the quantity and quality of care provided, may be profound.

It has been argued that the medical staff's role in allocating hospital resources is a major determinant of hospital behavior. To whatever extent the medical staff dominated the hospital's administration in the past, it seems less likely this will be the case in the present environment. Shortell (1985, p. 4) points out that "physicians are now more affected by the organizational structure of hospitals than the reverse." He lists the following four important reasons for the increase in the hospitals' relative power:

☐ Regulatory and reimbursement systems, such as PPS, intended to slow health care cost inflation
☐ Increased competition among providers
☐ A possible trend toward the "corporatization" of American health care
☐ Changes in patient demographics and technology which may lead to the delivery of health care by teams of professionals

The net result of the growth in hospitals' relative power is that changes in hospital reimbursement are likely to have a direct impact on physician behavior.

Our purpose is to describe conceptually a model of hospital-medical staff interactions that may be used to gain inferences about observed input and output phenomena under different hospital reimbursement mechanisms. The model may then be used for deriving health policy implications. The following section reviews the literature on two heretofore separate research tracks: (1) the relationship between hospitals and physicians and (2) the switch from cost-based to PPS reimbursement of hospitals. In addition, a model that synthesizes these two approaches is described. Policy implications are discussed and an agenda for future research is presented. The final section contains conclusions.

Conceptual Model

A number of authors (Pauly and Redisch 1973; Harris 1977; Shortell 1983; Benson and Mitchell 1986) have investigated the relationship between hospitals and physicians. The hospital provides the physical plant and ancillary inputs for inpatient care. The medical staff allocates these inputs in the treatment of their patients. Physicians usually neither own the hospital nor pay directly for the hospital inputs. Furthermore, the hospital and the physician bill their services separately and often face different reimbursement mechanisms. Hospitals, reacting to the new financial incentives produced by PPS, are likely to try to persuade medical staff physicians to reduce length of stay, which will enable hospitals to reduce the amount of ancillary services. Physicians may react by investing their own time and money to replace the lost inputs to the production of health care.

Other researchers have developed models that capture the switch from cost-based to PPS reimbursement of hospitals. Foster (1985) considers the case of a profit-maximizing hospital as the only decision-making agent. His basic result is that the effects of a shift to PPS depend on the shape of the cost curves. He has the hospital initially on the declining section of the average cost curve. The shift to PPS will cause hospital output (in terms of admissions) to *expand*. Foster notes a potential offset to this prediction: if the prospectively determined price is less than the rate paid under cost-based reimbursement, as might be the case with the simultaneous switch from a "patient day" basis of payment to an "admission" basis, the hospital will have an incentive to reduce the average length of hospital stay. This could more than completely offset the admission effect, in which case Medicare patient volume would fall. Ellis and McGuire (1986) also have considered provider behavior under PPS. They model the physician as the sole decisionmaker, with respect to the allocation of hospital patient care resources. The unit of analysis is a particular episode of care. The physician maximizes his or her utility function, the arguments of which are (1) the patient's benefit from hospital services and (2) hospital profits. Hence, the physician acts as the agent of both the hospital and the patient. Ellis and McGuire argue that the physician is likely to be biased in favor of the hospital, which leads to a *reduction* in the volume of services delivered to the individual patient following a switch to PPS. Since they do not consider the aggregate inpatient stock, which may rise, the implied effect on hospital inputs is ambiguous.

Our chapter departs from previous research in several respects. In contrast to Foster and Ellis and McGuire, we model both the physician and the hospital as decision-making agents. To accomplish this, we posit that the hospital and the medical staff health care decisions are dependent upon each other's actions. Further, we simultaneously consider the nature of interactions between the medical staff and the hospital under alternative behavioral assumptions, a factor as yet unexplored in the health care field to the best of our knowledge.

Our basic model is now described. Physicians, hospitals, and patients interact in a market for health care services. For the most part, we concentrate on services rendered to the Medicare population. Health care services can be viewed as outputs of a production process. We assume there are three factors of production: physician time, physician office inputs, and hospital inputs. The physician controls the allocation of the first two, while control of hospital inputs is shared by the physician and the hospital in a way to be described below.

Exactly what a unit of health care is deserves some discussion. Since "health" is difficult to measure, we choose to describe a mythical unit of health care and posit a direct relationship between the seriousness of an episode of illness, volume of inputs, and health care output. Physicians employ office inputs, hospital inputs, and their own time to produce a basic homogeneous unit of health care. They then allocate those units of health care across episodes of illness. Episodes requiring more intensive care are allocated more units of health care. Thus, the physician's fee schedule can be condensed to one price, and the fact that physicians charge more for an appendectomy than an office visit is explained by the greater number of health care units needed to produce an appendectomy relative to an office visit.

The physician's objective is the maximization of net income. Income is generated by treating Medicare patients. Collectively, all physicians comprise a homogeneous hospital medical staff. The hospital maximizes profit, net revenue, or "surplus," all of which are assumed to be identical concepts.

A thorny issue is the nature of input supply functions. It probably does little violence to reality to assume most factors of production are competitively supplied, and there are simplifying analytical gains in doing so. It is not realistic to make such an assumption for the physician's professional services, the supply price of which undoubtedly rises with quantity supplied. This exception notwithstanding, the analysis below assumes fixed input prices.

The price of hospital output depends on the reimbursement system. Under a PPS, the price is fixed by the regulatory body and is invariant with respect to output changes. In contrast, a cost-based reimbursement system requires the price to be an increasing function of average cost; in other words, the greater the output, the higher is the unit price (average revenue), so long as average cost increases. We model the cost-based output price as rising at a decreasing rate, with respect to average costs.

While this assumption abstracts from reality, it has several attractive features. First, it generates a finite optimum. A reimbursement system that provides a constant or increasing markup over average cost would have led the hospital to incur infinite costs. Second, although in actuality cost-based reimbursement did place some limits on the hospital's reimbursement levels, those limits were determined by areawide average costs and subject to frequent revision. It would be inappropriate to model hospitals as being constrained in the long run by these limits. Finally, the hospital's ability to exploit cost-based reimbursement was constrained by patients with other third-party reimbursement mechanisms. Although we have not directly modeled them here, the demand of paying consumers for hospital services is reduced as costs increase. Initially, we omit these types of patients from our model for tractability, but our description of the hospital's average revenue captures the effect of these patients on hospital decision making.

So far we have discussed how health care is produced. We now consider the demand for health care by patients. It has frequently been observed that consumption may not be very elastic with respect to price. There are a couple of reasons for this. First, the existence of health insurance drives a wedge between the actual and effective prices. Second, there is an asymmetry of information between patients and physicians concerning diagnosis and treatment. Thus, in their dual roles as agents and providers, physicians may have incentives to select more costly courses of treatment than patients would if they had the same information. These two factors have led many health care researchers to assume physicians can manipulate the demand for their services. There are several problems with this approach. It assumes consumers face no costs for health care other than the actual fees paid to physicians and hospitals. If patients are to face other costs, such as lost income, the ability of physicians to induce demand will be limited. From an analytical point of view, assuming physicians can induce demand limits the prediction value of any model of physician behavior. Demand inducement is consistent with almost every pricing and supply strategy. Moreover, there is empirical evidence that physicians are constrained by demand (Custer 1986; McCarthy 1985).

In our basic model, in which physicians sell their output in a single market, we assume they face a perfectly elastic demand curve. We assume a zero co-insurance rate for hospital services. In this model, the results are not qualitatively different if we posit a downward-sloping demand curve. However, if the physician faces more than one market differentiated either by patient reimbursement type or by treatment site, the cross-elasticity of demand will play an important role in determining the new optimum after a exogeneous shock, such as the switch to PPS from cost-based reimbursement for hospitals.

The roles of physicians and hospitals in the allocation of hospital resources have been widely discussed. Theoretical models revolve around the issues of the objective function of hospitals and the degree of control over hospital inputs by physicians. The profit maximization objective for the hospital has been analyzed by several researchers (Newhouse 1970; Feldstein 1983), as has been an output maximizaton assumption (Klarman 1965; Long 1964). An extension of this line asserts that the utility of the hospital manager, which includes both the quantity and quality of output, is the objective function (Newhouse 1970). All three types of models have implications that are at odds with observed phenomena in the hospital sector, not the least of which is failure to account for physician influence in hospital decision making. Pauly and Redisch (1973) attempted to deal with some of these shortcomings by using a model in which physicians control decision making in the hospital. Many of the anomalies in the health field are explained by this approach. However, the omission of hospital influence altogether would appear to render deficient such an extreme approach. Benson and Mitchell (1986) incorporate the objectives and controls of both parties in a hospital decision-making model. While providing a role for both physicians and the hospital, their model does not take account of the shift to PPS reimbursement or *any* form of Medicare payment to the hospital.

Our approach to hospital resource allocation allows a role for both physicians and the hospital. Our benchmark model posits independent decision making. The physician decides on the amounts of his or her own time and office inputs to use for a given level of hospital inputs. The hospital determines the quantity of its input to employ, given the amount of physician inputs. In this version, the hospital maximizes profits and has complete control over its inputs. Other versions allow for alternative types of hospital input control, culminating in a cartel model, in which there is joint decision making with respect to *all* inputs.

An issue that deserves attention, and one that is not considered here, is the difference between short-run and long-run input adjustments. This is especially important for the hospital where capital investment decisions have consequences that reach far into the future. The traditional view is that the hospital provides the "capacity," and the physicians determine the degree of utilization of that capacity. Allowing for both parties to have a say in investment decisions may provide insights and explanations lacking in traditional models.

Given this simple model of hospital and physician behavior, some of the implications of a switch from cost-based reimbursement to a prospective reimbursement system may be explored. We demonstrate that the impact of PPS on physician and hospital depends on the nature of the hospital–medical staff relationship. We analyze three forms of this relationship based on the duopoly literature.

Independent Decision Making

As a benchmark case, we assume the hospital and its medical staff are engaged in a noncooperative game represented by a Cournot-type model. In the Cournot model, each side chooses its optimal course of action, assuming its opponent's course of action is fixed. Thus, the medical staff chooses its optimal physician time and office inputs for a given amount of hospital inputs. Likewise, the hospital chooses its optimal quantity of hospital inputs for fixed amounts of physician time and office inputs. If either is surprised at the other's choice, successive rounds of adjustment take place. The Cournot equilibrium is characterized by a set of input quantities such that neither physicians nor the hospital wish to change their decision.

We assume the physician produces health care according to the following production function:

$$N = N(o,t,z) \quad \text{with} \quad N_o, N_t, N_z > 0, \quad N_{oo}, N_{tt}, N_{zz} < 0 \tag{1}$$

where

N = number of units of inpatient health care produced;
o = vector of physician office inputs;
t = amount of physician time;
z = vector of hospital inputs.

The physician is assumed to take the price of a unit of health care (P), the vector of office input prices (k) and the opportunity cost of his or her time (w) as given. The physician chooses o and t to maximize his or her income (Y).

$$Y = PN(o,t,z) - wt - ko \tag{2}$$

The hospital's medical staff is assumed to be composed of V identical physicians. The hospital is reimbursed at the rate H per unit of health care produced and faces total costs $C = C(VN,z)$. The hospital chooses z to maximize profits.

$$\pi = HVN(o,t,z) - C(z) \quad \text{with} \quad C_z > 0, \quad C_{zz} > 0 \tag{3}$$

Under a PPS, H is fixed for the hospital by the regulatory body. In contrast, a cost-based reimbursement system requires that H be an increasing function of average costs.

$$H = H\left(\frac{C(z)}{VN}\right) \quad \text{with} \quad H' > 0, \quad H'' < 0 \tag{4}$$

Given this simple model of hospital and physician behavior, some of the implications of a switch from cost-based reimbursement to a prospective reimbursement system may be explored.

Consider health care output or admissions from the hospital's perspective under cost-based reimbursement. Implicitly, this involves the choice of the optimal quantity of the hospital input vector, given the medical staff's choice of physician inputs. The optimal amount of hospital input equates marginal revenue product and marginal factor cost (which is identical to factor price). However, due to the nature of the reimbursement structure, marginal factor cost exceeds the value of the marginal product because marginal revenue is greater than output price under the type of prospective reimbursement structure we have posited.

Next, consider a switch to a prospectively determined hospital output price. The regulatory body chooses a fixed output price. For the purpose of comparing the Cournot solutions under cost-based reimbursement and PPS, we assume the regulatory body chooses a budget-neutral price—a price identical to that obtained in equilibrium under cost-based reimbursement. The relevant input demand schedule for the hospital now becomes the value of the marginal product. If output and hospital input remain at their cost-based levels following the change in reimbursement methods, then marginal factor cost will exceed the value of the marginal product, as was noted in the previous paragraph. This will encourage the hospital to supply fewer inputs, resulting in a reduction in output relative to that under cost-based reimbursement. In effect, a subsidy for additional output will have been removed. This is not the final equilibrium because the medical staff physicians will react by changing the supply of their inputs. The direction of change depends on the signs of the crossmarginal products between the inputs. For example, if physician and hospital inputs are "complements," physicians would reduce their input supplies, reinforcing the initial effect of decreasing output. If, on the other hand, physician and hospital inputs are "substitutes," more physician inputs would be supplied, offsetting the output-reducing effect of the decline in hospital inputs. It is highly unlikely output would actually increase in the latter case, however. The new equilibrium following the switch to PPS will be characterized by less hospital inputs and admissions, with the direction of change in physician inputs unclear.

Our results are not sensitive to such assumptions as a single setting of health care and a single type of patient. To show this, let the physician produce outpatient care according to a production function with the same characteristics as the inpatient production function; further, suppose the physician receives a fixed price per unit of outpatient care. The hospital's optimization problem is the same as before. Hence, a switch from cost-based to prospective payment still leads the hospital to supply less inputs. The marginal revenue product of physician inputs in the inpatient market is changed. However, the marginal revenue product is unaffected in the outpatient market. Therefore, the physician's optimal response will involve the entire adjustment taking place in the inpatient market. In contrast, if we were to relax the assumption of constant input prices and let physicians face an upward-sloping supply curve for their inputs, then the adjustment to a change from cost-based reimbursement to PPS can be shown to affect both the inpatient and outpatient markets. Consequently, the impact will be smaller in the inpatient market when factor costs are rising, compared with the case when input prices are fixed. Moreover, by incorporating an upward-sloping marginal factor cost curve, it is possible to show that a switch to PPS will lead physicians to devote fewer inputs to the outpatient market since an increase in inputs purchased for one market increases the marginal factor cost in both markets.

The analysis presented so far is based on a simple model of physician and hospital behavior. The model depicts the physician and hospital delivering a single specific service to only one type of patient—Medicare patients. This abstracts from some important elements of the health care system and can be expanded to better capture the current health-sector environment. We have extended the model along several important dimensions. First, in order to examine the issue of uncompensated/charity care, we can change both the physician and hospital objectives functions from profit to utility maximization. Second, we can increase the number of services the hospital and physician deliver. Finally, we can incorporate both a Medicare and a non-Medicare market. Overall, our general result holds: a budget-neutral switch to prospective payment leads hospitals to reduce their supply of inputs, inducing physicians to substitute their own inputs in the production of health care. The results now, however, depend upon the demand and cost structure of the various markets. For example, in the case where there are two markets, one for private pay patients and the other for Medicare patients, we find the hospital employs less inputs after the switch to PPS, causing physicians to substitute their own inputs in the production of health care. In this extension, it is interesting to note that the reduction in inputs by the hospital occurs in both the Medicare and non-Medicare markets. The magnitude of the adjustment depends on the relationship between the reimbursement rates and the marginal costs in the two markets.

Semicooperative behavior

A slightly different result is obtained if the hospital-medical staff relationship is similar to the Stackelberg model of duopoly behavior. In comparison to the Cournot model, which had each participant taking the other's actions as given, the Stackelberg model assumes one firm takes the other firm's reactions as given. For example, let us assume firm A is dominant in the sense that it knows how firm B will react to firm A's output choices.

If the hospital is dominant, then the hospital's problem is to maximize profits subject to the medical staff's reactions. The medical staff's optimization problem is the same as in the Cournot model. If the crossmarginal products between hospital inputs and both physician inputs are equal to zero, then the Stackelberg and Cournot equilibria are identical. The difference between the Cournot and Stackelberg equilibria depends on the sign of the crossmarginal products. As long as they are nonzero, the hospital will be better off in the Stackelberg case. If both crossmarginal products are negative ("substitutes"), the hospital will reduce its input, but the medical staff will provide more physician inputs. The effect is most likely a reduction in health care output. If the crossmarginal products are both positive ("complements"), the hospital will use more inputs, raising the marginal products of physician inputs and inducing an increase in their use. More health care is produced.

The Stackelberg solutions under the two reimbursement schemes can be compared by assuming the regulatory body again chooses a budget-neutral output price, following the switch to prospective payment. Our model suggests the hospital will supply less inputs under PPS for the same reason as before: marginal revenue product falls relative to marginal factor cost in the vicinity of the cost-based optimum. Since the hospital could have chosen the original quantity of its inputs and achieved the same profits under PPS as were achieved under cost-based reimbursement, profits must be higher at the new equilibrium under PPS. Physicians, on the other hand, find it optimal to replace hospital inputs with costly (to them) office and time inputs if they are substitutes; otherwise, less physician inputs will be supplied. However, atypical input crossmarginal products notwithstanding, health care output and physician income both fall.

A similar result is found if the roles are reversed and the medical staff is dominant in the Stackelberg model. We omit the technical details and an extended discussion. However, it can be shown that the medical staff produce less output at greater personal cost and, hence, earn smaller profits under PPS than under cost-based reimbursement, even though physicians dominate the hospital in the Stackelberg sense.

Full cooperation

In this model, it is assumed the medical staff and the hospital collude; that is, they cooperate to maximize the sum of their net incomes. They form a cartel, in effect. The single objective function is the sum of hospital profits and medical staff net income. It is important to note that although the optimum maximizes the cartel's net income, the individual partners in the cartel may be winners or losers in a move from the Cournot equilibrium to the cartel optimum. In such a case, the winners must make side payments to the losers or the cartel will unravel. It should be noted that the full-cooperation solution is Pareto superior to either of the other two, given side payments.

However, it can be shown that under cost-based reimbursement the cartel will produce more units of health care than were produced at the Cournot equilibrium. This follows from the fact that the Cournot quantities leave marginal revenue product in excess of marginal factor cost for all inputs. Some or all inputs must be increased to reach the cartel's optimum. Therefore, so long as the inputs have positive marginal products, the total number of health care units produced must increase.

Again, choosing a budget-neutral output price, total output will fall after a switch to PPS because marginal factor cost will exceed marginal revenue product for all inputs at the cost-based input quantities. The cartel's profits, on the other hand, will rise. Since PPS was designed to yield the same revenue per unit of health care as at the cartel's cost-based optimum, they could have achieved at least the same profits under PPS as were gained under cost-based reimbursement. The fact that the PPS optimal input vector differs from the cost-based optimal input vector indicates that an increase in cartel profits occurs under prospective payment.

To briefly summarize: our analysis has yielded three major insights. First, we show that the overall objective of the Medicare PPS of reducing hospital costs is achieved by reducing the hospital's optimal supply of inputs. Second, this reduction in hospital inputs causes physicians to change their practice patterns by altering their own input combinations. The exact changes depend upon the production function for health care, but a likely result is for physicians to increase their time and office inputs. Since these inputs are costly to physicians, the net result is likely to be a fall in the total number of health care units that are produced and, consequently, physician income. Finally, our analysis indicates a motivation for medical staffs to enter into cooperative agreements with their hospital due to prospective payment. Physicians are better off when the hospital takes their welfare into consideration. Although the hospital's incentive to collude under PPS has been noted, it takes both sides to agree.

Our results may be compared with the institutional literature on the expected effects of PPS on various dimensions of health care inputs and outputs (see Lohr et al. 1985; Roe and Gong 1986; and U.S. Congress 1985). It was generally expected that one measure of hospital output—admissions—would rise following the shift to PPS. This contradicts our prediction. On the other hand, it was expected that two measures of hospital input would fall, including the average length of a hospital stay and the quantity of inpatient services utilized. Further, the literature predicted a shift of services away from the inpatient setting. Our model predicts a reduction in hospital inputs, but whether outpatient service usage rises or falls depends on the signs of the crossmarginal products.

Summary statistics from the American Medical Association (1985) and the American Hospital Association (AHA) (Hospital Research and Education Trust 1986) sources, supplemented by other research findings, provide confirmation for many of our theoretical results. The following compares the first year or so of PPS-era experience with the late pre-PPS period. Hospitals reduced their use of inpatient inputs. Full-time-equivalent employees and staffed beds both declined. The average length of a hospital stay declined substantially from the historical trend for Medicare patients but hardly at all for non-Medicare patients. This finding is also confirmed by Guterman and Dobson (1986) and Chesney et al. (1985). In contrast to what had been anticipated, total Medicare admissions declined, even though the population sixty-five and over grew, which has also been reported by Guterman and Dobson (1986) and Rosenbach and Cromwell (1985). A majority of physicians reported they were urged by hospitals to limit diagnostic testing or to cut costs by conducting fewer procedures (Rosenbach and Cromwell 1985). In response, they ordered fewer unnecessary tests and procedures but also reported more instances of more short staffing, inappropriate generic drug substitutions, and postponement of new technology by hospitals (American Society of Internal Medicine 1985). The percentage of cases with at least one consultation during the hospital stay rose slightly for both Medicare and non-Medicare patients in 1984, which may be interpreted as physicians not "cutting corners" to get Medicare patients out of the hospital quicker (Chesney et al. 1985). Although hospitals experienced lower occupancy rates, their profits increased (Guterman and Dobson 1986).

Hospitals produced less output following the introduction of prospective payment. The number of weekly discharges per physician fell for Medicare patients, while remaining steady for non-Medicare patients. Physicians felt pressure from hospital management to discharge patients earlier than they did prior to diagnosis-related groups (DRGs) (U.S. Senate 1985). This was especially true for physicians other than radiologists, anesthesiologists, or pathologists (nonRAPs), physicians with high Medicare caseloads, and nonsalaried physicians (Rosenbach and Cromwell 1985). Some of these earlier discharges were considered to be medically premature by physicians, resulting in increased mortality and morbidity (American Society of Internal Medicine 1985). Furthermore, there is evidence that physicians felt pressure from hospital management to "sequence" patients—discharging, then readmitting them for a second diagnosis, which went untreated during the initial hospitalization (American Society of Internal Medicine 1985). Despite this pressure, there was no significant change from the trend in readmissions for either Medicare or non-Medicare patients (Chesney et al. 1985).

Hospitals altered their service patterns after the reimbursement structure for Medicare inpatients changed. There was a drastic increase in hospital outpatient visits, which are not subject to prospective pricing coincident with the decrease in Medicare inpatient activity.

Physicians have responded to the decrease in hospital inputs by supplying more of their own inputs since PPS. Weeks practiced per year accelerated its rate of increase, as did hours per week spent in patient activities. Encounters with hospital inpatients declined, as evidenced by a reduction in the average number of weekly hospital-round visits with Medicare patients. The slack was taken up by increased office activity. Both total office hours and the number of visits per week increased for the typical physician.

Policy Implications

The predicted reduction in the supply of hospital inputs resulting from the switch to PPS reimbursement has serious potential consequences for the quality of and access to care for Medicare beneficiaries, as has been observed by many analysts.

What has not received much attention is the ideal form of physician-hospital relationship. We observed that collusive interaction generates the greatest potential gains to providers under PPS. However, health care output was predicted to decline to the detriment of patients. From a social perspective, the ideal form of relationship takes the net benefits of both consumers and producers into account. Any form of insurance on the demand side favors socially excessive consumption. The form of hospital reimbursement does not affect this distortion. Cost-based reimbursement exacerbates the overproduction of health care by subsidizing excessive use of hospital inputs. Switching to a fixed, prospectively determined price eliminates the supply distortion and reduces output closer to the social optimum. Judged by this criterion, PPS is seen to be a superior hospital reimbursement method. In textbook examples, cartels are generally found to undersupply output compared with the social ideal. Such examples do not typically include the type of demand-side subsidies inherent in health insurance. With such distortions present, cooperation between hospitals and physicians may well move output closer to the social optimum than noncooperative relationships.

Research Agenda

The theoretical model may be extended farther. So far we have considered the case of a single hospital operating within a competitive hospital sector. Real-world hospitals face competitive pressures, but it would be more accurate to model the hospital as possessing some degree of market power in the output market. We have assumed all physicians are identical. Allowing for a diversity of physician types would be a useful extension, for example, office-based and hospital-based physicians. Another extension would be to examine the internal dynamics of the medical staff, for example, allowing for different objectives and constraints among physicians and determining whether the medical staff acts as a monopolist vis-à-vis the hospital or as independent decision-making agents. Our analysis has not made a distinction between the short run and the long run, nor has it captured the time dynamics of the transition to a new reimbursement system. Accounting for such factors as these may yield fruitful additional insights.

Another obvious and needed elaboration is the inclusion of multivariate empirical analysis. The data used to examine the implication of our theoretical model may be drawn from two sources. Physician data may be taken from the American Medical Association Socioeconomic Monitoring System (SMS) surveys, which are annual telephone interviews of a random sample of approximately 4,000 nonfederal patient care physicians each year. Most major practice characteristics are available from this survey, including the percentage of gross revenue accruing from care of Medicare patients, practice expense data, and utilization information. Although this survey is not a panel per se, approximately one-third of each year's respondents are reinterviewed in the following year. Hospital data are available from the AHA Annual Survey of Hospitals, which is an ongoing survey of all U.S. hospitals. For the purpose of this survey, a hospital is defined as the organization or corporate entity registered as a hospital by a state to provide diagnostic and therapeutic patient services by a variety of medical conditions, including both surgical and nonsurgical services. The 1982 and 1984 surveys may be used here as examples of pre-PPS and PPS years and merged to create a two-period panel. In addition, the 1984 SMS survey contains a hospital identifier for the principal hospital at which the physician admits the majority of his or her patients. Hence, when applicable, 1984 SMS physician data can be linked with hospital characteristics.

The objectives of the data analysis include: (1) determining the signs of the crossmarginal products of the health care production function, (2) searching for input and output effects following the switch to PPS, and (3) evaluating the validity of the various models of medical staff–hospital interactions.

Conclusion

We have employed a simple model of hospital and physician behavior to analyze the impacts of a switch to a PPS for hospital Medicare reimbursement. We found that PPS reduces the hospital's optimal supply of inputs to the production of health care. As a result, physicians substitute inputs that are costly to them for the nominally free hospital inputs. This is likely to result, depending on the production function for health care, in less health care being produced and lower physician incomes.

These results raise a number of issues. First, does PPS make the input mix in the production of health care more efficient? The general notion is that it has since cost-based hospital reimbursement essentially acted as a subsidy for hospital inputs. The actual answer is likely to vary by diagnosis and availability of alternative inputs, however. Second, our analysis indicates the amount of health care produced is likely to fall. We could easily interpret these results as being a reduction in the quality of health care delivered, rather than a reduction in the number of patients treated. Alternatively, it may be that, previously, too much quality was delivered in the sense that procedures with low marginal benefit were performed, but this point may need further investigation. Finally, collusive arrangements between hospitals and their medical staff add a new dimension to the physician's medical decision making. Resolving the hospital-medical staff conflict may introduce conflict into the physician-patient relationship.

Notes

The views and opinions expressed in this paper do not necessarily reflect the official policy of the AMA. The authors wish to thank Mark Pauly for much of the motivation for this chapter and for many helpful comments on earlier drafts.

References

American Medical Association, *Socioeconomic Characteristics of Medical Practice*, Chicago, IL: 1985.

American Society of Internal Medicine, *The Impact of DRGs on Patient Care*, Washington, DC: American Society of Internal Medicine, 1985.

Benson, B. L., and J. M. Mitchell, "A Partial Reconciliation of Hospital Decision-Making Model," mimeographed, 1986.

Chesney, J., S. Desharnais, E. Kobrinski, M. Long, S. Fleming, and R. Ament, *The Impact of the Prospective Payment System on the Quality of Inpatient Care*, mimeographed, November 19, 1985.

Custer, W. S., "Hospital Attributes and Physician Prices," *Southern Economic Journal*, 52(4):1010–1027, April 1986.

Ellis, R. P., and T. G. McGuire, "Provider Behavior Under Prospective Reimbursement," *Journal of Health Economics*, 5(2):129–151, June 1986.

Feldstein, P., *Health Care Economics*, New York: John Wiley & Sons, 1983.

Foster, R. N., "Cost-Shifting under Cost Reimbursement and Prospective Payment," *Journal of Health Economics*, 4(3):261–271, September 1985.

Glandon, G. L., and M. A. Morrisey, "Redefining the Hospital-Physician Relationship Under Prospective Payment," *Inquiry*, 23(2):166–175, Summer 1986.

Guterman, S., and A. Dobson, "Impact of the Medicare Prospective Payment System for Hospitals," *Health Care Financing Review*, 7(3):97–114, Spring 1986.

Harris, J. E., "The Internal Organization of Hospitals: Some Economic Implications," *Bell Journal of Economics*, 8(2):467–481, Autumn 1977.

Hospital Research and Education Trust, *Economic Trends*, 2(2), Summer 1986.

Klarman, H. E., *The Economics of Health*, New York: Columbia University Press, 1965.

Lohr, K. N., R. Brook, G. Goldberg, M. Chassin, and T. Glennan, *Impact of Medicare Prospective Payment on the Quality of Medical Care: A Research Agenda*, Santa Monica, CA: The Rand Corporation, March 1985.

Long, M. F., "Efficient Use of Hospitals," in *The Economics of Health and Medical Care*, Ann Arbor, MI: University of Michigan Press, 1964.

McCarthy, T. R., "The Competitive Nature of the Primary Care Physician Services Market," *Journal of Health Economics*, 4(2):93–118, June 1985.

Newhouse, J., "Toward a Theory of Nonprofit Institutions: An Economic Model of a Hospital," *American Economic Review,* 60(1):64–74, March 1970.

Pauly, M. V., and M. Redisch, "The Not-for-Profit Hospital as a Physicians' Cooperative," *American Economic Review,* 63(1):87–100, March 1973.

Roe, W., and J. Gong, *The Potential Impact of Prospective Payment on the Quality of Care,* Washington, DC: Lewin & Associations, Inc., March 1986.

Rosenback, M. L., and J. Cromwell, *Physicians' Perceptions about the Short-Run Impact of Medicare's Prospective Payment System: Final Report,* Needham, MA: Health Economics Research, Inc., November 14, 1985.

Shortell, S., "Physician Involvement in Hospital Decision-Making," in B. H. Grey, ed., *The New Health Care For-Profit: Doctors and Hospitals in a Competitive Environment,* Washington, DC: Institute of Medicine, National Academy of Sciences, 1983.

———, "The Medical Staff of the Future: Replanting the Garden," *Frontiers of Health Services Management,* 1(3):7–48, February 1985.

U.S. Congress, Office of Technology Assessment, *Medicare's Prospective Payment System: Strategies for Evaluating Cost, Quality, and Medical Technology,* OTA-H-262, Washington, DC: U.S. Government Printing Office, October 1985.

U.S. Senate, Special Committee on Aging, Staff Report, *Impact of Medicare's Prospective Payment System on the Quality of Care Received by Medicare Beneficiaries,* Washington, DC: U.S. Government Printing Office, September 26, 1985.

10. Capitation and Medicare: Past, Present, and Future

JUDITH D. KASPER, GERALD F. RILEY,
AND JEFFREY S. MCCOMBS

Despite the relatively small number of Medicare beneficiaries currently enrolled in health maintenance organizations (HMOs), interest in capitation as a mechanism for payment for the full Medicare benefit package is intense. It is an explicit goal of the present administration to promote options in addition to fee-for-service providers of health care and to increase HMO enrollment among Medicare beneficiaries. Other mechanisms to increase full capitation of Medicare benefits are being explored as well, including contracting with employer and union groups to provide Medicare benefits to retirees for a prospective per capita payment. This chapter provides an overview of the issues surrounding full Medicare capitation and, where relevant, provides data from two HMOs that enrolled Medicare beneficiaries under a Health Care Financing Administration (HCFA) demonstration.

This chapter is organized into three sections. The first provides a brief historical review of the enrollment of Medicare beneficiaries in HMOs. As concerns about the costs of Medicare mounted in the early 1970s, HMOs were increasingly viewed as desirable settings for delivering care to beneficiaries. Not until 1982, with the passage of the Tax Equity and Fiscal Responsibility Act (TEFRA), which provides for purely prospective payment to HMOs by Medicare, were there sufficient incentives to the HMO industry to actively enroll Medicare beneficiaries.

The second section, on the present status of Medicare and full capitation, first discusses the promise and pitfalls of capitated delivery systems for Medicare beneficiaries and then focuses on the experience of two early efforts to enroll beneficiaries in HMOs. Capitation is believed to be a successful means of reducing health care costs. Primarily by limiting inpatient hospital use, HMOs appear to deliver care at lower cost than the fee-for-service sector. The promise of capitation may fall short, however, if HMO savings result not from efficiency but from enrolling a healthy population (biased selection). Proponents of HMOs have long argued as well that this type of delivery system provides more preventive care, encourages care-seeking at earlier stages of illness, and delivers greater continuity of care. Empirical evidence to support these claims is sparse, but the theoretical possibility of improved access under prepayment retains a strong appeal. The pitfalls of capitation relate to the potential adverse impact on access and quality of care of a delivery system that rations services, mainly by controlling access to expensive care, such as inpatient hospitalizations and specialty services.

The experience of two HMOs that enrolled beneficiaries is used to address three questions under the heading "Can the promise be realized?" First, will beneficiaries enroll and stay enrolled? Second, will HMOs attract those who could benefit most from their potential to improve access and provide greater continuity of care? Third, will HMOs save money for the Medicare program? The third section of this chapter turns to issues likely to affect the future of Medicare and capitation.

Medicare and HMOs—the Past

Prepaid group practices predate the Medicare program by several decades. The oldest and largest practices in the country were developed in the 1930s and 1940s, often to serve specific employee or consumer populations. Among these are the Kaiser-Permanente Medical Care Program, the Group Health Cooperative of Puget Sound, and the Health Insurance Plan of Greater New York. While HMOs vary substantially in their characteristics, Luft (1981) has defined their key features as (1) assuming contractual responsibility to provide health services, (2) serving a defined population that voluntarily enrolled in the plan, (3) payment by enrollees of a fixed amount for care independent of use, and (4) assuming some risk or gain for the cost of providing services. Luft points out as well that any description of HMOs may soon be outdated by the continuing changes in HMOs. This observation is borne out by the emergence of entities such as preferred provider organizations (PPOs) and the increasingly blurred distinctions between HMOs and PPOs.

Programmatic changes in Medicare treatment of HMOs can be grouped under three headings—types of services capitated, reimbursement methods, and eligibility restrictions. These are summarized in Table 10.1.[1] When Medicare was

TABLE 10.1
Changes in Services Capitated, Reimbursement Methods, and Eligibility Restrictions for HMOs under Medicare, 1966 to the present

Year	Services capitated	Reimbursement methods	Eligibility restrictions
1966	Part B services only	Retrospective adjustment of monthly payments based on costs (cost-based reimbursement)	
1972 (Section 1876, implemented 1976)	Capitation of all Medicare benefits (Part B and inpatient services)	Risk option introduced	Restricted to federally qualified HMOs
		Retrospective adjustment using the AAPCC and actual HMO costs	
		HMO at risk for losses, retains 50% of savings up to 10% of AAPCC	
1980 and 1982 HCFA demonstrations		HMO retains savings (difference between AAPCC and ACR), which must be used to expand benefits or reduce cost sharing	
		HMO paid a percent of AAPCC; retrospective adjustment eliminated	
1982 (TEFRA amends Section 1876, implemented April 1985)		HMO paid 95% of AAPCC	Eligible plans expanded to include CMPs

enacted in 1966, HMOs with enrolled beneficiaries could receive monthly capitated payments to provide physician and related services covered by Part B of Medicare. These payments, however, were subject to adjustment at the end of the year to 80 percent of the reasonable cost of providing services (a requirement to make payments comply with Part B regulations). Payments for hospital, skilled nursing, and home health services for these same beneficiaries were made directly to the institutions providing care. Thus, serving Medicare beneficiaries presented difficulties for HMOs, in contrast to their younger enrollee population. First, while payments were prospective, the retrospective adjustment meant reimbursement was actually cost based. Collection of requisite cost and use data for services provided to Medicare enrollees posed administrative difficulties for organizations in which the norm was prepayment. Second, HMOs were not paid directly to provide hospital inpatient care, whereas evidence now suggests that HMO savings may be greatest in this area (Luft 1981; Manning et al. 1984).

Several legislative efforts began in the early 1970s that eventually resulted in major changes. One was an attempt to introduce into the Medicare program a Medicare "Part C," which would have allowed beneficiaries to enroll in HMOs on an at-risk basis as an alternative to regular Medicare (Brown [1983] provides a detailed portrayal of this effort and the development of the 1973 HMO Act). While the addition of a Medicare Part C to the already existing Parts A and B never materialized, major changes in all three areas—services capitated, reimbursement methods, and eligibility restrictions—were embodied in the 1972 legislation (see Table 10.1). When the regulations were issued in 1976, this legislation (Section 1876) introduced the option of enrolling beneficiaries at risk and provided for capitation of the total Medicare benefit package, both outpatient and inpatient services. However, it restricted participation to federally qualified HMOs (as determined under the HMO Act).

Intended as a tool to stimulate development of HMOs, the process of federal qualification necessary to enjoy the benefits of the legislation was regarded by many HMOs as onerous. Among the requirements for qualification were provision of a minimum benefit package under a community rating, at least one thirty-day open enrollment period each year, and no more than 50 percent of enrollees who are Medicare/Medicaid beneficiaries. In return for these restrictions, federally qualified HMOs received access to loans and grants and, in areas where federally qualified HMOs existed, employers of at least twenty-five people were required to offer to their employees the option of enrollment (Brown 1983; Trieger et al. 1981). Restricting at-risk contracting to federally qualified HMOs was a reflection of legislative concern that if HMOs were encouraged to enroll Medicare or Medicaid beneficiaries, beneficiaries in return should be protected by requiring HMOs to meet certain standards believed to ensure good care.

(Some justification for this concern was provided by the questionable practices of prepaid plans with Medicaid contracts in California in the mid-1970s.)

Despite the changes introduced in Section 1876, the legislation did not lead to substantial increases in HMO enrollment of the elderly. Between 1976 and 1982 four HMOs signed at-risk contracts to serve Medicare beneficiaries (about 45,000 elderly were enrolled in these HMOs in 1982 when TEFRA was enacted). For many HMOs, the opportunity to enroll Medicare beneficiaries was not sufficient incentive to undergo the process of becoming federally qualified. In addition, while all Medicare-covered services could be capitated and paid for prospectively, the payments were still subject to retrospective adjustment. Actual costs were compared with the adjusted average per capita costs (AAPCC), an estimate of what the cost of providing services to a specific HMO's enrollees would be under fee-for-service. A significant aspect of the 1972 legislation was the introduction of the AAPCC as a means of determining HMO capitation payments. If actual costs exceeded the AAPCC, the HMO absorbed the loss. If costs were less than the AAPCC, the HMO was allowed to retain 50 percent of the "savings" but only up to 10 percent of the AAPCC.

In 1980, HCFA initiated a demonstration project to test alternative ways of reimbursing HMOs for Medicare beneficiaries enrolled at risk. The initial round of demonstrations involved eight plans that began enrolling Medicare beneficiaries in HMOs in 1980 and 1981 (data on the experience of two of these plans—Fallon Community Health Plan of Massachusetts and Greater Marshfield Community Health Plan of Wisconsin—are presented in this chapter). A second group of HMOs, under the rubric of the Medicare Competition Demonstration, began in 1982 with twenty-six HMOs participating by the end of 1984 (Medicare Competition Demonstration 1986a). The major purpose of these demonstrations was to further modify reimbursement methods under risk contracting and expand HMO enrollment of Medicare beneficiaries. Rather than retrospectively adjusting payments using audited cost reports, HMOs were paid 95 percent of a prospectively determined AAPCC and allowed to retain any savings between this amount and the HMO's estimate of the cost of providing coverage of Medicare benefits in the HMO (the adjusted community rate [ACR]).[2] Savings could be used in three ways: (1) to expand benefits beyond those covered by Medicare (e.g., prescribed drug coverage), (2) to reduce or eliminate deductibles associated with Part A and Part B coverage (currently $520 per admission for Part A and $75 annually for Part B) and the 20 percent coinsurance for Part B services, or (3) to reduce for Medicare enrollees the HMO's usual premiums or copayments.[3]

In 1982 the reimbursement methods used in the HCFA demonstrations were adopted into law under TEFRA. This legislation also allowed prepaid health plans, other than federally qualified HMOs, to be eligible for a Medicare contract if they qualified as a competitive medical plan (CMP).[4] HCFA began signing TEFRA risk contracts with HMOs in April 1985.

In November 1986, 2.7 percent of Medicare beneficiaries nationwide were enrolled in HMOs on an at-risk basis (Table 10.2). All states with more than 10,000 at-risk enrollees are shown in the same table. Florida had the highest number (169,548) and Minnesota had the highest percentage (25.1 percent) of at-risk enrollees, followed by Hawaii (18.1 percent). Cost-based reimbursement remains an option under TEFRA (as of November 1986, 41 cost contracts were in effect, covering 99,462 Medicare beneficiaries). This type of reimbursement reduces but does not eliminate an HMO's risk, since HMOs under cost contracts are limited to costs or 100 percent of the AAPCC, whichever is less. When cost-based enrollees are added in, the percentage of beneficiaries receiving care from prepaid plans exceeds 3 percent.[5]

TABLE 10.2
Medicare Beneficiaries and Capitated HMO Enrollment by State: November 1986[a]

State	Medicare beneficiaries[b]	At-risk HMO enrollees	Percent of beneficiaries enrolled at risk
Total Medicare population	29,125,563	789,227	2.7
Florida	1,928,444	169,548[e]	8.8
California	2,777,748	158,476	5.7
Minnesota	534,227	134,231	25.1
Massachusetts	785,676	53,003	6.8
Illinois	1,386,304	51,587	3.7
Michigan	1,096,217	35,497	3.2
Oregon	361,218	21,619	6.0
Pennsylvania	1,759,865	20,833	1.2
Hawaii	95,327	17,204	18.1
New York	2,314,347	15,416	0.7
Nevada	95,462	14,530	15.2
New Jersey	992,522	13,629	1.4
Kansas	333,212	13,057	3.9
New Mexico	141,502	12,139	8.6
Arizona	390,865	11,545	3.0
Other states with at-risk enrollees[c]	9,126,064	461,913	0.5
States with no at-risk enrollees[d]	5,006,563	—	—

[a]Counts of at-risk enrollees as of November 1986. Counts of Medicare beneficiaries as of March 1986.
[b]All beneficiaries with both HI and SMI. The total numbers of beneficiaries with HI and/or SMI is 31,082,801.
[c]States with fewer than 10,000 at-risk enrollees.
[d]Twenty states have no at-risk enrollees.
[e]127,055 or 75% of all enrollees are in one HMO.

Medicare and HMOs—the Present

The promise and pitfalls of capitated delivery systems

As the costs of the Medicare program have risen, the search for ways to control costs has intensified. One significant change in provider payment has been implemented—paying hospitals for inpatient care on the basis of diagnostic category (diagnosis-related groups [DRGs]) rather than number and types of services rendered. Several proposals for large-scale reform of the Medicare program, aimed at expanding benefits as well as controlling costs, have appeared recently (e.g., Harvard Medicare Project 1986; Davis and Rowland 1986). Encouraging enrollment of Medicare beneficiaries in HMOs has a role in many of these proposals. Some are more optimistic than others about the importance of the role HMOs will play. Taylor and Kagay (1986), for example, predict high levels of HMO enrollment across all segments of the population, while others suggest preferences for HMOs as sources of health care may be more limited (Davis and Rowland 1986; Brown 1983; Mechanic 1985).

Leaving aside for the moment predictions of the levels of HMO enrollment, the promise and pitfalls of capitation involve three broad areas: cost containment, access, and quality of care. The issues in each of these areas as they affect the Medicare population are addressed below.

Cost containment. The reputation of HMOs as more cost-efficient organizations for delivering care is based primarily on their use of fewer inpatient services. Lower rates of hospitalization among HMO enrollees were documented by Luft in his comprehensive review of HMO research (1981), and more recent studies continue to support these findings (Manning et al. 1984; Reidel et al. 1984).

Evidence on provision of ambulatory services and related cost savings is mixed. Some studies suggest similar levels of physician services among HMO and fee-for-service patients (Manning et al. 1984); others suggest that ambulatory use rates are higher in HMOs (Hirshfield and Meyers, in Reidel et al. 1984). There is conflicting evidence as well regarding fluctuations in levels of ambulatory use early in enrollment and later on (Griffith and Baloff 1981; Baloff and Griffith 1981; Mullooly and Freeborn 1979).

If lower use of inpatient care is the major source of HMO savings, the question often posed is how do HMOs achieve these lower levels of use. Two types of explanations are generally offered. One relies on organizational characteristics of the HMO, for example, the mix of services offered, the types of physicians recruited to HMO practice and their mode of practice, the incentives to providers, and the utilization controls employed by HMOs. The other explanation looks more to the types of persons who enroll in HMOs, who may be different from nonenrollees in ways that affect patterns of use (e.g., healthier individuals or those with less propensity to use care).

Potential savings to Medicare from HMO enrollment of beneficiaries cannot be predicted reliably until there is more evidence both about the characteristics of persons who enroll in HMOs and the organizational aspects of HMOs as they affect delivery of care to the elderly. If HMOs' lower costs are due in large part to enrollment of persons who use services at lower levels (favorable selection), Medicare may not realize savings because of the way the current payment mechanism is structured. Further discussion of this payment mechanism (AAPCC) follows later in this chapter.

Access to care. Under the Medicare program, access to physician care has improved substantially. For example, in 1963 (prior to Medicare), only 68 percent of the elderly saw a physician, compared with 82 percent in 1980. Differences in use have also declined between lower-income and better-off elderly and between minority elderly persons and others (Ruther and Dobson 1981; Kasper 1986a; Aday et al. 1984). Nonetheless, barriers to access still exist. The elderly are believed by some to delay seeking care, for reasons including financial, with serious consequences for their ability to function independently (Branch and Nemeth 1985; Besdine 1982).

Although Medicare coverage reduces the financial liability of the elderly, beneficiaries must bear the costs of deductibles, coinsurance, and expenses for noncovered services, such as drugs and dental care. In addition, liability due to unassigned claims for Medicare-covered services is rising (McMillan, Lubitz, and Newton 1985). Many elderly have responded by purchasing "Medigap" insurance. It has been found that those elderly with no supplemental coverage still use less care than others, even when their health is poor (Kasper 1986b).

The absence of large out-of-pocket payments at the time of service in HMOs has long been cited by advocates of prepayment as likely to lead to better access to care. Most TEFRA risk HMOs charge a premium of $20 or more a month (85 percent in November 1986; 15 percent charged no premium). This may still be substantially less than the out-of-pocket costs associated with fee-for-service care, taking into account the deductible for Medicare benefits, liability for unassigned claims, and lack of drug coverage. In addition, HMOs may contribute to improved access through coverage of services not included under current Medicare benefits. As of November 1986, 69 percent of TEFRA risk plans were offering vision care, 70 percent drug coverage, and 15 percent coverage of dental services to Medicare enrollees. None of these services are covered under Medicare in the fee-for-service sector. (Coverage of drugs above an annual deductible of $500 to $600, with a 20 percent coinsurance above that amount, may be included in 1988 legislation to provide catastrophic coverage under Medicare.) HMOs may, in addition, cover preventive and "wellness" promotion services not covered by Medicare. Offering expanded benefits helps HMOs attract enrollees.

It also offers one of the few opportunities to obtain coverage beyond the current benefit package, barring rare expansions of benefits, such as catastrophic coverage or hospice care.

The argument that HMOs may achieve more timely access to care is usually tied to their potential for case management. Bonanno and Wetle (1984) suggested that HMOs provide better coordination of service use across hospital, ambulatory, and home health care for elderly enrollees than occurs when the elderly use a variety of independent providers in the community. It has also been suggested, however, that currently HMOs do not have the incentive and often lack an orientation toward care of chronically ill or elderly patients (Schlesinger 1986). This same article suggests HMOs limit coverage of chronic illness, such as psychiatric care. One supporting example is provided by the General Motors Corporation, which became dissatisfied with mental health and substance abuse care provided by many of the HMOs serving their employees and retirees. Problems included restricted hours for providing this type of care, long waits for referrals, and reluctance by some primary care physicians to refer patients. In response to pressure from General Motors, the HMOs under contract made substantial changes in the way these services were delivered (from remarks by Beach Hall, National Health Policy Forum 1986).

If HMOs ration services to constrain costs (Mechanic 1985), as opposed to providing care more efficiently (the point at which efficiency becomes rationing may be difficult to detect), access may suffer. Aggressive utilization controls focused on high users could disproportionately affect the elderly, compared with younger enrollees. Elderly people, in general, consume more acute care resources than younger people. In addition, the prevalence of chronic disease requiring long-term management is greater among the older population (Manton 1982; Rice and Feldman 1983).

HMOs typically employ a number of utilization review procedures to control levels of use, including monitoring specialty referrals and admission decisions by physicians.[6] A number of other characteristics associated with more bureaucratically organized health delivery systems may reduce or deter utilization as well. Longer waiting times for appointments and restricted availability of specific physicians are characteristic of many HMOs (Mechanic et al. 1980). One study suggests that physicians working in bureaucratic settings are more likely than solo practitioners to regard their patients' problems as trivial (Mechanic 1976). Since the elderly often present with nonspecific symptoms that require more time to assess and diagnose (Rowe 1985), they may be especially vulnerable to such characterization.

Medicare beneficiaries can leave an HMO and return to the fee-for-service sector at any time. One response by high-use Medicare beneficiaries to unforeseen explicit and implicit mechanisms for controlling use and costs may be to disenroll. Alternatively, such measures may discourage prompt care-seeking when ill. Utilization controls and "gatekeeping" functions, with regard to appointments and specialty referrals, may be necessary from the HMO's point of view to maintain financial viability and to monitor service use, but there is little understanding of their impact on Medicare enrollees. New utilization controls have often accompanied enrollment of the elderly as HMOs begin serving this population (Carpenter 1985).

Discussions of the effects of HMO enrollment on access to care for Medicare beneficiaries thus far remain largely theoretical. Research in different treatment settings is needed, particularly for those who are chronically ill. Among the questions that should be addressed are the following:

1. Is case management of the elderly an effective strategy in HMOs—and, if so, what are the organizational characteristics and techniques associated with success?
2. Are special outreach programs or health assessments needed to ensure access for the elderly in more complex health delivery settings?
3. What do patterns of disenrollment suggest about ease of access and quality of care in HMOs?

Quality of care. Quality of care covers a broad and complex set of issues. Federal regulations require that HMOs and CMPs make organizational arrangements for quality-assurance programs if they wish to participate in Medicare risk-based contracting. The legislation states these programs should "stress health outcomes to the extent consistent with the state of the art," collect and review data on patient care, and include mechanisms for action in the case of "inappropriate or substandard" provision of services (Section 1301(c)(7) of the Public Health Service Act). The quality-assurance programs developed in response to these regulations span a wide range—from a small committee reviewing selected cases to sophisticated data systems maintained by a few large plans. Often, HMOs lump together utilization controls and quality assurance, so that it becomes difficult to separate the utilization control components from those concerned with quality of care.

There is no consensus on the appropriate methods for assessing quality of care or on techniques for assuring quality, either in the fee-for-service sector or HMOs. Further, it is difficult to differentiate factors influencing quality of care from those affecting access. (For example, case management is believed to ensure continuity in treatment and thus better quality medical care but may also provide a regular point of entry to the health care system, thus improving access.) Most studies to date indicate that quality of care in HMOs is as good as that provided in the fee-for-service sector (Luft 1981, Brown 1983; Brook 1973; Koepsell and Soroko, in Reidel et al. 1984). There are, however, still few empirical studies of quality of care in HMOs.

One recent study does raise some concern. Ware and his colleagues examined health outcomes for persons randomly assigned to receive care from the fee-for-service sector or a prepaid health plan (Ware et al. 1986). At the end of the three- to five-year study period, low-income enrollees who were initially in poor health appeared to be worse off than their fee-for-service counterparts, while high-income enrollees were in better health than a comparison group in the fee-for-service sector. As measured by health outcomes, at least some enrollees received poorer quality care than might have been the case in the fee-for-service sector. In interpreting the data, the authors suggest that the poor may be less adept at coping with barriers to access in HMOs, such as difficulty in making appointments or arranging transportation to sites of care. These findings suggest that for some people, perhaps those who are less aggressive in seeking care or less skillful in dealing with complex organizations, prepaid groups may deliver poorer care.

Increasing effort is being spent to monitor and evaluate quality of care for the Medicare population. The 1986 budget reconciliation bill added HMOs to the oversight responsibilities of professional review organizations that already monitor the quality of inpatient care to Medicare beneficiaries in the fee-for-service sector. There is, however, still little knowledge about the organizational attributes of prepaid or fee-for-service settings that may affect quality. The theoretical incentives for better or poorer quality of care in prepaid groups, as for improved or diminished access, have been described briefly here, but empirical evidence remains scarce.

Can the "promise" be realized?
Whether enrollment of Medicare beneficiaries in HMOs will result in lower program costs and better medical care for enrollees depends on several factors. This section is structured around three questions intended to advance our understanding of these factors. These questions focus on enrollment and disenrollment, cost savings, and characteristics of enrollees. Findings presented in this section are from two of the original eight Medicare demonstrations sponsored by the HCFA in 1980 and 1981—Fallon Community Health Plan of Worcester, Massachusetts, and Greater Marshfield Community Health Plan of Marshfield, Wisconsin.[7]

Fallon and Marshfield are best regarded as case studies. They began serving Medicare beneficiaries at a time when few prepaid plans had experience with this population. Both plans initially underestimated levels of use, had problems with out-of-plan use by enrollees, and implemented new utilization controls to stem cost overruns during the demonstration (Carpenter 1985; Bonanno and Wetle 1984; Greenlick and Lamb 1985). Fallon continues to serve Medicare enrollees under a risk contract. Marshfield discontinued enrollment of the elderly in their prepaid plan after the two-year demonstration but continues to serve this population on a fee-for-service basis.

Plan descriptions. Fallon is a group model HMO established in 1977 and co-sponsored by the Fallon Clinic and Blue Cross of Massachusetts. It was the first Medicare demonstration to begin operation (in April 1980) and the first HMO to sign a TEFRA risk contract. Currently, there are about 12,000 Medicare beneficiaries who are capitated enrollees with Fallon's senior plan. About 16 percent of the plan's membership is elderly, and 40 percent of the 1986 budget was designated for care to senior plan enrollees (from remarks by Christy Bell 1986b).

Marshfield Clinic was established in 1916. In 1971 the Marshfield Clinic, St. Joseph's Hospital, and Blue Cross/Blue Shield United of Wisconsin jointly established a prepaid health care program called the Greater Marshfield Community Health Plan. The prepaid health plan is often described as an Independent Practice Association (IPA) type or network HMO.

Marshfield Clinic is a large (173 physicians in 1980) multispecialty group practice, serving a rural population in north central Wisconsin. The clinic is the major provider of physician services, but the group has developed relationships with other local physicians to provide a broader delivery system for prepaid plan members and to give members better geographic access. These physicians are paid a percentage of their charges out of the clinic's capitation payment. As a result, most providers in the area participate in the prepaid plan, and patients often do not have to change providers to join the prepaid plan. The prepaid component forms about one-third of the clinic's business, and physicians in the clinic are usually unaware of whether they are treating prepaid or fee-for-service patients (Broida and Lerner 1975). The Marshfield Medicare demonstration began in June 1980 and ended in September 1982.[8]

Claims data. Two data sources are used in this chapter. The first consists of use and expenditure data obtained from the Medicare Statistical System and, for enrollees during the demonstration period, from the HMO sites.[9] Data on characteristics of enrollees and controls are limited to those found in the Medicare files (e.g., age, sex, and type of entitlement).

For Marshfield these data run from January 1979 through September 1982 for about 8,600 enrollees and a sample fee-for-service comparison group of about 14,400. Both enrollees and controls have a maximum of one year of data in the preenrollment period and a maximum of 27 months of data in the postenrollment or demonstration period. Marshfield began enrollment of Medicare beneficiaries in June 1980; 56 percent of those who joined enrolled in that month. At Fallon data cover the period January 1979 through December 1983 for about 5,300 enrollees and a comparison group of about 14,500. Both enrollees and controls have a maximum of one year of preenrollment data and a maximum of 33 months of demonstration period data. Fallon began enrollment in April 1980 and enrolled 18 percent of total enrollment in the first month and 54 percent in the first three months.

Charges for HMO enrollees are fee-for-service equivalents (both Marshfield and Fallon serve fee-for-service patients, in addition to prepaid plan members) obtained from the two plans. To ensure comparability between enrollee and control group charge data, several adjustments were necessary.

First, charges for some services were removed from control group data and from enrollee data for the period prior to enrollment, because data on charges for these services were not available for the enrollee group after enrollment. For Part A charges, skilled nursing facility (SNF) charges were excluded. For Part B charges, charges associated with home health services and hospital outpatient department (OPD) emergency room (ER) charges were excluded.[10]

Second, each year of charge data was adjusted for inflation, using the medical care component of the consumer price index. This averaged about 11 percent a year from 1979 to 1982. All charges in these analyses are in constant 1982 dollars.

Third, two adjustments were made to Part B charges for enrollees for the period of enrollment. Charges obtained from the HMOs were total charges, without application of the fee screen reduction applied to Medicare Part B charges under fee-for-service. The Medicare Statistical System retains only these reduced fee-for-service charges and retains no charges for beneficiaries who do not meet their annual deductible. During the demonstration period, this reduction in Part B fee-for-service charges averaged 21 percent in Massachusetts and 25 percent in Wisconsin. Total submitted Part B charges for Fallon and Marshfield enrollees have been reduced accordingly. Following the fee screen reduction, charges for any enrollee whose Part B charges were less than the Part B deductible ($60 until 1982, $75 since) were reduced to zero.

The analyses of enrollee admissions and charges often are divided into a preenrollment period and a demonstration or postenrollment period. To create a preenrollment and demonstration period for the fee-for-service control group, a random start date was assigned to these beneficiaries, based on enrollment dates of the HMO population (stratification variables used to assign dates to controls were age, sex, and a geographic variable, McDevitt 1984). Analyses of admission and charge data also adjust for differing lengths of preenrollment and demonstration period experience.

Survey data. The second source of data used in this chapter is a survey conducted in the fall of 1982 of 307 enrollees and 322 controls at Fallon and 303 enrollees and 392 controls at Marshfield. Data were collected on health status, income, education, attitudes toward providers, ambulatory care use, and other characteristics. The age-sex distribution of people in the enrollee and fee-for-service samples were matched (equal numbers in each of ten age-sex cells, male and female, with five age groups beginning at sixty-five).

Will beneficiaries enroll and will they stay enrolled? The steady increases in HMO enrollment among the elderly and the rising number of plans with TEFRA risk contracts indicates considerable interest on the part of both beneficiaries and HMOs in beneficiary enrollment (trends in enrollment are reported in McMillan, Lubitz, and Russell 1987). Table 10.3 indicates characteristics and attitudes related to enrollment at Marshfield and Fallon (when possible, variables are mea-

TABLE 10.3
Attitudes and Characteristics Related to Enrollment (Logistic Regression, 1 = Enrolled): Survey Data, Fall 1982[a]

Attitudes and characteristics	Fallon		Marshfield	
	b	p value	b	p value
Intercept	0.313	0.233	−0.528	0.029
Attitudes[b]				
Worries about health			0.468	0.043
Avoids going to doctor	−0.461	0.018		
Health status				
Needs help with self-care	−1.285	0.015		
Needs help walking				
Unable to do routine chores	−0.593	0.030	−0.947	0.001
Previous insurance				
Private insurance	0.561	0.001	−1.771	0.001
Medicaid				
Demographics[b]				
Married	0.410	0.015		
Low income			−0.706	0.002
High income			−0.115	0.553
Low education				
High education				
Prior use				
Usual source of care	−0.681	0.005	0.675	0.007
Hospital admissions				
Part B charges			0.009	0.001
Other				
Formerly disabled				
More than 4 years at address				

Note: Variables with no coefficients were included in a preliminary stepwise regression but were not significant at the 0.05 level and were excluded from the logistic regression.
[a]The sample design controlled for age-sex differences between the enrollee and control populations.
[b]The attitude and demographic variables are at the time of the survey for both enrollees and controls. Health status for enrollees was measured at time of enrollment. Income was for calendar year 1981.

sured at time of enrollment; otherwise, they reflect characteristics at the time of the survey). A stepwise ordinary least-squares regression was used to select significant variables for the model. A logistic regression model was then developed with those variables.

At enrollment, Fallon enrollees were less likely than controls to need help with activities of daily living (ADLs) or to be unable to do routine chores. Enrollees also were more likely to be married and to have private insurance and less likely to have a usual source of care. Although there was no difference in needing help with ADLs between enrollees and controls at Marshfield, as at Fallon, enrollees were less likely to be unable to do routine chores. In contrast to Fallon, enrollees at Marshfield were more likely to have a usual source of care and less likely to carry private health insurance. In addition, Medicare claims data showed that enrollees at Marshfield had higher Part B charges prior to enrollment than did controls. Many enrollees at Marshfield were able to join the prepaid plan without changing physicians (see the earlier description of the Marshfield Clinic) and may have joined at the suggestion of their physician. Early findings from the Medicare Competition Demonstration (1986a) indicate 50 percent of enrollees in IPA plans did not have to change doctors to join the plan, as against 6 percent of enrollees in the group model plans, most of whom had to change doctors to join.

As suggested by studies of younger enrollees (Merrill et al. 1985), these data indicate different factors may influence the enrollment decision for different types of HMOs. Under the style of prepaid group typified by Marshfield, in which enrollment does not require changing physicians, having a tie to a physician may increase likelihood of enrollment since the physician is in a position to recruit people into the plan. Marshfield, however, like many older IPAs, does not put individual physicians directly at risk for the costs of patient care. Newer style IPAs may be more likely to do so, perhaps leading to different recruitment behavior by physicians. Berenson (1986) provides a thoughtful discussion of the potential conflict of interest for physicians as HMO recruiters. On the one hand, they must consider the financial advantages to chronically ill patients of HMO enrollment; on the other, they must weigh the financial consequences of adverse selection for themselves and their fellow HMO physicians. Although most of the health status variables in Table 10.3 (as well as Tables 10.5 and 10.6) do not indicate selection bias at Marshfield, lack of private insurance coverage, and higher Part B charges prior to enrollment were associated with enrollment. If enrollees do not have to change doctors, financial considerations may play a larger part in the decision to enroll.

At Fallon the greater likelihood of enrollment among those with no usual source of care adds to the evidence that group model HMOs are more likely to attract enrollees without existing ties to a physician.[11] Among the elderly, these individuals are likely to be healthier (with universal Medicare coverage and greater health needs, the elderly are less likely than younger people to be without a usual source of care). The health status measures in Table 10.3 (and more convincingly those in Tables 10.5 and 10.6) indicate those who chose to enroll at Fallon were healthier than those who did not.

While understanding the elements that affect enrollment decisions by Medicare beneficiaries is important, of equal importance is understanding who chooses to leave an HMO after enrolling and why. Disenrollment from HMOs is of concern from the HMO's point of view because high levels of disenrollment can lead to administrative expense and may indicate problems in delivery of care. Who disenrolls may also indicate access problems or pressures on selected patients to leave because they are troublesome or expensive to serve. Finally, disenrollment may reflect the extent to which individuals, having tried an HMO, prefer alternative forms of health care delivery.

Medicare beneficiaries have the right to disenroll from an HMO with thirty days' notice (younger group enrollees usually can choose to enroll or disenroll only once a year). For this reason and others, including the higher levels of use characteristic of elderly people, factors in disenrollment may be different for Medicare beneficiaries than for the younger population.

Different HMOs have experienced very different rates of disenrollment among the elderly. Only a small percentage disenrolled (both voluntary and involuntary disenrollment, excluding deaths) during the demonstration period at Fallon (4.9 percent) and Marshfield (2.5 percent). In the Medicare Competition Demonstration (1986a), of those enrolling during 1984, 22.9 percent disenrolled within one year. Disenrollment rates were at 10 percent or less in eight of the ten market areas, but in six HMOs in the other two market areas disenrollment ranged from 20 to 40 percent. About 45 percent of all disenrollment in this study occurred within three months of joining the plan. However, some Medicare Competition Demonstration HMOs experienced constant rates of disenrollment during the year, and others had higher levels of disenrollment among those enrolled six months or longer than among those more recently enrolled.

Table 10.4 compares characteristics of enrollees and disenrollees at Fallon and Marshfield. At both sites, those who disenrolled had higher rates of hospital admissions in the period prior to enrollment than once they joined the HMO. At Fallon total Part B charges were significantly higher in the preenrollment period for disenrollees but once in the HMO were no different for disenrollees and those who stayed enrolled.

While disenrollment at Fallon and Marshfield was rare, those who later disenrolled appear to have been higher users of services prior to enrollment than those who stayed. There are at least two hypotheses concerning these disenrollees. One

TABLE 10.4
Comparison of Disenrollees with Those Who Remained Enrolled—Hospital Use and Physician Charges Prior to and During Enrollment

Hospital use and physician charges	Fallon		Marshfield	
	Disenrolled	**Stayed** [a]	**Disenrolled**	**Stayed** [a]
Unweighted population[b]	264	5,045	221	8,389
Percent	4.9%	95.1%	2.5%	97.5%
Mean age	71.4	71.5	73.1	72.2
Percent male	43.6%	48.5%	43.2%	47.0%
Mean admissions per 1,000 person-years				
Preenrollment	303[d] (36)	187 (8)	313[d] (56)	192 (6)
Enrollment period	373 (65)	271 (9)	454 (91)	390 (11)
Mean hospital days per person-year				
Preenrollment	3.6[d] (0.6)	1.8 (0.1)	2.6 (0.5)	1.7 (0.1)
Enrollment period	4.2 (1.2)	2.4 (0.1)	4.3 (0.9)	3.6 (0.1)
All Part B charges per person-year[c]				
Preenrollment	418[d] (54)	295 (10)	330 (42)	344 (9)
Enrollment period	301 (41)	369 (8)	795 (120)	845 (17)

Note: Standard errors appear in parentheses.

[a] Includes persons who died during the demonstration period.

[b] Includes persons who enrolled at age 65 and have no data for the preenrollment period.

[c] In constant 1982 dollars.

[d] Indicates a statistically significant difference between those who disenrolled and those who stayed at the 0.05 level or greater.

is that they are in poorer health, as reflected by their higher prior use. Disenrollees in the Medicare Competition Demonstration (1986a) were older, poorer, more worried about their health, and more likely to report their health status was poor at time of enrollment. The other is that these individuals have a propensity for higher levels of use and find unsatisfactory the relatively reduced level of services provided to them by the HMO. Buchanan and Cretin (1986) found higher claims among disenrollees under sixty-five years of age in the first year following disenrollment, which might be used to support either hypothesis. It does appear, however, that persons who disenroll may have different patterns of service use before and after HMO membership than those who remain enrolled.

A variety of reasons were given for disenrollment in the Medicare Competition Demonstration (1986a). About 19 percent disenrolled because they did not realize they had to switch doctors in order to enroll. Thus, many beneficiaries appear to be unclear about the restrictions associated with HMO enrollment. Additional reasons for disenrollment were moving from the service area (9 percent), feeling the HMO was too expensive (5.7 percent), and lack of availability of a particular service or specialty (6.4 percent).

With regard to the restrictions associated with HMO membership, out-of-plan use was a significant problem in the early demonstrations as well. Kaiser had greater problems with out-of-plan use among the oldest enrollees (remarks by Sara Lamb 1986; Greenlick and Lamb 1985) and urgent care services were increased at Fallon to reduce unauthorized use of hospital outpatient facilities (remarks by Christy Bell 1986b).[12] As the number of HMOs increases and beneficiaries become more knowledgeable about HMOs, levels of disenrollment related to such misunderstandings may decline. In areas where several HMOs compete for Medicare enrollees, disenrollment may turn out to be linked to switching among HMOs, as well as for the reasons mentioned here.

Will HMOs reach those who could benefit most from improved access and continuity of care? One of the major issues surrounding HMO enrollment of Medicare beneficiaries is that of biased selection—whether HMO enrollees are healthier or sicker than average. Eggers and Prihoda (1982), using Medicare claims data, showed that on one measure of health status, prior use of services, enrollees were healthier than controls at two Medicare HMOs, Fallon and Kaiser-Portland, although not at Marshfield. The data from Fallon and Marshfield provide additional health status measures that bear on this issue.

Table 10.5 compares enrollees and controls on several self-reported health status indicators. Enrollees at Fallon were more likely than controls to report themselves in better health than others their age and less likely to need help with self-care or to be unable to do routine chores. There were no differences between enrollees and controls at Marshfield. Table 10.6 shows selected conditions reported by enrollees and controls and whether they were receiving care for these

TABLE 10.5
Measures of Health Status for Enrollees and Controls: Survey Data, Fall 1982

	Fallon		Marshfield	
Health status measures	**Enrollees**	**Controls**	**Enrollees**	**Controls**
Reports fair or poor health	21.8%[a]	28.6%	35.3%	39.0%
Reports health "better or much better than others my age"	78.5[a]	64.0	62.4	61.2
Needs help with self-care	4.6[a]	8.7	8.6	5.1
Needs help walking	9.1	11.2	13.2	12.0
Unable to do routine chores	13.7[a]	19.6	22.4	28.1
Aware of problem needing care when enrolled	1.6	—	2.0	—

[a]Chi-square test indicates enrollee population is different from the control population at 0.05 level or better.

conditions. Unlike the measures of overall perception of health and daily functioning (see Table 10.5), there were almost no differences in prevalence of conditions between enrollees and controls at either site. The exception is the higher percentage of enrollees with a vision problem; likelihood of treatment for this condition was higher among enrollees as well. This undoubtedly reflects coverage of routine vision exams at both HMOs, not a covered benefit under Medicare. (Fallon also initially covered one pair of glasses every twelve months, and, from 1982 on, one pair every twenty-four months.) It is worth noting that the condition data do not provide evidence of biased selection at Fallon, as do the other measures of health status. The development of measures of function for the elderly has been spurred in part by the need for better measures of overall health status than diagnosis or condition (Katz and Akpom 1976). Furthermore, the relationship between diagnosis and function is not well understood (Besdine 1984).

Table 10.7 provides a third measure of health status differences—mortality rates among enrollee and control populations. At both Fallon and Marshfield, mortality rates per 1,000 persons were lower among men and women who enrolled than among those who did not. Differences were greater at Fallon. Across all age groups at Fallon, mortality rates among enrollees were less than half those of controls. At Marshfield, mortality rate differences were least between male enrollees and controls.

Taken together, the data in Tables 10.5 to 10.7 appear to indicate favorable selection among enrollees at Fallon; however, only the mortality rate data suggest favorable selection at Marshfield. There is no indication of adverse selection.

Most observers agree that there is currently little financial incentive for HMOs to enroll sicker beneficiaries (McClure 1984; Lubitz et al. 1985). Although this is

TABLE 10.6
Presence of and Care for Conditions Among Enrollees and Controls: Survey Data, Fall 1982

Selected conditions at time of survey	Fallon				Marshfield			
	Has condition		Receiving care for condition		Has condition		Receiving care for condition	
	Enrollees	Controls	Enrollees	Controls	Enrollees	Controls	Enrollees	Controls
Arthritis or rheumatism	44.6%	49.7%	45.3%	50.6%	59.4%	52.6%	32.2%	28.2%
High blood pressure	42.7	40.1	97.0[a]	89.9	34.7	36.0	93.3	87.9
Heart trouble	24.1	28.0	90.5	88.9	28.1	23.5	95.3[a]	85.9
Circulation trouble in arms or legs	22.5[a]	33.2	65.2	51.4	30.7	30.1	39.8	34.8
Diabetes	9.1	11.5	82.1	73.0	10.6	11.2	81.3	90.9
Digestive disorders such as ulcers, gallbladder trouble, other liver, stomach, intestinal problems	11.7	13.4	75.0	60.5	12.9	15.1	38.5	42.4
Urinary tract disorders	9.1	11.8	57.1	65.8	14.9	14.8	42.2	39.7
Effects of stroke	3.3[a]	8.1	50.0	55.6	6.3	7.7	57.9	53.3
Hearing impediment or impairment	29.3	25.5	33.3	47.6	41.9[a]	30.4	36.2	40.3
Vision impediment or impairment	88.6[a]	70.5	97.8[a]	87.7	79.9[a]	67.1	89.7[a]	79.9
Periods of anxiety or depression	17.3	15.2	9.4[a]	28.6	22.8	22.5	18.8[a]	8.0

[a] Chi-square test indicates enrollee population is different from the control population at 0.05 level or better.

TABLE 10.7
Mortality Rates per 1,000 Persons During the Demonstration Period[a]

Sex by age[b]	Fallon			Marshfield		
	Enrollees	Controls	Ratio E/C	Enrollees	Controls	Ratio E/C
Total	42.8	102.4	0.42	63.3	106.2	0.60
Male						
65–66	33.4	71.1	0.47	52.1	57.4	0.91
67–74	59.1	120.8	0.49	74.2	81.3	0.91
75–84	66.7	175.2	0.38	105.7	134.3	0.79
85 or over	124.5	285.4	0.44	167.9	236.5	0.71
Female						
65–66	11.4	33.8	0.34	20.5	34.8	0.59
67–74	31.4	74.6	0.42	38.9	46.8	0.83
75–84	44.0	92.9	0.47	58.1	73.0	0.80
85 or over	97.9	202.3	0.48	114.9	196.8	0.58

[a]For thirty-three months at Fallon and twenty-seven months at Marshfield.
[b]Age at enrollment (or random start date for controls).

a group that theoretically could benefit from organizational features of HMOs that improve access and continuity of care, current payments to HMOs from Medicare do not provide higher amounts for such people (see Eggers and Prihoda [1982] for the AAPCC as presently calculated). One means of encouraging HMOs to enroll sicker beneficiaries is generally agreed to be the inclusion of a health status measure in the calculation of the AAPCC. This would pay HMOs for the added costs of serving high-use individuals. It would also protect the Medicare program from overpayment in the case of biased selection of healthy people into HMOs.

Several types of health status adjustments to the AAPCC have been explored. These include incorporating measures of prior use or diagnostic information (Ash et al. 1986); functional health status measures (Thomas and Lichtenstein 1986); or using clinical risk factors, such as high blood pressure. Both the predictive strength and administrative feasibility of some of these measures is currently being studied (Lubitz [1986] provides an extensive discussion of the current state of research into health status adjustors for the AAPCC).

With larger numbers of enrollees, potential losses to Medicare due to favorable selection increase, and an improved AAPCC becomes more urgent. There are other approaches to capitation, however, that circumvent the need for basing the AAPCC on the fee-for-service population, such as putting a large employer or union group at risk for covering retirees.[13] Under such an arrangement, employers would be paid a capitated rate to cover Medicare benefits for all retirees but could offer a choice of plans with varying benefits (HMOs and other options). The capitated rate, rather than relying on the AAPCC, could be based on the group's claims experience. (An unintended incentive to control claims might develop, however.) Biased selection would not be a problem for the Medicare program if employers had to cover all retirees and retirees could not opt out of the system. However, biased selection could be a problem for the employer or union that offered a choice among plans that included both HMO and fee-for-service options.

Enrollment under such capitation arrangements potentially could be extensive. In 1977 a little less than a quarter of the elderly (36 percent of all those with private insurance) held some type of group insurance, almost all of which was related to present or former employment (Cafferata 1984). This type of coverage was more likely among those sixty-five to sixty-nine than among those seventy-five or older, an indication it is now more common. A sizable number of beneficiaries could be covered under this type of approach, exceeding perhaps the number of beneficiaries that would enroll in HMOs in the current environment. Many beneficiaries could not be included in such a system, however. This group may consist of people in the poorest health—those not in the labor force (some for health reasons) and those who work in jobs that do not provide private insurance coverage.

Will HMOs save money for the Medicare program? The presumption that HMOs can provide care at lower costs is central to arguments that beneficiaries should be encouraged to enroll in prepaid plans. But it remains unclear how much of the reduced use among enrollees is attributable to the workings of the HMO and how much to favorable selection of enrollees.

HMOs continue to be concerned about adverse selection. Several have discontinued participation in risk contracting, and others express concern about potential losses (*Modern Healthcare* 1986). Studies in the 1970s on the population under sixty-five years of age suggested that HMOs would attract people who had more serious health problems or who anticipated increased use of services in the near future (Bice 1975; Tessler and Mechanic 1976). More recent studies indicate healthier people enroll (Jackson-Beeck and Kleinman 1983; Eggers and Prihoda 1982). Since HMOs are paid by Medicare in a way that assumes enrollees are representative with regard to costs and use of services, enrolling a healthier group of beneficiaries results in greater profits for the HMO. If prepaid plan enrollees become a significant proportion of Medicare beneficiaries, under conditions of favorable selection payments to HMOs would be based on an increasingly smaller and sicker fee-for-service population.

In addition to the health status measures examined earlier, use and charges prior to enrollment provide some indication of biased selection between those who enroll in HMOs and others. Again, the experience at Fallon and Marshfield is instructive. Charges for Part B and inpatient services were consistently lower for enrollees at Fallon, both prior to and after enrollment compared with the control group of fee-for-service beneficiaries (Table 10.8). At Marshfield, however,

TABLE 10.8
Mean Charges per Person-Month (in Constant 1982 Dollars) for Enrollees and Controls in the Preenrollment Period and Demonstration Period [a]

Type of expense	Preperiod			Demonstration period		
	Enrollees	Controls	Ratio	Enrollees	Controls	Ratio
Fallon						
Total Medicare dollars	88 [b]	151	0.58	130 [b]	306	0.43
Total Part A dollars	63 [b]	116	0.54	100 [b]	242	0.41
Total Part B dollars	25 [b]	35	0.71	30 [b]	64	0.47
Marshfield						
Total Medicare dollars	76 [b]	96	0.79	182	170	1.07
Total Part A dollars	48 [b]	69	0.70	111	123	0.90
Total Part B dollars	29	28	1.04	70 [b]	47	1.49

[a] Weighted to control for age and sex differences between enrollees and controls.
[b] Significantly different from control group at the 0.05 level or better.

TABLE 10.9
Mean Hospital Admissions per Person per 1,000 Person-Years[a]

	Fallon			Marshfield		
	Enrollees	Controls	Ratio	Enrollees	Controls	Ratio
Population[b]	5,309	14,546		8,630	14,432	
Total						
One year preenrollment	195	307	0.64	200	230	0.89
One year postenrollment	267[d]	431[d]	0.62	355[d]	331[d]	1.07
Second year postenrollment	228[d]	397[d]	0.57	337	339	0.99
Survivors						
One year preenrollment	184	256	0.72	175	184	0.95
One year postenrollment	227[d]	288[d]	0.79	255[d]	205[d]	1.24
Second year postenrollment	178[d]	299	0.59	249	246[d]	1.01
Decedents[c]						
One year preenrollment	420	773	0.54	530	635	0.83
One year postenrollment	1,167[d]	1,808[d]	0.64	1,838[d]	1,509[d]	1.22
Second year postenrollment	1,819[d]	2,134[d]	0.85	2,642[d]	2,068[d]	1.28

[a]Weighted to control for age and sex differences between enrollees and controls.

[b]Population counts during first year postenrollment.

[c]Deaths during demonstration were: Fallon enrollees, 227; Fallon controls, 1,492; Marshfield enrollees, 546; Marshfield controls, 1,536.

[d]Significantly different from previous one-year period at 0.05 level or better.

while inpatient and total Medicare charges were lower for enrollees in the pre-enrollment period, following enrollment these charges were similar for enrollees and controls. Charges for physician services were higher after enrollment among Marshfield plan members compared with controls. The increase in charges between the preenrollment period and demonstration reflects the higher costs associated with deaths in the demonstration period.

Table 10.9 shows hospital admissions for one year prior to enrollment (or random start date) and two years after. The ratio of enrollee to control group admissions at Fallon indicates consistently fewer admissions among enrollees in each one-year period. Ratios were similar in the year preenrollment (0.64) and the first year postenrollment (0.62). Further reductions in enrollee admissions relative to controls appear to have been achieved in the second year postenrollment (from 0.62 to 0.57, among survivors from 0.79 to 0.59).

At Marshfield enrollee admission rates were below those of controls one year prior to enrollment. But in the first year following enrollment, enrollee rates exceeded those for the control group. Admission rates were virtually identical for the two groups in the second year postenrollment, although admission rates for enrollee decedents remained higher than control group decedents in the second year.

The Part B charge data (Table 10.10) show a similar pattern. Fallon enrollees were lower users of Part B services prior to enrollment and remained so after joining the HMO. Fallon appears, however, to have achieved a further reduction in use for their enrollee group in the second year following enrollment (ratio of enrollee to control charges dropped from 0.61 to 0.54 for all enrollees, 0.85 to 0.66 for survivor enrollees). Marshfield enrollees and controls had similar levels of Part B charges in the year prior to enrollment. In the first year postenrollment, however, enrollee Part B charges were 1.7 times those of the control group. Enrollee charges remained higher in the second year postenrollment as well.

Fallon and Marshfield were among the first HMOs to provide services to Medicare beneficiaries under risk contracting. Some of what they experienced may be attributable to lack of experience among prepaid plans in serving the elderly. However, these data support the conclusion that enrollees at Fallon were a healthier group than those who did not join the HMO. They suggest as well, however, that Fallon achieved further reductions in both hospital admissions and Part B use among their enrollees. For Marshfield, the picture is more complex. Using only prior use data, Marshfield enrollees appear to be similar or slightly lower users of services than controls. Once enrolled, however, both admission rates and Part B use in the first year was higher for enrollees than controls. In the second year, admission rate levels among enrollees fell to that of controls, but Part B charges remained 40 percent higher.

TABLE 10.10
Mean Part B Charges per Person per Person-Year in Constant 1982 Dollars[a]

	Fallon			Marshfield		
	Enrollees	Controls	Ratio	Enrollees	Controls	Ratio
Total						
One year preenrollment	$311	$437	0.71	$364	$353	1.03
One year postenrollment	385[b]	634[b]	0.61	787[b]	458[b]	1.72
Second year postenrollment	328[b]	612	0.54	751	528[b]	1.43
Survivors						
One year preenrollment	298	371	0.80	330	299	1.10
One year postenrollment	373[b]	437[b]	0.85	647[b]	313	2.06
Second year postenrollment	314[b]	476[b]	0.66	637	409[b]	1.56
Decedents						
One year preenrollment	592	1,047	0.57	825	823	1.00
One year postenrollment	657	2,536[b]	0.26	2,853[b]	1,821[b]	1.57
Second year postenrollment	756	3,031[b]	0.25	3,755[b]	2,752[b]	1.36

[a]Weighted to control for age and sex differences between enrollees and controls.
[b]Significantly different from previous one-year period at 0.05 level or better.

One explanation suggested for the Marshfield experience is that beneficiaries withheld their use of services in anticipation of enrollment in order to reduce their out-of-pocket expenses.[14] The pattern of Part B charge data (i.e., Part B charges increased substantially after enrollment) lends credence to this argument. In addition, Eggers and Prihoda found that the ratio of enrollee Part B reimbursements to fee-for-service Part B reimbursements was lower in the year prior to enrollment than in any of the three previous years. We cannot ascertain from our data whether this explanation is correct.

HMOs and Medicare—the Future

Enrollment of Medicare beneficiaries at risk under TEFRA increased between February and November of 1986 from around 500,000 to almost 800,000, representing nearly 3 percent of Medicare beneficiaries. About 8 percent of the U.S. population is currently enrolled in HMOs and among federal employees who have had an HMO option for many years, 16 percent were enrolled in 1985. Both the recent increases and experience with other populations suggest there may be considerable room for increased HMO enrollment among the elderly. In addition, as the population ages, more younger people for whom an HMO is their usual source of care will reach retirement age. Regardless of whether there is some upper limit of HMO enrollment, the search for mechanisms to increase capitation of beneficiaries will continue. It is conceivable that many beneficiaries may also eventually be enrolled under alternative capitation arrangements such as employer-at-risk programs.

Concerns about quality of care in HMOs and ease of access will continue as well, prompted by the evidence that these organizations control costs through reduced utilization. More than one health care analyst has suggested it is not possible to implement stringent cost controls and simultaneously maximize access and quality of care (Feder 1986; Mechanic 1985). There is still little research to illuminate the trade-offs among costs, quality, and access for patients cared for by HMOs (the HMO industry often argues these relationships are no better understood in the fee-for-service sector). Awareness of these concerns by the HMO industry can be seen in the efforts of organizations such as the Group Health Association of America and the American Medical Care Review Association (bodies whose memberships are largely group model HMOs and IPAs, respectively) to establish an independent quality review body.

Diversity in the HMO industry is increasing. HMOs now vary in terms of ownership with for-profit HMOs increasing in enrollment and numbers faster than nonprofit HMOs (McMillan, Lubitz, and Russell, 1987). Organizational characteristics differ as well, such as how physicians are selected and paid, how care is managed through "gatekeepers," and how processes of care are monitored and controlled. Most HMO research has focused on mature, established HMOs such as Kaiser, Group Health of Puget Sound, and the Marshfield Clinic. But these established HMOs may differ from newer organizations, and a recent national HMO census indicated more than a quarter of all HMOs in 1985 were less than a year old (Interstudy 1986). The same survey showed IPAs now represent just over half of all HMOs. How these new HMOs differ from older organizations and each other is not well understood, nor are the implications of such diversity for service delivery. The environment within which HMOs operate is changing as well. Competition among HMOs is occurring in some areas of the country, and the fee-for-service sector is responding with new alternatives such as PPOs. Given these developments, it may no longer be useful to view HMOs as homogeneous systems for delivering care.

One of the major resources for understanding patterns of use and expenditures of Medicare beneficiaries, and examining issues of ease of access and quality of care, is the Medicare Statistical System. This data base consists of claims submitted by fee-for-service providers of care. As beneficiaries are prospectively capitated, their utilization experience disappears from the Medicare data base. While there is concern about burdening HMOs by requesting data, many keep data on visits and admissions for internal management purposes. In addition, many large companies with HMO contracts are beginning to ask for cost and use data to evaluate company health expenditures for employees enrolled in HMOs. It seems clear that many of the questions about Medicare HMO enrollment cannot be addressed without such data.

Despite the optimism of some policymakers and HMO advocates, it is unlikely that HMOs will be the optimal solution for all beneficiaries for the combined problems of containing costs and maintaining or improving access and quality of care. Today, HMOs are especially popular for their perceived ability to control costs. In the past, advocates stressed the HMO's ability to improve access and shift the focus of services from acute to preventive care. Under what circumstances HMOs, and more broadly capitation, are most likely to meet these goals and who can benefit most from participation in these types of delivery systems are among the issues for future research.

Notes

This chapter benefited from the review and comments of James Lubitz, Arnold Epstein, Sue Levkoff, Marian Gornick, and Paul Eggers.

1. This review draws on several versions of the legislative history of capitation and Medicare. Among them are Trieger, Galblum, and Riley (1981); Bonanno and Wetle (1984); and Langwell and

Hadley (1986). A detailed account of the evolution and outcome of the HMO Act of 1973 is found in Brown (1983).

2. The ACR is based on a plan's community rate—the per capita average premium for the HMO's non-Medicare line of business. This community rate is then adjusted for the expected level of use and costs of the elderly and differences in the benefit package offered for those under and over sixty-five. In the early demonstrations, data from Kaiser, which had experience serving the elderly, were used to calculate the initial ACR (Carpenter 1985). Once an HMO has experience serving the elderly, the ACR can be calculated using the HMO's own experience.

3. As of December 1986, 20 of 145 plans with Medicare risk contracts charged no premium to Medicare enrollees.

4. Competitive medical plans are organizations that offer prepaid delivery systems but are not federally qualified HMOs. As of November 1986, 17 of 145 Medicare risk contracts were with CMPs, covering 46,740 beneficiaries.

5. As of May 1986 another 2 percent of beneficiaries were in cost-based Part B plans.

6. An example of the types of utilization controls implemented by HMOs is provided by Health Plans of Michigan, Inc., an IPA-type HMO, which lists the following among its utilization control procedures (from remarks by Gerald Landgraf, National Health Policy Form 1986):

□ Member selection of a primary physician
□ Primary physician control (has responsibility for management of care and costs with incentive systems for rewarding efficiency, as well as risk to penalize inappropriate practice patterns)
□ Controlled in and out of plan referrals
□ Precertification of elective hospitalization and concurrent review of all hospitalization
□ Physician credentialing process
□ Utilization and cost management reporting
□ Review process for over- and underutilization, with required physician participation in the review process
□ Aggressive quality-assurance programs
□ Enforcement and disciplinary procedures

7. These analyses are restricted to the elderly, although some disabled beneficiaries were enrolled as well.

8. Descriptions of the Marshfield Clinic are found in Mechanic et al. (1980) and Carpenter (1985). Carpenter (1985) also provides a detailed explanation of the rate-setting procedures and assesses the fiscal performance during the demonstration of Marshfield, Fallon, and Kaiser.

9. Both Fallon and Marshfield Clinic serve fee-for-service enrollees. Marshfield maintains data on services and associated charges for all patients whether fee-for-service or prepaid. Charges for Fallon enrollees are fee-for-service equivalents from encounter forms completed for patients. Inpatient charges for enrollees were taken from claims, which continued to be filed as though these patients were fee-for-service.

10. For the period prior to enrollment (or prior to the random start date for controls) the excluded charges per person-month were as follows:

	Enrollees		Controls	
	Marshfield	Fallon	Marshfield	Fallon
SNF	$0.3	$0.9	$0.5	$2.8
Home health	0.6	1.0	0.8	3.2
Hospital OPD/ER	2.1	4.8	3.1	7.5

The control group sample was drawn to be representative of both the total Medicare fee-for-service population residing in the demonstration area, as well as the composition of the HMO-enrolled population, depending on the weight used. The sample was stratified by age, sex, and a residential indicator (see McDevitt 1984).

11. Garfinkel et al. (1986), using these same data, also reported persons who had to change providers to enroll were less likely to enroll.

12. Fallon implemented several educational measures to control out-of-plan use as well. They mailed "friendly reminders" to elderly enrollees about what to do in an emergency and reinforcing that they come to Fallon for all care. In addition, they sent enrollees phone stickers, introduced a senior newsletter, and mailed out wallet holders for Medicare and Fallon health plan cards (Christy Bell, personal communication 1986).

13. Competitive bidding among HMOs to provide services to Medicare beneficiaries is another approach. One advantage to competitive bidding is that it should save the government money in a situation where competition among HMOs would result in a price lower than the AAPCC. But breaking the link with fee-for-service expenditure levels (which is the basis for the AAPCC) raises other issues. The government would have to determine what its contribution toward premiums would be. If payment to HMOs under a competitive bidding system were substantially lower than the AAPCC, there would be pressure to reduce fee-for-service payments. This might lead to lower payments to physicians and hospitals. Or it might lead to a mandatory voucher system, in which all beneficiaries would choose a health plan and would have to contribute a share out-of-pocket for plans whose premiums were higher than the base amount the government would pay. Either scenario would represent a major change in the basic philosophy of the Medicare program as a service benefit program.

14. There was a gap of three to four months between much of the marketing effort at Marshfield and the beginning of the demonstration. There is anecdotal evidence of cancellations of appointments for examinations among fee-for-service patients at the clinic who planned to join the prepaid plan. Anecdotal evidence of physicians and patients postponing elective procedures is mentioned as well (Gregory Nycz, personal communication 1986). Some of these circumstances are unique to Marshfield and unlikely to recur. Buchanan and Cretin (1986), however, found the families in their study who joined HMOs withheld use prior to joining.

References

Aday, L., G. Fleming, and R. Andersen, *Access to Medical Care in the U.S.: Who Has It, Who Doesn't,* Chicago, IL: University of Chicago, Center for Health Administration Studies, Pluribus Press, 1984.

Ash, A., F. Porell, L. Gruenberg, E. Sawitz, and A. Beiser, "An Analysis of Alternative AAPCC models using data from the Continuous Medicare History Sample," working paper, Heller Graduate School, Brandeis University, August 1986.

Baloff, N., and M. J. Griffith, "Reply to Comments: Membership duration and Utilization Rates in a Prepaid Group Practice," *Medical Care,* 24(12):1233–1238, December 1981.

Bell, C., Fallon Community Health Plan, personal communication, 1986a.

———, Remarks to the National Health Policy Forum, Session entitled "HMOs and the Elderly: Bright Future or False Promise?" July 1986b.

Berenson, R., "Capitation and Conflict of Interest," *Health Affairs,* 5(1):141–153, Spring 1986.

Besdine, R., "The Data Base of Geriatric Medicine," in J. Rowe and R. Besdine, (eds.), *Health and Disease in Old Age,* Boston, MA: Little, Brown and Co., 1982.

———, "Functional Assessment in the Elderly: Relationship between Function and Diagnosis," paper presented at the Annual Conference of the Maryland Gerontological Association, October 1984.

Bice, T. W., "Risk Vulnerability and Enrollment in a Prepaid Group Practice," *Medical Care,* 13(8):698–703, 1975.

Bonanno, J. B., and T. Wetle, "HMO Enrollment of Medicare Recipients: An Analysis of Incentives and Barriers," *Journal of Health Politics, Policy, and Law,* 9(1):41–62, Spring 1984.

Branch, L., and K. Nemeth, "When Elders Fail to Visit Physicians," *Medical Care,* 23(11):1265–75, November 1985.

Broida, J., and M. Lerner, "Knowledge of Patient's Method of Payment by Physicians in a Group Practice," *Public Health Reports,* 90(2):113–118, April 1975.

Brook, R. H., "Critical Issues in the Assessment of Quality of Care and Their Relationship to HMOs," *Journal of Medical Education,* 48:114–134, 1973.

Brown, L. D., *Politics and Health Care Organization: HMOs as Federal Policy,* Washington, DC: The Brookings Institution, 1983.

Buchanan, J. L., and S. Cretin, "Risk Selection of Families Electing HMO Membership," *Medical Care,* 24(1):39–51, January 1986.

Cafferata, G. L., "Private Health Insurance Coverage of the Medicare Population," Data Preview 18, National Center for Health Services Research, National Health Care Expenditures Study, Rockville, MD: U.S. Department of Health and Human Services, Publication No. (PHS) 84-3362, September 1984.

Carpenter, B., *Analysis of Medicare Risk Contractors' ACR Development,* Contract No. 500-81-0017, Prepared for Health Care Financing Administration, Rockville, MD: Jurgovan and Blair, Inc., August 1985.

Davis, K., and D. Rowland, *Medicare Policy—New Directions for Health and Long Term Care,* Baltimore, MD: Johns Hopkins University Press, 1986.

Eggers, P. W., and R. Prihoda, "Pre-Enrollment Reimbursement Patterns of Medicare Beneficiaries Enrolled in 'At-Risk' HMOs," *Health Care Financing Review,* 4(1): 55–73, September 1982.

Feder, J., "Juggling Goals in Nursing Home Reimbursement Policy," paper presented at the Annual Meetings of the Association for Health Services Research, Boston, June 1986.

Friedlob, A., and J. Hadley, *Marketing Medicare in a Competitive Environment,* Health Care Financing Special Report, Baltimore, MD: Office of Research and Demonstrations, August 1985.

Garfinkel, S. R., W. E. Schlenger, K. R. McLeroy, et al., "Choice of Payment Plan in the Medicare Capitation Demonstration," *Medical Care,* 24(7):628–640 July 1986.

Greenlick, M. R., and S. J. Lamb, *A Demonstration of Alternative Models for Prepaid Capitation of Health Care Services for Medicare Recipients,* prepared for the Health Care Financing Administration under Contract 500-78-0078, August 1985.

Griffith, M. J., and N. Baloff, "Membership Duration and Utilization Rates in a Prepaid Group Practice," *Medical Care,* 19(12):1195–1210, December 1981.

Hall, B., General Motors Corporation, Remarks to the National Health Policy Forum, Session entitled "HMOs and the Elderly: Bright Future or False Promise?" July 1986.

Harvard Medicare Project, *Medicare: Coming of Age, A Proposal for Reform,* Cambridge, MA: Center for Health Policy and Management, J. F. Kennedy School of Government, Harvard University, March 1986.

Hirshfeld, S. B., and S. M. Myers, "Use of Ambulatory Services," in Reidel, et al., eds., *Use of Health Care Resources,* Ann Arbor, MI: Health Administration Press, 1984.

Interstudy, *National HMO Census 1985,* Excelsior, MN, 1986.

Jackson-Beeck, M., and J. Kleinman, "Evidence for Self-Selection Among Health Maintenance Organization Enrollees," *Journal of the American Medical Association,* 250(20):2826–2829, 1983.

Kasper, J. D., *Perspectives on Health Care: United States, 1980,* Washington, D.C. Office of Research and Demonstrations, Health Care Financing Administration, 1986a.

———, "Health Status and Utilization: Differences by Medicaid Coverage and Income," *Health Care Financing Review,* 7(4):1–17, Summer 1986b.

Katz, Sidney and C. Amechi Akpom, "A measure of primary sociobiological functions," *Intl. Journal of Health Services,* Vol. 6, No. 3, 1976.

Koepsell, T., and S. Soroko, "Appropriateness of Hospital Admission. Appropriateness of Inpatient Care," in Reidel, et al., eds., *Use of Health Care Resources,* Ann Arbor, MI: Health Administration Press, 1984.

Lamb, S. J., Kaiser Foundation Health Plan of the Northwest, remarks to the National Health Policy Forum, Session entitled "HMOs and the Elderly: Bright Future or False Promise?" July 1986.

Landgraf, G., Health Plus of Michigan, remarks to the National Health Policy Forum, Session entitled "HMOs and the Elderly: Bright Future or False Promise?" July 1986.

Langwell, K., and J. P. Hadley, "Capitation and the Medicare Program: History, Issues, and Evidence," *Health Care Financing Review,* 1986 Annual Supplement, HCFA Office of Research and Demonstrations.

Lubitz, J., "Health Status Adjustments for Medicare Capitation," Draft Report, Baltimore, MD: Office of Research and Demonstrations, Health Care Financing Administration, July 1986.

Lubitz, J., J. Beebe, and G. Riley, "Improving the Medicare HMO Payment Formula to Deal with Biased Selection," *Advances in Health Economics and Health Services Research,* 6:101–122, 1985.

Luft, H., *Health Maintenance Organizations: Dimensions of Performance,* New York, NY: John Wiley and Sons, Inc., 1981.

———, "Health Maintenance Organizations and the Rationing of Medical care," *Milbank Memorial Fund Quarterly,* 60(2):268–306, 1982.

Manning, W., G. Leibowitz, W. Goldberg, W. Rogers, and J. Newhouse, "A Controlled Trial of the Effect of a Prepaid Group Practice on Use of Services," *New England Journal of Medicine,* 310(23):1505–1530, 1984.

Manton, K., "Changing Concepts of Morbidity and Mortality in the Elderly Population," *Milbank Memorial Fund Quarterly/Health and Society,* 60(2):183–244, 1982.

McClure, W., "On the Research Status of Risk-Adjusted Capitation Rates," *Inquiry,* 21(3):205–213, 1984.

McDevitt, R., "Sampling and Weighting Methodologies Used in Constructing Utilization and Expenditure Files for the Medicare HMO Capitation Evaluation," unpublished, September 1984.

McMillan, A., J. Lubitz, and M. Newton. "Trends in Physician Assignment Rates for Medicare Services: 1968–1984," *Health Care Financing Review,* 7(2):59–76, Office of Research and Demonstrations, Health Care Financing Administration, Winter, 1985.

McMillan, A., J. Lubitz, and D. Russell, "Medicare Enrollment in Health Maintenance Organizations" *Health Care Financing Review,* 8(3):87–94, Office of Research and Demonstrations, Health Care Financing Administration, Spring 1987.

Mechanic, D., *The Growth of Bureaucratic Medicine,* New York, NY: John Wiley and Sons, Inc., 1976.

———, "Cost Containment and the Quality of Medical Care: Rationing Strategies in an Era of Constrained Resources," *Milbank Memorial Fund Quarterly,* 63(3): 453–475, 1985.

Mechanic, D., J. R. Greneley, P. D. Cleary, et al., "A Model on Rural Health Care: Consumer Response Among Users of the Marshfield Clinic," *Medical Care,* 18(6): 597–608, June 1980.

Medicare Competition Demonstration, *Enrollment and Disenrollment in Medicare Competition Demonstration Plans,* Mathematica Policy Research Inc. for the Health Care Financing Administration under Contract 500-83-0047, 1986a.

———, *Report on the Implementation of the Medicare Competition Demonstrations,* Mathematica Policy Research Inc. for the Health Care Financing Administration under Contract 500-83-0047, 1986b.

Merrill, J., C. Jackson, and J. Reuter, "Factors That Affect the HMO Enrollment Decision: A Tale of Two Cities," *Inquiry,* 22:388–395, Winter 1985.

Modern Health Care, "Government Spending Cuts Force HMOs to Walk Payment Tightrope," September 12, 1986.

Mullooly, J., and D. Freeborn, "The Effect of Length of Membership upon the Utilization of Ambulatory Care Services: A Comparison of Disadvantaged and General Membership Populations in a Prepaid Group Practice," *Medical Care,* 17(9): 922–937, 1979.

Nycz, G., Greater Marshfield Community Health Plan, personal communication, 1986.

Reidel, D., D. Walden, S. Meyers, and R. Wilson, *Use of Health Care Resources: A Comparative Study of Two Health Plans,* Ann Arbor, MI: Health Administration Press, 1984.

Rice, D., and J. Feldman, "Living Longer in the United States: Demographic Changes and Health Needs of the Elderly," *Milbank Memorial Fund Quarterly/Health and Society,* 61(3):362–376, 1983.

Ruther, M., and A. Dobson, "Equal Treatment and Unequal Benefits: A Reexamination of the Use of Medicare Services by Race, 1967–1976," *Health Care Financing Review,* 2(3):55–84, Winter 1981.

Rowe, J. W., "Health Care of the Elderly," *New England Journal of Medicine,* 312(13): 827–837, March 1985.

Schlesinger, M., "On the Limits of Expanding Health Care Reform: Chronic Care in Prepaid Settings," *Milbank Memorial Fund Quarterly: Health and Society,* 64(2): 189–215, 1986.

Taylor, H., and M. Kagay, "The HMO Report Card," *Health Affairs,* 5(1):81–89, Spring 1986.

Tessler, R., and D. Mechanic, "Consumer Response in Varying Practice Settings," in D. Mechanic, ed., *The Growth of Bureaucratic Medicine*, New York, NY: John Wiley & Sons, 1976.

Thomas, J. W., and R. Lichtenstein, "Functional Health Measure for Adjusting Health Maintenance Organization Capitation Rates," *Health Care Financing Review*, 7(3): 85–95, Spring 1986.

Trieger, S., T. W. Galblum, and G. Riley, "HMOs: Issues and Alternatives for Medicare and Medicaid," *Health Care Financing Issues*, Office of Research and Demonstrations, Health Care Financing Administration, April 1981.

Ware, J. E., R. H. Brook, W. H. Rogers, et al., "Comparison of Health Outcomes at a Health Maintenance Organization with Those of Fee-for-Service Care," *The Lancet*, 1017–1022, May 3, 1986.

11. Direct Physician Capitation Under the Medicare Program: Evidence and Feasibility

□ □ □

KATHRYN LANGWELL, LYLE NELSON,
AND SHELLY NELSON

Introduction

There has been considerable attention in recent years to the high annual rate of
increase of payments for physician services under the Medicare program and to
the examination of a number of physician payment reform alternatives that might
constrain future increases (Reinhardt 1984; U.S. Senate 1984; U.S. Congress.
Budget Office 1986; U.S. Office of Technology Assessment 1986; Jencks and
Dobson 1984; Langwell and Nelson 1986; Sloan and Hay 1985; Wilensky and
Rossiter 1985; Pauly and Langwell 1986). These approaches have been limited in
two ways. First, they have assumed that the objective of the reform of the physician payment system is to constrain future increases in expenditures for physician
services alone. However, recognition of the key role of physicians in generating
expenditures for all health services suggests that potential reforms of the physician payment system should be examined to establish the impact of the change on
all health services expenditures. Indeed, it may be appropriate to include that
total impact as one of the criteria for choosing the method of paying physicians. There is evidence that the usual, customary, and reasonable (UCR) system
created incentives for physicians to use more of all services; it will be important
to consider whether alternative payment mechanisms would have similar effects.

Second, there has been an assumption that it is necessary to choose one
system for paying all physicians, or at least one system for paying all physicians

of a particular class (e.g., hospital-based physicians or physicians providing services related to a hospital stay). The present Medicare system, and the direction of the current administration, suggests this view is too limited and limiting. The direction of Medicare policy is toward increasing competition and expanding the choices that Medicare beneficiaries are offered in this market, in order to facilitate competition. A diverse physician payment system would result in increased competition and create incentives for physicians to use all health services efficiently. It would permit beneficiaries to elect to receive services from physicians receiving fee-for-service payments (based, perhaps, on a relative value scale [RVS] established fee schedule) or to elect to receive services from a primary care physician who acts as a case manager and who is financially at risk for services rendered. While some physicians would face direct financial incentives to constrain excessive resource use, others would face competitive pressures to reduce out-of-pocket costs to beneficiaries or lose patients to capitation systems. Other payment mechanisms might be in place for hospital-based physicians and for hospital-related services provided by not-at-risk physicians, in order to influence physician decision making, with respect to use of nonphysician services.

In this chapter, we explore the feasibility and evidence for expanding the choices of Medicare beneficiaries to include physicians who are at financial risk for all or a subset of Medicare-covered services. This *physician* capitation is to be distinguished from the *full* capitation paid to a health maintenance organization (HMO). The potential benefits of direct physician capitation include the following:

☐ Reductions in out-of-pocket costs for Medicare beneficiaries to the extent that at-risk physicians reduce cost sharing and add benefits (e.g., preventive services) to attract patients
☐ Reductions in expenditures for all health services provided to beneficiaries participating in the physician-at-risk program
☐ Greater budget control for the Medicare program for prospectively paid beneficiaries
☐ More rapid expansion of the benefits of competition, since, while HMOs are entering the Medicare market under the Tax Equity and Fiscal Responsibility Act of 1982 (TEFRA) regulations, the limited number of HMOs and their limited geographic distribution constrain their competitive effects
☐ Lower explicit transactions costs

On the negative side, putting physicians at risk may raise several concerns:

☐ The financial incentive may result in some physicians providing too little care or care of lower than acceptable quality
☐ Some physicians may try to discourage sicker patients from participating and/or may try to "dump" high-cost patients

☐ To the extent that physicians recruit their existing patients into the risk program, there may be a potential for favorable selection that may result in higher direct costs to the Medicare program

In the next section, we provide a conceptual framework for the examination of direct physician capitation under the Medicare program. The issues of concern include quantity, quality, access, costs, and competitive effects. Potential impacts are discussed, and administrative and other mechanisms that might be useful in addressing undesirable effects are suggested.

The remaining sections of this chapter include a review of the literature on physician practice patterns, the role of information and administrative rules in altering practice patterns, and the effect of economic incentives on physician practice patterns. Then, we examine the structure of existing capitation arrangements with physicians to identify sets of services for which physicians are accepting financial risk and the stop-loss limits in place in these arrangements. Finally, we summarize and discuss the evidence and feasibility of direct physician capitation under the Medicare program.

Issues of Quality, Access, Cost, and Competition

A direct physician capitation program could potentially be designed to permit participation by existing or specially organized medical groups, as well as individual physicians who agree to act as primary care gatekeepers. Under such a program, Medicare would pay a fixed amount per beneficiary to the medical group or individual physician, who in return would assume responsibility for providing all services covered under the capitation payment during a specified period of time. The set of services included in the capitation contract could either be limited to a subset of Medicare services, such as all those covered under Part B, or could include both Part A and Part B services. In this section, we provide a conceptual framework for assessing the feasibility and potential impacts of expanding the Medicare program to include a physician capitation option.

Expected impacts on the quantity and quality of services provided
A major limitation of fee-for-service reimbursement is that if the fee exceeds marginal cost, physicians have clear incentives to increase the quantity of services provided. Under a capitation system, these incentives for overutilization are eliminated since the physician is under financial risk for costs of services provided. As stated above, the advantage of a physician capitation program is that it would introduce incentives into the Medicare market that are expected to result in reductions in the use of services. The potential disadvantage of such a system is that the incentives created may result in physicians providing too little care or

care of unacceptably low quality. This potential undesirable effect and possible mechanisms for mitigating it are addressed below.

The nature and extent of the incentives facing physicians to constrain service use under a capitation system depend on the specific characteristics of the system under consideration. One critical issue to consider in designing a physician capitation program is the degree of financial risk to be placed on the recipient of the capitation payment. Pauly and Langwell (1986) have noted that for a physician capitation program to be feasible, there must be a mechanism for pooling or limiting financial risks. Otherwise, the recipient of the capitation payment (i.e., the medical group or individual physician) could face an excessively powerful financial incentive to constrain services for cases that are so catastrophically expensive that the cost would greatly compromise the recipient's financial viability. They, therefore, argue that payment recipients should have the potential of enrolling a fairly large number of beneficiaries, that reinsurance policies be available, and that proof of solvency be required.

The size of the entity receiving the capitation payment will have an important effect on the extent to which financial risks can be pooled. For example, in considering the implications of capitating individual physicians, it should be recognized that the Medicare patient load of individual physicians will generally be too small to permit much risk spreading. Therefore, if individual physicians are to be capitated for a broad range of Medicare services, fairly extensive stop-loss insurance must be available. However, appropriate stop-loss policies may not be available in the private insurance market or may be quite expensive.

One approach pointed out by Pauly and Langwell that would permit greater risk spreading and facilitate reinsurance arrangements would be for individual physicians and/or medical groups to join together to form an independent "umbrella" entity similar to an Independent Practice Association (IPA)-HMO, which would act as the financial intermediary between the Health Care Financing Administration (HCFA) and the individual physicians and medical groups. If this entity were staffed by individuals with HMO experience, it would offer the additional advantage of providing technical assistance in the development and implementation of appropriate utilization review and quality-control programs.

The incentives facing physicians to constrain service use under a capitation program, and the extent of financial risk to which they are exposed, will depend on the specific services covered under the capitation payment. The covered services could range from all Part A and Part B services to some subset of Medicare services, such as all those covered under Part B. If capitation covers all Medicare services, the at-risk physicians would face strong incentives to constrain the use of hospital services. However, the incentives regarding ambulatory care are mixed. On the one hand, physicians would have an incentive to encourage the use of ambulatory care if such care can serve as a substitute for more expensive inpatient care. On the other hand, however, capitation provides an incentive to reduce the use of all services, including those provided on an ambulatory basis. Thus, while a full capitation system would be expected to reduce the use of hospital care, the impact on ambulatory service use cannot be predicted a priori.

If the capitation payment covers only a subset of Medicare services, physicians would have an incentive to constrain the use of capitated services and to shift patients out of capitation. For example, if only Part B services are covered under the capitation agreement, physicians would have an incentive to shift care from an outpatient to an inpatient setting. This suggests that some type of risk-sharing arrangement may be needed for noncapitated services. For example, under a system in which medical groups and/or individual physicians are capitated for Part B services, a mechanism could be established to permit physicians to share in the "savings" if Part A costs for their capitated enrollees do not exceed a prespecified target.

As discussed above, some mechanism for pooling of financial risks would be necessary under a physician capitation program to prevent physicians from having too powerful a financial incentive to provide too little care or care of unacceptably low quality. Additional factors that would tend to offset the potential incentive to skimp on care under a capitated system include the threat of malpractice litigation, the threat of losing clients, and the professional ethics of physicians.

Expected impact on access to care

Implementation of a direct physician capitation option under the Medicare program would presumably expand beneficiaries' access to capitated care as an alternative to fee-for-service care, as long as the payment level was set high enough. Currently, regulations authorized by TEFRA permit HMOs and competitive medical plans (CMPs) to enroll Medicare beneficiaries on a capitated basis. An important advantage of capitated care to the Medicare population is that HMOs and CMPs have reduced or eliminated cost-sharing requirements and added benefits such as preventive care in order to attract enrollees. It is expected that at-risk physicians would offer similar benefits and/or reduced cost sharing to attract enrollees under a physician capitation program.

While capitated care has proved to be popular among Medicare beneficiaries in some areas of the country, the access to such care is currently limited by the fact that HMOs are distributed very unevenly throughout the country and are concentrated primarily in metropolitan areas. Introduction of a direct physician capitation program would expand the access of Medicare beneficiaries to the financial advantages of capitated care in geographic areas not currently served by an HMO.

One approach to direct physician capitation that would be expected to significantly reduce access to care would be to make such a program mandatory. This effect would be most pronounced if the level of per capita payment was set at a price below the price available to physicians when they treat non-Medicare patients, or if physicians perceived that the degree of financial risk was too high. Such a mandatory capitation program could lead to a situation in the Medicare program similar to that which exists in the Medicaid program, where fee schedules are set sufficiently low to deter many physicians from participating.

Expected impacts on the costs of care

Interest in direct physician capitation as a payment option under the Medicare program is based largely on the presumption that physicians operating at risk will be able to provide Medicare services in a more cost-effective manner than the fee-for-service sector. The effects of physician capitation on the costs of providing services to beneficiaries who enroll in the program may be viewed from three perspectives: (1) total costs to society, (2) costs to enrollees, and (3) government costs.

The incentives created by physician capitation are expected to reduce the total costs of providing Medicare services to enrollees by reducing the utilization of services as described above and by encouraging physicians to be more efficient in the use of resources. Furthermore, if a large umbrella entity is formed to act as intermediary between HCFA and medical groups and/or individual physicians, that entity may have sufficient market power to negotiate significant price discounts from hospitals and other providers. This source of cost savings is likely to be much less relevant for medical groups acting independently, however, due to insufficient market power.

As discussed above, it is expected that medical groups and/or individual physicians who choose to participate in a physician capitation program would offer beneficiaries reduced cost sharing and/or expanded benefits, such as preventive care, in order to increase their share of the Medicare market. Such behavior has been observed among HMOs and CMPs that are currently permitted to enroll Medicare beneficiaries on a capitated basis under TEFRA (Langwell et al. 1986). Thus, a direct physician capitation program would be expected to reduce out-of-pocket health care costs among enrollees.

If physicians who are at risk are able to reduce the overall cost of providing Medicare services, the government has the potential of sharing in the cost savings by setting capitation payments at a level below the cost it would have experienced for enrollees in the fee-for-service sector. While conceptually this is straightforward, in practice the task of setting capitation rates to achieve a target level of government savings per enrollee may be quite challenging because (1) there may be biased selection of enrollees and providers into the program and (2) the government may have insufficient information to adequately account for biased selection in setting rates.

Biased selection could be either "adverse" or "favorable." That is, enrollees may be either sicker or less sick than nonenrollees, where "sick" refers to the need or demand for services and the costliness of these services. Furthermore, the bias can arise from physician behavior in advertising or screening of applicants or from the choice behavior of enrollees. If physician behavior causes biased selection, it is likely to be in the form of favorable selection, since the profit motive is best served by enrolling the least sick clients in any reimbursement category and rejecting the sickest individuals. The choice behavior of beneficiaries, however, may lead to bias in either direction. Beneficiaries who choose to enroll may be those who are in most need of insuring themselves (heavy users) or, alternatively, those choosing to enroll may be those individuals who are unconcerned about being restricted to a given set of providers.

The critical issue for the government is whether capitation rates can be set to account adequately for the nature and extent of any biased selection that occurs. This problem may be particularly difficult among the class of beneficiaries who "roll over" into capitation without changing physicians, since physicians will be in a position to selectively target those individuals who are "least sick" within any reimbursement category. Two potential mechanisms for mitigating this problem are as follows:

☐ Requiring that physicians who participate in the capitation program do so for a full set of designated patients, rather than permitting physicians to elect capitation on a patient-by-patient basis

☐ Requiring that physicians enroll a specified number of "switchers" under capitation for every rollover, where switchers are defined as beneficiaries who either had no prior source of care or who changed providers to enroll

Finally, in assessing the potential impact of introducing physician capitation on government costs, it is important to consider the costs of the additional bureaucracy that would be required for the review, approval, and monitoring of medical groups and/or individual physicians who participate in the capitated system. Such costs would be higher the greater the number of separate entities required to be approved and monitored under the program. This suggests that the concept of an independent umbrella entity discussed above, which would act as an intermediary between HCFA and medical groups and/or individual physicians, should be given serious consideration as a method of minimizing government administrative costs.

Expected competitive effects

Our discussion thus far has focused on the expected impacts of direct physician capitation on the quantity, quality, and costs of care among Medicare beneficiaries who participate in the program. However, introduction of a physician capitation option may have significant competitive or "spillover" effects on the Medicare market, in particular, and the health care market, in general.

Physicians who participate in the capitation program would be expected to alter their practice patterns and become more efficient in the use of resources in response to the incentives created by capitation. Unless physicians identify capitated and noncapitated patients and treat them differently, these altered practice patterns would be expected to lead to more cost-effective treatment of non-Medicare patients and any Medicare patients treated under fee-for-service. Furthermore, introduction of a physician capitation option would stimulate competition for Medicare patients between physicians participating in the program and those remaining exclusively in the fee-for-service sector. One consequence of this competition may be a greater willingness on the part of fee-for-service physicians to accept assignment, which would lower out-of-pocket costs facing patients. Finally, introduction of a physician capitation option under the Medicare program may encourage other major insurers and employers to implement similar programs, which could increase the degree of competition in the entire health care market.

Review of the Literature on Physician Practice Patterns and Economic Incentives

The benefits from putting physicians at financial risk for Medicare beneficiaries are dependent upon several assumptions:

1. There are variations in practice patterns of physicians that are the result of custom or uncertainty, rather than quality differences.
2. Existing practice patterns can change if physicians are better informed, administrative rules are put in place, and/or economic incentives are offered.
3. Physicians respond to economic incentives but do not respond so strongly that poor quality of care results.

In this section, we review the evidence on these issues in order to assess the potential impacts of direct physician capitation under the Medicare program.

Evidence of variations in practice patterns

For a direct physician capitation system to be effective in reducing total Medicare services use, it is necessary that prior medical practice patterns, including hospital and other nonphysician services, be susceptible to change without diminishing quality of care. Recent studies of geographic variations in use of hospital and other services suggest that there is substantial variation in practice patterns (Wennberg and Gittelsohn 1982; McPherson et al. 1982; Connell et al. 1984; Roos and Roos 1981). The underlying cause of variations in practice patterns is not well understood.

Brook et al. (1984) suggest that such variation may reflect uncertainty of the decisionmakers about the appropriate clinical choice when presented with symptoms that are consistent with multiple diagnoses or when alternative therapies are available. Geographic variation also may reflect real variations in health needs and characteristics of the population. Wennberg et al. (1977) and Roos and Roos (1981) examine the contribution of measures of patient health needs to geographic variations in use patterns and conclude that measured differences in illness rates cannot provide an adequate explanation of differences in hospitalization rates seen in small area studies. Wennberg et al. (1984) examine the evidence on physician discretion as a source of variation in hospital admissions and suggest the evidence supports a conclusion that much of the variation in per capita rates of hospitalization is due to differences in physician practice styles. Brook et al. (1984) point out that there is at present insufficient evidence to conclude that patients in high use areas are receiving unnecessary services—there may be beneficial effects of higher use. In fact, patients in low use areas may be receiving inadequate amounts of care.

Several studies provide evidence on physicians' abilities to change practice patterns when provided with information on differences in admission rates for selected procedures (Dyck et al. 1977; Wennberg et al. 1977). Relatively low rates of hospital use in many HMOs, for Medicare beneficiaries as well as for younger patients, strongly suggest physicians can be encouraged to reduce variations in hospital use. The methods used by HMOs include education and feedback to physicians on their own practice patterns, administrative rules (e.g., prior authorization requirements for hospital admissions and specialty referrals), monitoring, and direct financial incentives to physicians (Nelson et al. 1986; Langwell et al. 1985).

Response to economic incentives
To the extent that physicians face direct financial incentives under a physician-at-risk system, there may be changes in the quantity, mix, or arrangements for care as a result. Physician responses to different payment policies have been investigated by a number of researchers. Langwell and Nelson (1986) surveyed this large body of literature on the effects of alternative payment systems on use and costs of services. The emphasis of most research in this area has been on the implications of changing from a fee-for-service system to a capitated system.

The alternative units of payments have very different implications for the incentives facing physicians (Reinhardt 1984; Mitchell and Cromwell 1984). A major limitaton of fee-for-service reimbursement is that physicians have incentives to increase the quantity of services provided, if price is above marginal (opportunity) cost. Thus, to the extent that physicians act as "agents" for patients and can induce additional utilization of their services, fee-for-service reimbursement encourages higher expenditures and, if price is not constrained, higher prices as well.

Under a capitation system, the physician receives a fixed payment for each case and thus has a strong incentive to minimize the resource cost of the treatment provided. In fact, the physician has an incentive to skimp on resources, although this incentive will be mitigated to an extent by the physician's sense of professional ethics, the patient's evaluation of the quality of care being provided, and the threat of malpractice. In addition to the incentive to skimp on resources, physicians also have an incentive to refuse to accept for treatment those patients for whom the expected cost of treatment exceeds the rate of payment.

The evidence on capitation and its effects on use and costs of services is substantial. Luft (1981) and Langwell and Moore (1982) summarize this extensive body of literature and conclude that HMOs, which are capitated for health services, save money for both third-party payers and enrollees. The total differential is apparently due to differences in utilization of medical care, particularly hospital services. Most studies suggest significant reductions in hospital admissions but report as great or greater utilization of ambulatory care when compared with fee-for-service experience. There is also evidence that there are differences among HMOs in the extent to which use and costs are controlled by capitated payment systems. The IPA-model HMOs, which have traditionally paid physicians on a discounted fee-for-service system, have been much less successful in controlling use and costs of services. Despite this extensive body of literature, Pauly and Langwell (1983) point out that there remain significant questions about the effects of capitated payments to HMOs on use and costs of services. In particular, the presence of favorable or adverse selection into HMOs requires more attention. Selection issues would also be present in a direct physician capitation program and would probably require some attention at an early stage of program development.

Evidence of the effect of capitation on quality of care
There is a considerable body of literature dealing with quality of care under capitated systems. Luft (1981) summarizes this literature and indicates that there is no evidence that HMO enrollees receive care of lower quality—in fact, some evidence suggests that HMO enrollees receive a more appropriate mix of services, under some conditions. However, he acknowledges that there remains a

variety of questions in this area that require additional research. LoGerfo et al. (1979), on the other hand, find that HMO enrollees are less likely to have surgery—even when it would be advised by generally accepted standards—and conclude that ". . . there is substantial evidence to support the contention of underprovision of surgical care in prepaid group practices as one explanation for observed differences in surgical rates" (p. 7).

It is also worthy of attention that many of the early studies of quality of care under capitated systems were of large, well-established HMOs that may be most likely to exhibit a long-range perspective that would lead to careful monitoring of quality of care. The experience of the California prepaid health plans reveals that entrepreneurs with short time horizons and strong profit motives may behave in ways that severely restrict both access and quality of care available to enrollees (Kimbell and Yett 1975). In addition, new HMOs and CMPs have proliferated in the past decade. These new plans exhibit a much greater variety of organizational structures and financial arrangements than was present in many of the older HMOs in which quality of care was studied. Studies of quality of care in organizations where individual physicians are capitated have not been conducted. Although HMOs and CMPs that capitate small medical groups and individual physicians may be aware of the potential consequences of these financial arrangements on quality of care—and frequently focus utilization review on ascertaining that adequate services are being provided (U.S. DHHS 1985; Mathematica Policy Research 1984)—no evidence is available.

Discussion

Although there is limited direct evidence of the effects of direct physician capitation on use, costs, and quality of care, indirect evidence suggests that putting physicians at risk will result in reductions in the use of services that physicians provide directly and services that are complementary to physician services. To the extent that quantity is reduced, expenditures for health services may also be reduced.

Organizations that contract with physicians have been able to affect practice patterns through administrative rules, as well as economic incentives. The relative strength of the administrative approach relative to economic incentives has not been explored. Under direct physician capitation, physicians would face financial incentives to constrain use of health services for participating beneficiaries—these economic incentives could cause these physicians to develop and put in place appropriate administrative rules to facilitate better management of health resources. These administrative rules might also extend to monitoring of utilization rates and formal quality of care review. There is little evidence that permits us to assess the potential impact of a physician-at-risk program on quality. However, it may be reasonable to assume that, with a stop-loss system in policy, quality effects may be no greater than the effects on quality of the fee-for-service system's incentives to order a greater quantity of services.

Evidence of Direct Physician Capitation Under the Medicare Program

Although there is no direct experience with physician capitation under the Medicare program, the financial arrangements between HMOs and physicians provide useful information on the feasibility of a physician-at-risk system and the administrative rules that would facilitate this approach. Under two separate contracts with the Department of Health and Human Services,[1] the authors have conducted case studies of the financial arrangements between HMOs and physicians. The issues of interest in these studies included organizational structures, economic incentives, and effects on use and costs of health services. During the studies, site visits were conducted to ten HMOs primarily serving an under age sixty-five enrollment and to nineteen HMOs that were participating in the Medicare Competition Demonstrations. Of these twenty-nine HMOs, sixteen had negotiated capitation agreements with the physicians who contracted to serve their members.[2]

In this section, we describe the characteristics of the capitation arrangements observed in these sixteen HMOs, including: (1) services for which physicians are directly at risk, (2) risk-sharing provisions for hospital and referral physician services, and (3) limits on financial risk. Then, we discuss the extent to which HMOs monitor quality of care in capitated systems and the role of utilization controls in capitated systems.

Financial arrangements between HMOs and physicians accepting capitation

Information on services covered under capitation arrangements, risk-sharing provisions for hospital and referral services, and (for the Medicare HMOs) limits on physician financial risk is presented in Table 11.1 and Table 11.2. We limited our examination to financial arrangements with primary care physicians, although some HMOs also have been able to negotiate capitation arrangements with specialist physicians. Of the sixteen HMOs reporting direct capitation arrangements with physicians, eight were IPA-HMOs, five were group model HMOs, and three were mixed model HMOs (two were staff IPA models, one was a group IPA model). The HMOs were geographically diverse: three each from Maryland and California; two each from Ohio, Florida, Michigan, and Massachussets; and one each in Colorado and Illinois. Thus, it appears that direct capitation of primary physicians is occurring in a variety of markets with different characteristics and environments.

TABLE 11.1
Financial Arrangements in HMOs that Capitate Primary Care Physicians or Physician Groups for Medicare Enrollees

HMO/model type	Services covered under capitation payment	Risk-sharing provisions for hospital and referral services	Limits on financial risk facing primary care physicians
HMO A—IPA	HMO capitates individual primary care for physicians Office visits In-office lab and X-ray services Coordination of all other medical services	$4 per member month "withhold" puts physician at risk for hospital and referral services; distribution of withhold is based on experience of individual physician patients; physicians receive bonus if targets for hospital and referral costs are met	Maximum risk for individual physicians for hospital services is $1,000 but no limitation for ambulatory and referral services; to reduce risk of adverse selection, physician may designate patient as "adverse risk" and exclude from risk pool
HMO B—IPA	Individual primary care physicians are capitated for Office visits Home visits Lab specimens for processing Stat lab work in office Chest and extremity X rays Physical therapy when performed in physician office Periodic physician exams Immunizations/injections Minor office surgery EKGs	Withhold equal to 10% of capitation amount places physicians at risk for referral services; distribution of withhold is based on individual physician referral rates; those with above-average referral rates forfeit part of withhold HMO created Medicare Primary Care Incentive program, which is based on overall profitability of its Medicare contracts; one-half of any surplus earned is divided among primary care physicians in proportion to their contribution to profit for year	
HMO C—IPA	Individual primary care physicians[a] are capitated for Office visits Physician hospital visits Injections/immunizations Periodic health exams Home care	Percentage withhold from capitation payment is used to offset any deficits in funds from which hospital and referral payments are made; if these funds experience surplus, physician receives entire withhold plus share of surplus	Withhold amount is maximum financial risk facing physicians for deficits in hospital and referral funds

TABLE 11.1 Continued
Financial Arrangements in HMOs that Capitate Primary Care Physicians or Physician Groups for Medicare Enrollees

HMO/model type	Services covered under capitation payment	Risk-sharing provisions for hospital and referral services	Limits on financial risk facing primary care physicians
	Emergency room visits (professional component) Outpatient hospital services Handling fees for lab and X-ray services	Physicians are organized into "risk pools" of roughly 14 each for purpose of sharing surpluses and deficits in hospital and referral funds	
HMO D—mixed	Affiliated groups are capitated for Physician services Lab and X-ray services Mental health counseling Prescribed medicines Limited DME/appliances Emergency room visits Speech therapy Occupational therapy Physical therapy	Affiliated groups receive incentive bonuses if hospital use meets negotiated target; groups are at risk for referral services through withhold from capitation payment	Maximum financial risk facing primary care physician is $5,000 per member per year
HMO E—IPA	Medical groups are capitated for Office visits, hospital visits, and consultation Ancillary medical services including lab, EKG, and X rays Miscellaneous services including diagnostic tests, therapy, injections, etc. Administrative costs Outpatient referrals to specialty physicians	Hospital costs and inpatient referrals are shared in 50/50 risk arrangement between HMO and each preferred provider group; funds are maintained in Health Care Management fund—preferred provider groups share surplus/deficit with HMO at end of year	
HMO F—mixed	HMO capitates IPA component for Office visits Output lab Routine chest and skeletal X rays Dermatological and anatomical pathology and histopathology	Physicians are placed at risk for hospital costs through withhold from capitation payment; physicians receive bonuses if hospital costs are within budgeted amount	

Outpatient diagnstic procedures
Inpatient and outpatient consultations
Mental health counseling

HMO G—group
HMO capitates medical group for
All ambulatory services
All member physician services associated with institutional care
Referral costs

If hospital expenditures are lower than budgeted, group receives 60% of surplus; similarly, group pays HMO 60% of any deficit incurred

HMO withholds referral care capitation and pays referral claims directly; if cost of referral services exceed risk pool for each quarter, loss is divided equally between HMO and medical group—same with any surplus

HMO H—group
HMO capitates medical group for all noninstitutional services, including
In-house physician services
Referral physician services
All other ambulatory care
Prescription drugs
Optical services

If HMO members use less than target number of hospital days annually, savings are split equally between HMO and group, up to dollar level negotiated annually; above that level savings are divided 40% to HMO and 60% to group

HMO I—mixed
In group model component, capitation covers
All physician services, including
Inpatient hospital care
Drug costs for injections/immunizations

In IPA model component, capitation covers
Office visits and procedures
Physical exams
Injections/immunizations, except for associated drug costs

Some groups are at risk for hospital costs through withhold from capitation payment; however, most groups, as well as entire IPA component, are not at risk

aPrimary care physicians have the option of receiving capitation for lab or X ray if they use their own facilities.

Source: Data collected by the authors through site visit interviews at HMOs that participated in the Medicare Competition Demonstrations (see note 1).

TABLE 11.2
Financial Arrangements in HMOs that Capitate Primary Care Physicians or Physician Groups for Non-Medicare Enrollees

HMO	Services covered under capitation payment	Risk-sharing provisions for hospital referral care
HMO AA—IPA	HMO capitates IPA for All general primary care services Lab and X-ray services IPA capitates each primary care physician	IPA withholds 20% of physician capitation, which is distributed to physician if revenues exceed costs at end of year Specialist physicians are paid from "specialty pool"; if pool of funds for specialist services is not exhausted, remaining funds are distributed to primary care physicians
HMO BB—IPA (network)	Group/individual physician is capitated for All ambulatory services, including ancillary and referral services Inpatient consultant fees	Medical group shares in any deficit or surplus in fund from which HMO pays hospital costs; if fund incurs deficit, group pays HMO up to 5% of its capitation payments for period
HMO CC—IPA (network)	HMO capitates medical groups for all ambulatory services, including ancillary service and for inpatient physicians services	HMO offers bonus to groups if hospital use remains under predetermined target level
HMO DD—IPA (network)	HMO capitates medical groups for all ambulatory physician and ancillary services	HMO establishes hospital claims pool; the end of year, funds retained in pool are distributed to groups
HMO EE—group	Capitation covers All ambulatory services Outpatient surgery Referral physician services Drugs Physical therapy Alcohol and drug treatment Ancillary services	Group practice is not at risk for inpatient care, although HMO offers bonus if hospital days per 1,000 are within prespecified amount
HMO FF—group	Capitation covers All ambulatory services Ancillary services Referral physicians services	Although group is not at direct risk for hospital expenses, HMO offers bonus if hospital days remain within prespecified target
HMO GG—group	HMO capitates medical group for Physician services Specialty referrals Emergency room visits Lab and X-ray services	

Source: Data collected by the authors through HMO site visit interviews (see note 1).

Services covered by capitation contracts. All of the financial arrangements examined put the individual physician or the contracting medical group at risk for office visits, including preventive care, and in-office lab and X-ray services, either by specifically mentioning these services or by including in their agreement that "all ambulatory services" were covered by the capitation. The definition of all ambulatory services is unclear across organizations, since some appear to exclude referral physicians, by mentioning them separately, while others appear to separate out "ancillary services" for contract purposes. Our interpretation is that the term all ambulatory services can be construed as covering at least primary care office visits and in-office ancillary services.

Other services for which primary physicians have agreed to accept risk include:

☐ Emergency room visits (3)
☐ Mental health visits (2)
☐ Referrals to specialists (9)
☐ Prescription drugs (4)
☐ Durable medical equipment (DME)/speech, physical, occupational therapy/ optical services (4)

Risk sharing for other services. None of the contractual arrangements examined put primary care physicians at direct financial risk for hospital services. However, the overwhelming majority placed physicians at some financial risk for hospital services. Table 11.3 summarizes the different risk-sharing arrangements in which physicians were participating. Only one HMO reported no physician risk sharing for hospital services. Two use indirect risk sharing by offering physicians a bonus related to overall HMO financial performance but impose no penalties for poor financial performance.

The largest number of HMOs (six) offered positive financial incentives through a bonus related to surpluses in the hospital pool, without any negative financial risk to the physicians. Another five plans limit physician risk sharing to the

TABLE 11.3
Summary of Physician Risk-Sharing Arrangements for Hospital Use

Hospital risk-sharing arrangement	Number
Withhold from capitation is forfeited if hospital costs exceed budget, no other incentive	1
Physicians share fully in excess hospital costs and hospital surpluses	2
Physicians receive bonus if surplus in hospital pool and share deficit through withhold	4
Physicians receive bonus for surplus but are not otherwise at risk	6
Physicians receive bonus if HMO total revenues exceed costs	2
No risk-sharing for hospital services	1

Source: Data collected by the authors through HMO site visit interviews (see note 1).

amount of a "withhold" from the physician capitation payment (typically 10–20 percent), and four of those plans also offer a bonus for meeting hospital use targets. Only two of the HMOs report that physicians share fully in the risk for hospital services; one of these HMOs is an IPA-HMO and one is a group model HMO. Risk sharing for referral physician services is explicitly reported by three of the seven HMOs that do not include referral services in the basic capitation agreement.

Although we would expect that capitation arrangements with primary care physicians would result in reductions of both physician services and complementary services, the risk-sharing arrangements reported by these sixteen HMOs suggest that there is a perception that there is a need to create financial incentives to control physician use of referral physician services and hospital services. In part, this may reflect the fact that referral physicians (when not covered by capitation) and hospital services may permit capitated physicians to shift patients out of capitation. In addition, physicians may give little attention to the financial impact of using these other services unless there are either financial incentives or administrative rules to focus their attention on this issue. In either case, it appears that, if physicians were to be capitated for less than the full set of Medicare Part A and Part B services, it might be necessary to consider introducing some degree of risk sharing for noncapitated services.

Limits on financial risk. While risk sharing is desirable, imposing too great a degree of risk sharing could have negative effects on physicians and beneficiaries. Physicians at risk for hospital services, for example, might respond to powerful financial incentives by not hospitalizing patients when hospitalization is appropriate care. Alternatively, physicians may refuse to participate or drop out of the capitation program if financial risk is too high. The issue of limiting financial risk is, therefore, a very important one for designing a feasible direct physician capitation system.

Among the sixteen HMOs examined in this study, only two set a dollar limit on physician risk:

☐ One IPA-HMO sets a maximum of $1,000 per patient for hospital risk to physicians and, in addition, permits the physicians to designate specific patients as "adverse risks" and exclude them from the individual physician's risk pool.
☐ Another IPA sets the maximum financial risk to primary care physicians at $5,000 per patient for all services.

Other HMOs do not set explicit dollar limits, but they do set the maximum risk at the level of the capitation withhold or at a proportional share of hospital and/or referral pool losses.

The lack of limits on financial risk for physicians accepting capitation payments for primary and ambulatory services suggests that this may not be a critical issue. Physicians participating in these HMOs have chosen to accept these risks and, for the Medicare HMOs, there does not seem to be a significant problem with high physician turnover in HMO participation.

Quality of care and utilization monitoring
Direct capitation of physicians, even when financial risk sharing is limited, might not be sufficient to control overall use of health services in the absence of administrative rules and information feedback to physicians. On the other hand, some physicians might respond excessively to these financial incentives. In either case, the capitating organization has an interest in encouraging appropriate practice patterns and in monitoring physician practice patterns. Evidence from the Medicare HMO evaluation provides some limited evidence on these issues.

Utilization controls and monitoring. HMOs that capitate physicians may be particularly concerned with utilization control and, consequently, may capitate physicians as one aspect of an overall utilization control strategy. Alternatively, HMOs may capitate physicians as a more direct route to utilization control, substituting direct financial incentives for administrative rules. Table 11.4 suggests the latter may be the case. While HMOs that capitate are likely to tie capitation to a primary care gatekeeper approach, these HMOs are less likely to require prehospitalization or prereferral authorization from physicians than are noncapitating HMOs.

The use of primary care physician profiles, on the other hand, is reported by all of the capitating HMOs but by only 60 percent of noncapitating HMOs. Physician profiles enable HMOs to determine individual physician practice patterns and to compare these practice patterns with those of comparable physicians. In a noncapitating HMO, physician profiles are a mechanism to identify physicians

TABLE 11.4
Utilization Control Activities Reported by Medicare HMOs, by Physician Payment Method

Utilization control	Percent of HMOs directly capitating physicians (N = 9)	Percent of HMOs not capitating physicians (N = 10)
Gatekeeper	78	50
Prehospital authorization	67	80
Prereferral authorization	11	30
Primary care physician profiles	100	60

Source: Data drawn from Brown (1987).

who have particularly costly practice styles (e.g., referring to specialists disproportionately). In capitated HMOs, the physician profile is more commonly used to monitor and identify the physician who is underutilizing on behalf of capitated patients. The profile typically includes number of specialist referrals, hospital use, ancillary services used, and office visits per patient for each physician. It is, therefore, of particular interest that this mechanism is used by all capitating HMOs and suggests that primary care physician profiles for these HMOs may represent quality monitoring, rather than a utilization control.

Quality assurance. Ensuring quality of care in capitated systems is often a joint responsibility of the HMO and its physicians (Brown 1987). When physicians are directly capitated by HMOs, quality-assurance may assume even greater importance since the HMO and physician incentives concur. In Table 11.5, several elements of HMO quality-assurance programs are examined for capitating HMOs and for noncapitating HMOs. For all three measures, capitating HMOs are more likely to report using the quality-assurance method than are noncapitating HMOs.

Discussion. Capitating HMOs use fewer utilization controls and more quality review mechanisms than do noncapitating HMOs. Although our sample is small and self-selected, these observations do suggest that (1) capitating physicians may make it less important to have in place a variety of utilization control mechanisms, and (2) assuring quality of care may be perceived as a greater concern when physicians are capitated. The implications for a direct physician capitation program under Medicare are mixed. Putting physicians at risk may be expected to result in reductions in services that are "unnecessary" (in some sense), without the need for an elaborate externally imposed utilization controls or monitoring. However, there is an issue of the feasibility of the Medicare program, assuming quality-assurance responsibility for medical groups or individual physicians receiving capitation payments. While the peer review organizations (PROs) have now been directed to review quality in Medicare HMOs, it is not evident

TABLE 11.5
Quality-Assurance Activities Reported by Medicare HMOs, by Physician Payment Method

Quality-assurance activity	Percent of HMOs directly capitating physicians ($N = 9$)	Percent of HMOs not capitating physicians ($N = 10$)
Periodic chart audits	100	80
Protocol development	78	60
Review patient complaints	67	40

Source: Data drawn from Brown (1987).

that PROs have sufficient funding to extend these reviews to the large number of medical groups that might participate in a Medicare direct physician capitation program. It may be feasible, however, to delegate external quality assurance to an existing organization involved in voluntary quality review of ambulatory services (e.g., National Committee For Quality Assurance [NCQA] or Accreditation Association For Ambulatory Health Care [AAAHC]), with participating medical groups absorbing the costs of this review.

Several points should be considered before concluding that quality monitoring is a barrier to direct physician capitation:

1. PROs will review hospitalized capitated patients and could be directed to report separately on patients who are capitated to physician groups.
2. A substantial number of HMOs delegate quality-assurance activities to their medical staff or group, rather than performing independent audits, which suggests that internal quality assurance may be sufficient in most cases.
3. Capitated patients would have two avenues of action available under the Medicare program. There is an established, well-publicized grievance system that permits the patient to carry unresolved grievances to Health and Human Services (HHS) regional offices. In addition, Medicare beneficiaries would, presumably, be able to disenroll from the medical group's capitated plan with thirty days or less of notice (as is the rule for TEFRA HMOs). While Medicare beneficiaries are not all able to assess adequacy of quality or quantity of care, higher than average disenrollments might be a trigger for a review by the HCFA Office of Prepaid Operations or other designated agency.

Quality-monitoring considerations, as well as risk-spreading considerations, may argue in favor of capitating only existing medical groups or groups organized particularly to receive capitation that agree to provide quality monitoring of its members.

Summary and Discussion

The purpose of this chapter has been to examine the desirability, feasibility, and evidence for direct physician capitation payments under the Medicare program. Our review of the existing evidence and economic theory suggests that putting physicians at risk for the costs of their practice decisions may result in a number of the following desirable changes in the market:

1. Physicians will face financial incentives to use services more carefully on behalf of Medicare beneficiaries for whom they are at risk. This will affect the use of both capitated and complementary noncapitated services.

2. The educational and informational aspects of physician capitated practice may be expected to lead to desirable changes in physician practice patterns, in general.
3. Since physicians will act as case managers for their capitated patients, participating Medicare beneficiaries will receive better coordinated and integrated services than may be the case under fee-for-service.
4. To the extent that capitated medical groups market a package of services with reduced cost sharing to attract Medicare beneficiaries, financial access to care will be facilitated.
5. Since medical groups are available in many geographic areas where HMOs are not presently available, Medicare beneficiaries would have greater opportunities to join capitated systems.
6. Competition between capitated organizations and fee-for-service providers would be enhanced by adding capitated medical groups to the existing Medicare HMOs in this market. "Spillover" effects on practice patterns and cost behavior of fee-for-service physicians might result.

Despite these beneficial aspects of a physician-at-risk program, several concerns remain, as follows:

1. Direct financial incentives to restrain service use may lead some physicians to skimp on services and/or to provide care below acceptable standards of quality.
2. To the extent that physicians are permitted to enroll existing patients into the capitated program, there is a potential for biased selection to become a problem that may offset any direct financial benefits to Medicare from the program.

Overall, the advantages of direct physician capitation as one component of a Medicare program that includes diverse payment arrangements, and permits beneficiaries to choose among a set of options, seem clear. Addressing the potential pitfalls of a physician-at-risk program moves into the area of feasibility. While a physician-at-risk program may be desirable in theory, its feasibility requires attention to a number of issues:

1. To obtain maximum benefits from the risk program, physicians must be at risk for the costs of a larger set of services than their own office-based services. Most HMOs include referral physician services in the capitation, and many put the medical group at risk for some amount of hospital costs.
2. To avoid putting physicians at risk for a disproportionately large portion of their potential annual revenues, there should be limits on financial risk. For large medical groups with a substantial number of Medicare patients, risk spreading may be sufficient. For smaller groups, the government should make available a stop-loss pool.
3. The stop-loss pool and careful consideration of the set of services for

which physicians are at risk will alleviate some concern about quality of care. In addition, a minimum group size to assure some degree of risk spreading could be specified. Administrative rules could specify minimum group quality-assurance activities. Similarly, reporting requirements should include utilization rates for, at least, office visits and hospital days, so that the HCFA can identify potential problem groups. Finally, offering and informing beneficiaries of a clear grievance procedure and permitting dis-enrollment with minimal time delays will protect beneficiaries to some extent against quality of care deficiencies.

4. To reduce the potential for biased selection into capitated medical groups, the Medicare program could impose a 2/1 (or 1/1) rule similar to that used to delay HMOs' conversion of cost contract enrollees to risk contracts. The specific conversion rule might be negotiated, but attention to this issue would be important during the design of a physician-at-risk program.

With careful consideration during the design period, it appears that direct physician capitation under the Medicare program may be a feasible, as well as desirable, option. To explore this option HCFA has supported a design effort[3] to develop a demonstration strategy that would be capable of implementation if, at some future time, HCFA decides to expand the capitation alternatives available to Medicare beneficiaries.

Notes

1. *Evaluation of Utilization Patterns and Physicians' Practice Arrangements* (ASPE), Contract No. HHS 100-82-0092, Spring 1985 and *Evaluation of the Medicare Competition Demonstrations* (HCFA), Contract No. 500-83-0047, October 1983–June 1988.

2. Although some HMOs capitate an IPA, we have not included these in our study unless the IPA capitates its member physicians.

3. Through Cooperative Agreement No. 95-C-98919/3-01, Design of a Demonstration of Medical Group Capitation Under the Medicare Program, with Mathematica Policy Research.

References

Brook, H. R., K. Lohr, M. Chassin, et al. "Geographic Variations in the Use of Services: Do they have Any Clinical Significance?" *Health Affairs*, 63–73, Summer 1984.

Brown, B., *Report on Quality Assurance Programs in Medicare HMOs*. Prepared under Contract No. 500-83-0047, with the Health Care Financing Administration, Washington, DC, February 1987.

Connell, F. H., L. A. Blaide, and M. H. Hanken, "Clinical Correlates of Small Area Variations in Population-Based Admission Rates for Diabetes," *Med Care*, 22(10): 929–949, October 1984.

Dyck, F. J., F. A. Murphy, J. K. Murphy, et al., "Effect of Surveillance on the Number of Hysterectomies in the Province of Saskatchewan," *New England Journal of Medicine*, 296:1326–1328, 1977.

Jencks, S. F., and A. Dobson, "Evaluating Options for Reforming Medicare's Physician Payment Process," Washington, DC: Office of Research Demonstrations, and Statistics, Health Care Financing Administration, August 1984.

Kimbell, L. J., and D. E. Yett, "An Evaluation of Policy-Related Research on the Effects of Alternative Health Care Reimbursement Systems," National Science Foundation Grant No. GI-39344. Los Angeles, CA: Human Resource Research Center, University of Southern California, 1975.

Langwell, K. M., et al., *Strategies and Operational Issues for HMOs and CMPs in the Medicare Market,* prepared under Contract No. 500-83-0047 with the Health Care Financing Administration, Washington, DC, January, 1986.

Langwell, K. M., and S. Moore, "A Synthesis of Research on Competition in the Financing and Delivery of Health Services," DHHS Publication No. (PHS) 83-3327, Washington, DC: U.S. Department of Health and Human Services, October 1982.

Langwell, K. M., and L. M. Nelson, "Physician Payment Systems: A Review of History, Alternatives, and Evidence," *Medical Care Review,* 43(1):5–58, Spring 1986.

LoGerfo, J. P., R. A. Efird, P. W. Diehr, and W. C. Richardson, "Rates of Surgical Care in Prepaid Group Practices and the Independent Setting: What Are the Reasons for the Differences?" *Medical Care,* 17:1–10, January 1979.

Luft, H. S., "The Operations and Performance of Health Maintenance Organizations; A Synthesis of Findings from Health Services Research," San Francisco, CA: San Francisco Institute for Health Policy Studies, School of Medicine, University of California, October 1981.

Mathematica Policy Research, "Implementation Case Studies of 20 Medicare Demonstration HMOs," Interim Reports to the HCFA under Contract No. 500-83-0047, Washington, DC: Mathematica Policy Research, 1984.

McPherson, K., J. E. Wennberg, O. B. Hound, P. Clifford, "Small-area Variations in the Use of Common Surgical Procedures; An International Comparison of New England and Norway," *New England Journal of Medicine,* 307:1310–1314, 1982.

Mitchell, J. B., and J. Cromwell, "Alternative Methods for Describing Physicians Services Performed and Billed," HCFA Contract No. 500-81-0054, Baltimore, MD: HCFA, May 1984.

Nelson, L., et al., *Final Report on the Analysis of Analysis of Aggregate Use and Cost Data from Medicare HMOs,* prepared under Contract No. 500-83-0047 for the Health Care Financing Administration, Washington, DC: Mathematica Policy Research, June 1986.

Pauly, M. V., and K. M. Langwell, "Research on Competition in the Financing and Delivery of Health Services, Future Research Needs," in L. F. Rossiter, ed., *Research on Competition in the Financing & Delivery of Health Services Future Research Needs,* HHHS Publication No. (PHS) Vol. 83-3328-2, Hyattsville, MD: National Center for Health Services Research, 1983.

———, "Physician Payment Reform: Who Shall be Paid?" *Medical Care Review,* 43(1):101–132, Spring 1986.

Reinhardt, U. E., "A Framework for Deliberations on the Compensation of Physicians." Statement before the U.S. Senate, Special Committee on Aging, Hearings on Physician Reimbursement, Washington, DC, March 16, 1984.

Roos, N. P., and L. L. Roos, "High and Low Surgical Rates: Risk Factors for Area Residents," *American Journal Public Health,* 71:591–600, 1981.

Sloan, F. A. and J. W. Hay, "Medicare Pricing Mechanisms for Physician Services: An Overview of Alternative Approaches," *Medical Care Review,* 43(1):59–100, Spring 1986.

U.S. Congress Congressional Budget Office. *Physician Reimbursement Under Medicare: Options for Change,* Washington, DC, April, 1986.

U.S. Congress Office of Technology Assessment, *Payment for Physician Services: Strategies for Medicare* (OTA-H-295), Washington, DC, February 1986.

U.S. Department of Health and Human Services, Office of the Assistant Secretary for Planning and Evaluation, Division of Health Resources and Services Policy, *Final Report: Evaluation of Utilization Patters of Physicians' Practice Arrangements,* prepared by Applied Management Sciences under Contract No. HHS 100-82-0092 and by the University of California, San Francisco, under Contract No. PHS 282-0700, Task No. 3, Springfield, VA: National Technical Information Service, U.S. Department of Commerce, Spring 1985.

U.S. Senate, Special Committee on Aging, "Medicare: Paying the Physician—History, Issues, and Options," S. PRT 98-153, Washington, DC: U.S. Government Printing Office, March 1984.

Wennberg, J. E., L. Blowers, R. Parker, and A. Gittlesohn, "Changes in Tonsillectomy Rates Associated with Feedback and Review," *Pediatrics,* 59:821–826, 1977.

Wennberg, J. E., and A. Gittelsohn, "Variations in Medical Care Among Small Areas," Scientific American, 246:120–129, 1982.

Wennberg, J. E., K. McPherson, and P. Caper, "Will Payment Based on Diagnosis-Related Groups Control Hospital Costs?" *New England Journal of Medicine,* 311(5):295–300, 1984.

Wilensky, G. R. and L. F. Rossiter, "Alternative Units of Payment for Physicians' Services: An Overview of the Issues." *Medical Care Review* 43(1):133–156, Spring 1986.

IV

Medicare Benefits and Private Burdens

12. Employers and Medicare as Partners in Financing Health Care for the Elderly

□ □ □

PAMELA FARLEY SHORT AND ALAN C. MONHEIT

Introduction

Medicare, Title XVIII of the Social Security Act, was enacted in 1965 to protect the elderly from major health expenses by providing insurance for hospital and physician care. The program was adopted during a period of sweeping economic and social change accomplished through federal legislation. At the time, when continued economic growth was expected, when budget deficits were less than 1 percent of the gross national product, when the cost of medical care was increasing by only 2.5 percent a year and the elderly were less than 10 percent of the population, the plans for funding Medicare through a mix of public and private financing mechanisms seemed quite adequate. Payroll taxes would go into a Hospital Insurance trust fund (Part A, covering hospital, skilled nursing facility, and home health care); premiums paid by beneficiaries and general tax revenues would finance Supplementary Medical Insurance (Part B, covering physician and other ambulatory services); and beneficiaries would also pay for their care directly, through deductibles and other cost-sharing provisions.

Twenty years later, the situation is changing. Sluggish economic growth has slowed the expansion of payroll and income tax revenues, the bulwarks of Medicare financing, at the same time that new medical technologies and more resource-intensive modes of treatment have expanded health care costs. In addition, there are increasingly fewer active workers paying into the system, compared with beneficiaries drawing out of it. Demographic projections indicate that the elderly will comprise 12 percent of the U.S. population in the year 2000 and 19 percent in 2030 (Davis and Rowland 1986). These trends, together with a political re-alignment that favors reduced public involvement in health care financing and a reduced role for the federal government more generally, are calling into question the assumptions of Medicare's current financing.

Is there a fairer or more efficient way, in the context of these changes, to maintain current levels of health insurance for the elderly? Of particular interest in this chapter is the role that employers can or should be expected to play. In 1965 the assumption was that health care for the elderly could not be financed satisfactorily through the employer-sponsored groups that insured most of the nonelderly population. Many fewer elderly persons were employed than nonelderly, and employers were generally unwilling to accept the liability of such a potentially sickly group of enrollees, based on past employment affiliations. At the time, about nine out of ten employees could expect to lose their group health insurance when they retired, although most could convert to a nongroup plan (Skolnik 1976). This, too, has changed since the advent of Medicare. According to the Bureau of Labor Statistics (1986), currently only 34 percent of full-time employees of medium and large firms have group plans that will not continue after retirement from the firm at age sixty-five. Over two-fifths of elderly beneficiaries with private insurance to supplement Medicare, a third of the elderly Medicare population overall, are now insured by current or former employers. An important difference, however, is the fact that health insurance groups are now responsible only for the expenses of elderly retirees that Medicare does not pay.

The federal government has already taken steps to expand the financing responsibilities of employers. The Tax Equity and Fiscal Responsibility Act of 1982 (TEFRA) required employers to offer the same insurance as they offer to younger employees to working beneficiaries aged sixty-five to sixty-nine and made Medicare the secondary payer. This reduced Medicare's liability to covered expenses not reimbursed by the employer's plan. In the Deficit Reduction Act of 1984 (DEFRA), the same rules were extended to the insurance of workers under sixty-five, covering a spouse on Medicare. Federal policy also permits employees to retire on Social Security when they are sixty-two but does not include them in Medicare until they are sixty-five. This gap is commonly filled by employers, with continuation of health benefits for early retirees. Even without any conscious public policy changes, as new Medicare enrollees with retiree benefits replace the old cohorts who stopped working before such benefits were common, the percentage of the Medicare population that is insured by employers will increase substantially over time.

Nevertheless, there are significant difficulties with the hope of a new partnership between employers and Medicare to preserve the health benefits of the elderly. Most importantly, employer health plans are in much the same situation as Medicare. Like Medicare, they operate on a pay-as-you-go basis, financing the health care of both active and retired employees from the current production of the active workforce. As employees retire earlier and the elderly population grows and lives longer, the higher ratio of retirees to workers raises the cost of retiree health benefits in relation to a firm's output and the wages of active workers (U.S. Senate Special Committee on Aging 1985). In addition, the sluggish performance of the economy means that employers and workers are not doing that well financially; they, too, have felt the pinch of health care inflation. Health insurance premiums paid by employers increased as a percentage of total labor compensation at a rate of 5 percent a year between 1970 and 1982 (Chollet 1984).

If the burden of Medicare on taxpayers is the issue, shifting the burden to employer-sponsored plans that rely on largely the same financing sources—namely, the wages of active workers and corporate profits—is not a solution. Moreover, the future burden on employer plans of paying for promised retiree health benefits is already substantial. As of 1983 unfunded employer liabilities associated with retiree health benefits were estimated by the Department of Labor to be $100 billion (U.S. Department of Labor 1986).

In addition to the already significant burden on employment-related health insurance groups in the future, there is an important difference between them and Medicare that is likely to make employers extremely cautious about accepting a larger role in insuring retirees. Unlike Medicare, according to recent court decisions, employers are not permitted to modify health benefits that they have either explicitly or implicitly promised to retirees (EBRI 1985; U.S. Senate Special Committee on Aging 1985; U.S. Department of Labor 1986). Thus, to offer benefits to a retiring employee is to risk a twenty- or thirty-year commitment in the face of an uncertain economic future and the uncertainties of medical inflation and future demand. Also, employers cannot control the future of Medicare itself, and cutbacks in Medicare could greatly increase the financial burden on their own plans.

Another problem is the uneven access to employer-sponsored plans among Medicare beneficiaries, which raises questions of fairness about the burdens distributed among the elderly themselves. Because the availability of retiree health benefits has expanded over time, the oldest beneficiaries (who are in the poorest health on average) are least often enrolled in group plans. Because of their historically lower rate of labor force participation, females are also less likely to be insured by employers. In the future, these differences will even out, as today's retirees with employer benefits grow older and the upward shift in female labor force participation is translated into an increase in female retirement benefits. However, there are also marked discrepancies in group enrollment between elderly whites and blacks, and the tight relationship between the lack of retirement income from prior employment (whether private pensions or Social Security) and poverty among the elderly means that the poor as a rule also lack health benefits from a former employer.

Despite emerging interest in the involvement of employers in insuring the elderly, there is not much factual information widely available. In this chapter, data from national surveys and other sources are assembled to provide a description of the employer-sponsored insurance of Medicare beneficiaries currently and to speculate on the future direction of retiree health benefits. In particular, the 1977 National Medical Care Expenditure Survey (NMCES) and the more recent Survey of Income and Program Participation (SIPP) are used to examine patterns and trends in enrollment. NMCES provides additional data concerning the payment of premiums by employers and retirees and the provisions of the insurance. (See Appendix 12.1 for more information about the data sources.) The estimates distinguish working Medicare beneficiaries from retirees who are covered by employer plans, as well as beneficiaries insured through their own employers from those insured through their spouses' employers. The former distinction has been important in recent legislation, and both are important in projecting the effects of changing demographics and labor force participation on enrollment in the future.

Current Retiree Benefits

Of the roughly 25 million persons aged sixty-five and over enrolled in Medicare in 1983, about 7.9 million or 31 percent also had employer-sponsored insurance (Table 12.1). In comparison, only a quarter of the 22 million Medicare elderly in 1977 (5.5 million) had employer-sponsored insurance six years before. This amounts to an increase in enrollment of about 6 percent per year. Retirees and their dependents (in contrast to workers and their dependents) accounted for roughly the same proportion of enrollment in 1977 and 1983 among those sixty-five and older. However, among those aged sixty-two to sixty-four there was a substantial shift in enrollment from active workers to retirees, reflecting the trend toward early retirement.

In 1977, in both age cohorts displayed in Table 12.1, employers insured about one dependent for every three retirees or employees. By 1983 this ratio was closer to one dependent for every two retirees or employees. In both years, employers insured roughly one dependent for every three retirees sixty-five and older, compared with the higher ratio of one to two for younger retirees sixty-two to sixty-four. The latter probably reflects the higher proportion of retirees aged sixty-two to sixty-four with a surviving spouse.

As noted earlier, the recent legislative trend is to declare Medicare the secondary payer for claims covered by the insurance of active employees. However,

TABLE 12.1
Enrollment in Employment-Related Plans by the Elderly

Enrolled in employment-related plans	1977[a]		1983[b]	
	Number (thousands)	Percent distribution	Number (thousands)	Percent distribution
Age 65+, with Medicare	5,469	100.0	7,865	100.0
Working primary insured	1,182	21.6	1,644	20.9
Primary insured	701	12.8	935	11.9
Dependent only	481	8.8	709	9.0
Retired primary insured	4,287	78.4	6,221	79.1
Primary insured	3,305	60.4	4,666	59.3
Dependent only	982	18.0	1,555	19.8
Age 62–64	3,313	100.0	3,777	100.0
Working primary insured	2,083	62.9	2,045	54.2
Primary insured	1,573	47.5	1,430	37.9
Dependent only	509	15.4	615	16.3
Retired primary insured	1,230	37.1	1,732	45.9
Primary insured	856	25.8	1,099	29.1
Dependent only	375	11.3	632	16.7

[a]NMCES, Health Insurance/Employer Survey.
[b]Survey of Income and Program Participation, wave 1.
Source: National Center for Health Services Research and Health Care Technology Assessment.

of the Medicare beneficiaries who were covered by employer plans in 1983, only 21 percent were either working themselves or were dependents of active workers. Most were either retirees or their dependents. Thus, even if this policy were carried out to its maximum extent, Medicare's liability for little more than a fifth of its beneficiaries would be affected. Indeed, if the decline in labor force participation of persons sixty-five and older over the last decade continues as expected, from 16.3 to 13.3 percent of males and from 7.5 to 7.0 percent of females between 1984 and 1995 (U.S. Bureau of the Census 1985), the relative effectiveness of this policy may be diminished somewhat. Further, the policy itself is likely to encourage the trend toward earlier retirement since firms can reduce their insurance costs by retiring employees who have Medicare.

National data are available only for 1977 with respect to the cost of the insurance provided by employers (Table 12.2). At that time, employers paid over $1.3 billion, 64 percent of the premiums, for coverage supplementing the Medicare benefits of employees and retirees. Projecting the average premium at the same rate of growth as private health insurance premiums per enrollee overall (13 percent a year between 1977 and 1983, HIAA 1985), while taking into account the growth in enrollment, yields an estimate of roughly $4 billion in 1983. Most employers offer the same insurance plan to retirees as to active workers (BLS 1986). However, the average total premium for retirees on Medicare ($498) was about $350 less than the average total premium for workers aged sixty-two

TABLE 12.2
Financing of Employment-Related Plans of the Elderly[a]

Primary insured persons	No. of primary insured (thousands)	Mean annual premium (dollars)	Percent distribution by source of payment		
			Family	Employer	Other
Age 65+, with Medicare	4,006	516	31.0	64.3	4.7
Working	701	601	36.9	60.5	2.6
Retired	3,305	498	29.5	65.3	5.3
Age 62–64	2,429	811	26.3	72.0	1.7
Working	1,573	852	26.4	72.0	1.6
Retired	856	736	26.0	72.0	2.0

[a]NMCES, Health Insurance/Employer Survey, 1977.
Source: National Center for Health Services Research and Health Care Technology Assessment.

through sixty-four in 1977, and the average difference in employer-paid premiums was nearly $300. In short, the cost of retiree health insurance was substantially less than the insurance of active workers under age sixty-five.

This difference is a function of several factors. The main difference, and presumably a major consideration in the willingness of employers to offer retiree health benefits since the introduction of Medicare, is the fact that Medicare and not the employer-sponsored plan is the primary payer for the claims of retired beneficiaries. These savings are reflected in the lower premium that is set for each Medicare beneficiary in the employer's plan. Because employee health benefits have improved over time, the lower average premium for all elderly retirees also reflects the lower premiums of older cohorts who retired some time ago with plans less generous than those currently offered. The increasing breadth of retiree health benefits over time is evident from Table 12.3, where the inclusion of selected services under the plans of primary insured persons in 1977 is compared by age. For example, only 62 percent of those seventy-five and older were insured for prescription drugs, an expense not covered by Medicare, compared with 68 percent of those aged seventy through seventy-four, and 74 percent of those aged sixty-four through sixty-nine. Employees and retirees between the ages of sixty-two and sixty-four most often had drug benefits (83 percent). Also, few elderly retirees have family coverage to insure their spouses, as noted earlier.

Although Medicare is the primary payer for all elderly retirees, there are several ways of specifying the supplementary benefits to be paid under an employer's plan. The beneficiary's out-of-pocket costs and the amount saved by the employer's plan depend on the method specified. A "carve-out" provision is apparently the most common (EBRI 1985). Under this arrangement, benefits under the employer's plan are first calculated without regard to Medicare and are then reduced by the amount that Medicare pays. For example, suppose the employer

TABLE 12.3
Breadth of Employment-Related Benefits by Age of Primary Insured [a]

Primary insured persons	Percent covered for service			
	Outpatient physician	Outpatient psychiatric	Prescribed medicines	Dental
Total	78.1	64.4	74.5	14.4
Age				
62–64	84.1	73.3	82.8	18.9
65–69	73.4	60.7	74.3	12.7
70–74	75.2	60.1	68.0	13.6
75+	76.0	54.8	61.7	7.9

[a]NMCES, Health Insurance/Employer Survey, 1977.
Source: National Center for Health Services Research and Health Care Technology Assessment.

has a major medical plan with a $50 deductible and 20 percent coinsurance. For a $500 physician bill, Medicare would pay $340 (80 percent of the amount in excess of the $75 Part B deductible), and the employer's plan would pay $360, ignoring Medicare (80 percent of the amount in excess of $50). The employer's benefit is reduced by the $340 paid by Medicare to $20, leaving the beneficiary to pay $140. In effect, the beneficiary is open to whatever cost sharing is specified by the employer's plan.

Under coordination of benefits (COB), the benefits under the employer's plan are again calculated without regard to Medicare but are available to offset any covered costs not reimbursed by Medicare. In the example above, $160 from the employer defrays all of the cost sharing left by Medicare, and the beneficiary pays nothing. Thus, in contrast to a carve-out, the beneficiary's out-of-pocket payments are reduced to zero at the private plan's expense. An "exclusion plan" falls somewhere in between, both with respect to the plan's savings and the beneficiary's out-of-pocket expenses. Here, the deductible and coinsurance provisions of the employer's plan are applied to the out-of-pocket expenses remaining after Medicare. The employer's plan would pay $88 in this example, 80 percent of the difference between the Medicare cost sharing of $160 and the plan deductible of $50. Finally, some employers offer reduced benefits to retirees (about 15 percent in medium and large firms, BLS 1986) compared with active workers, often along the same lines as the "Medigap" plans marketed directly to the Medicare population that specifically cover the program's various deductibles and copayments.

An indirect effect of increasing Medicare's cost-sharing requirements would be to shift more of the financial burden to the employer plans that cover beneficiaries. Under all of the arrangements described above, except for the exclusion plan, the employer's plan would probably pick up the entire difference.[1] But who would end up paying the increase in premiums that would result from the increase in benefit payments? If the present shares were maintained, Medicare beneficiaries would pay about a third and employers or active workers would pay the rest. However, conceivably any distribution of the burden of payment among beneficiaries, younger workers, and employers could result.[2]

Similarly, the Medicare program could probably also be cut back at the expense of employer-sponsored plans by postponing the age of Medicare eligibility, with the expectation that employers would continue to provide insurance to young retirees. As noted earlier, continued group coverage is already offered by many employers of any significant size to early retirees, those between sixty-two and sixty-five years of age who are eligible for Social Security but are not eligible for Medicare (BLS 1986). In fact, more employers offer continued coverage to early retirees than to those who retire at age sixty-five, when they are eligible for Medicare. Employers insured 1.7 million early retirees and their dependents in 1983 and 1.2 million in 1977 (see Table 12.1). They also paid 72 percent of the premiums in 1977, the same share as for active workers, at a cost of $0.6 billion (see Table 12.2). One could argue that employers expect to insure employees until they are sixty-five and, consequently, are willing to do so even if the employee retires. However, to insure all employees for several additional years beyond age sixty-five is a somewhat different proposition, perhaps unacceptable to employers without a reduction in plan benefits or the employer's share of the premiums. Here, too, especially in the short run, the issue is how much elderly beneficiaries, active workers, and employers would each end up paying.

Uneven Access to Employer-Sponsored Insurance

The other reason for not hoping for too much from employers is the uneven access of beneficiaries to employer-sponsored plans. Most Medicare beneficiaries lack employment-related insurance (Tables 12.4 and 12.5), despite an increase in the proportion of covered beneficiaries from 25 percent in 1977 to 31 percent in 1983. About 40 percent of elderly Medicare beneficiaries purchased private supplementary insurance directly from insurance companies in 1983, down slightly from 43 percent in 1977, and about 30 percent had no private insurance at all. Some of those without private insurance are covered by Medicaid, but 20 percent of the Medicare population have no supplementary insurance (Cafferata 1984). They would bear the full brunt of either a cutback in Medicare benefits or a postponement of eligibility in terms of higher out-of-pocket expenses, as would nongroup enrollees in terms of higher premiums (Taylor, Farley, and Horgan forthcoming).

Coverage of the elderly Medicare population by employment-related health insurance varies systematically, with a number of demographic and economic variables. The extent of employer-sponsored coverage is inversely related to age, with 42 percent of persons sixty-five through sixty-nine having coverage in 1983, compared with only 31 percent of those seventy to seventy-four and about 22 percent of those seventy-five and older. The oldest age groups are somewhat more likely to purchase other private insurance, but this only partly compensates for their lack of employee coverage. About 36 percent of persons seventy-five and older and about 27 percent of those seventy to seventy-four lacked private supplementary insurance in 1983, compared with less than a quarter of the sixty-five through sixty-nine age group.

Disparities between males and females reflect historical differences in labor force participation and employment experience. Twenty-seven percent of elderly females on Medicare had employer-sponsored insurance in 1983, about 12 percent as the dependent of an active worker or retiree. About 37 percent of elderly males on Medicare had employer-sponsored insurance in 1983, 26 percent as a result of their own employment. By the same token, married females were almost twice as often insured by employers as females who were not married (including the widowed and divorced). The rise in the proportion of beneficiaries obtaining employment-related coverage since 1977 is evenly distributed by sex, with both groups experiencing an increase of 6 percentage points.

Racial differences in the employment-related insurance of the elderly, as well as in supplementary private insurance more generally, are quite pronounced but have narrowed somewhat since 1977. In that year, roughly twice the proportion of whites had employment-related insurance as blacks (28 percent compared with 15 percent). In 1983, 32 percent of whites had employment-related coverage compared with 21 percent of blacks. As of 1983 whites and blacks had almost the same probability of obtaining employment-related insurance as a retiree (19 percent of whites, 14 percent of blacks), while in 1977 white retirees were almost four times as likely to receive such benefits. Just 17 percent of blacks purchased other private insurance, compared with 43 percent of whites, leaving almost two-thirds of elderly blacks without private insurance to supplement Medicare.[3]

Among the elderly, as among the younger working population (Farley 1986), income and employment-related insurance are tied closely together. Social Security benefits, as well as pension benefits, are important income sources that reflect prior employment experience. Prior employment, in turn, is a necessary prerequisite for enrollment in an employer-sponsored plan. As a consequence, those best able to supplement Medicare out of their own pocket are the most likely to have comprehensive, employer-subsidized insurance, and those least able to pay for uncovered expenses have the least employment-related insurance. Over 50 percent of the Medicare elderly with high family incomes in 1983 were insured through employers, compared with about 20 percent of those with low

TABLE 12.4
Private Health Insurance of the Medicare Elderly (SIPP)[a]

All Medicare elderly	Number of persons (thousands)	Percent distribution by category with employment-related insurance					Other private insurance	No private insurance
		Total	Active worker	Dependent of active worker	Retiree	Dependent of retiree		
Total[b]	25,329	31.1	3.7	2.8	18.4	6.2	39.6	29.2
Age								
65–69	8,461	42.0	6.6	5.3	21.1	9.1	34.1	23.8
70–74	7,051	30.7	3.5	2.2	18.3	6.7	42.8	26.5
75 and over	9,818	21.9	1.4	1.1	16.2	3.2	42.1	35.9
Sex and marital status								
Male	10,306	36.9	6.1	2.4	25.7	2.7	35.5	27.6
Not married	2,403	20.6	3.1	0.2c	17.1	0.2c	32.9	46.3
Married	7,903	41.8	7.0	3.1	28.3	3.4	36.3	21.9
Female	15,023	27.1	2.0	3.1	13.4	8.5	42.5	30.4
Not married	9,221	20.3	2.5	0.5c	17.3	0.1c	44.3	35.3
Married	5,803	37.7	1.3	7.2	7.3	21.9	39.5	22.7
Race								
White	22,489	32.4	3.7	2.9	19.2	6.5	42.5	25.1
Black	1,974	20.7	3.1	0.9c	14.2	2.5	17.4	61.7

Family income, adjusted for family size								
Poor	3,080	4.7	0.8[c]	0.1[c]	3.7	0.1[c]	29.7	65.6
Near poor	2,358	8.9	0.8[c]	0.4[c]	6.7	0.9[c]	41.3	49.8
Low	5,621	19.8	1.0[c]	0.6[c]	15.3	2.9	48.0	32.2
Middle	9,504	41.7	4.0	3.1	24.9	9.7	39.9	18.1
High	4,765	51.0	9.6	7.7	24.3	9.4	34.8	14.2
Family pension benefits								
Yes	7,739	56.9	4.2	1.7	46.5	4.5	28.5	14.5
No	17,590	19.7	3.5	3.3	6.1	6.9	44.5	35.7
Region								
North	5,747	33.1	4.1	3.8	19.0	6.3	38.6	28.1
North central	6,202	36.2	3.6	2.8	22.4	7.4	40.7	23.2
South	8,948	26.5	3.5	2.2	15.5	5.4	39.9	33.6
West	4,435	30.4	3.5	2.8	18.0	6.1	39.1	30.3

[a]SIPP: wave 1, 1983.

[b]Includes persons of Hispanic and other ethnic origin or unknown race and unknown pension status not shown separately.

[c]Relative standard error exceeds 30% of estimate.

Source: National Center for Health Services Research and Health Care Technology Assessment.

TABLE 12.5
Private Health Insurance of the Medicare Elderly (NMCES)[a]

All Medicare elderly	Number of persons (thousands)	Percent distribution by category with employment-related insurance					Other private insurance	No private insurance
		Total	Active worker	Dependent of active worker	Retiree	Dependent of retiree		
Total[b]	21,766	25.1	3.2	2.2	15.2	4.5	43.1	31.8
Age								
65–69	7,276	35.9	6.5	3.2	20.4	5.9	38.7	25.4
70–74	6,075	25.0	3.0	2.4	14.0	5.6	44.2	30.8
75 and over	8,415	15.8	0.5c	1.3c	11.5	2.5	46.1	38.1
Sex and marital status								
Male	8,897	31.0	5.5	1.8	21.6	2.1	38.9	30.1
Not married	2,044	19.8	4.3	1.2c	13.9	0.4c	29.3	50.9
Married	6,853	34.4	5.9	2.0	23.9	2.6	41.8	23.9
Female	12,869	21.0	1.6	2.5	10.8	6.2	46.0	33.0
Not married	8,260	14.8	1.7	1.5c	11.1	0.4c	49.2	36.0
Married	4,608	32.3	1.4c	4.2	10.1	16.6	40.3	27.5
Race								
White	16,933	27.8	3.3	2.1	17.5	5.0	47.9	24.4
Black	1,632	15.3	5.1	4.8	4.6	0.7c	19.8	65.0

Family income, adjusted for family size							
Poor	3,476	6.9	0.4c	0.2c	5.5	0.8c	37.4	55.7
Near poor	2,052	10.2	0.8c	0.2c	8.0	1.2c	41.3	48.5
Low	5,025	19.9	1.7c	0.3c	13.6	4.3	46.2	33.8
Middle	6,670	32.1	4.0	3.4	18.5	6.2	46.1	21.8
High	4,543	41.3	7.0	5.0	22.7	6.6	40.3	18.4
Family pension benefits							
Yes	5,175	44.2	3.5	2.5	27.9	10.2	42.6	13.2
No	13,999	19.7	3.3	2.2	11.7	2.5	45.4	34.9
Region							
North	5,021	24.7	4.0	3.8	14.0	2.9	47.8	27.5
North central	5,789	28.6	4.0	2.5	15.9	6.1	47.8	23.7
South	6,639	20.8	2.5	1.3c	13.3	3.6	39.6	39.7
West	4,316	27.8	2.2	1.4c	18.6	5.7	36.8	35.5

[a]NMCES, Health Insurance/Employer Survey, 1977.

[b]Includes persons of Hispanic and other ethnic origin or unknown race and unknown pension status not shown separately.

[c]Relative standard error exceeds 30% of estimate.

Source: National Center for Health Services Research and Health Care Technology Assessment.

incomes and just 5 percent of the poor. The connection created by the dual role of employment as a source of income and as a source of insurance is evident in the 57 percent of Medicare beneficiaries with employment-related insurance in families with pension income, almost three times the rate of families without a pension. This proportion has increased markedly since 1977 in families with pension income (47 percent receiving health insurance benefits in 1983, compared with only 28 percent in 1977) and reflects the increased growth in retirement benefits since that time.

Note that the situation is made even more favorable for the wealthy by the exclusion of noncash benefits from taxable employee income, an implicit subsidy that increases in value as income increases. The retirement benefits of highly paid workers are consequently the most highly subsidized. There is also an incentive to substitute health insurance benefits from a former employer for taxable pension income.

Finally, there appear to have been substantial increases in the employment-related insurance of the elderly in the South and West between 1977 and 1983 that were reflected in a decline in the percentage of Medicare beneficiaries without supplementary insurance. The latter figure stayed roughly the same in the north central region and in the Northeast, but there was a shift to employment-related plans from other private insurance.

Looking into the Future

Continued enrollment in an employer-sponsored health insurance plan is an attractive retirement benefit. Such plans generally supplement Medicare far more generously than a plan purchased directly from an insurance company at about the same cost (Cafferata 1984). Not only do employers pay a substantial share of the premiums, but group insurance also offers marketing and administrative economies and safeguards against adverse risk selection that result in lower rates. Furthermore, retiree health benefits receive favorable tax treatment in comparison to nongroup premiums that have to be paid out of taxable retirement income.

Employers are playing an increasingly significant role in supplementing Medicare, a trend that will continue if present economic and demographic forces are allowed to have their effect. Although employers now insure just 31 percent of the entire elderly Medicare population, 36 percent of recent Medicare enrollees have employment-related insurance. Approximately two-thirds of today's full-time employees are promised private insurance to supplement Medicare, and an even larger number work for firms that offer continuing coverage until age sixty-five for employees who retire before they are eligible for the program. Enrollment of the Medicare population in employer-sponsored plans will also increase as a result of the dramatic increase in the labor force participation of women, who comprise 60 percent of the Medicare population and will qualify for retiree benefits in increasing numbers.[4] Despite recent court decisions that have limited the flexibility of employers in adjusting retiree benefits to reflect changing economic circumstances, there is no sign as yet of a retrenchment by employers (BLS 1984; BLS 1986).

The employment-related insurance of Medicare beneficiaries is expanding in terms of the amount of coverage as well as enrollment. Because most employers offer the same benefits to retirees as they offer to active workers, the continuing expansion of employee benefits over time is mirrored in the private insurance of retirees. For example, the proportion of the population aged sixty-five through sixty-nine with insurance for prescribed medicines was 20 percent greater in 1977 than the proportion of persons seventy-five and older. As older retirees die and are replaced by new retirees with more generous insurance, the benefits paid by employer plans will increase.

"Employer-provided health benefits for retirees are a vital part of the developing three-legged stool in health coverage for older Americans—government, employers and individuals," observed Chairman John Heinz during hearings held in July 1985 by the Senate Finance Subcommittee on Savings, Pensions, and Investment Policy. "Instead of growing, though, the employer leg may be on the verge of collapsing. We need desperately to find a way to encourage employers to provide retiree health benefits before the tremendous burden of costs for older Americans is dumped entirely on the government and the elderly themselves" (Kosterlitz 1985, p. 1746).

In other words, although a conscious policy decision to shift even more of Medicare's financial burden to employer-sponsored plans is appealing at first glance, employers are already uneasy about their present level of commitment. There are also questions of equity and efficiency to be addressed before relying too heavily on this public-private partnership. The 50 percent increase in the ratio of retirees to active workers that is projected in the next fifty years creates the same problem for employers as it does for Medicare and raises the same questions about the burden on younger workers and taxpayers, since both employers and Medicare finance retiree health benefits on a pay-as-you-go basis. Furthermore, unlike the health insurance benefits of active workers, which can be modified from year to year, retiree benefits commit an employer to a specified plan for as many as twenty to thirty years into the future. Not only is this a significant long-term liability, but its actual amount depends uncertainly on future inflation, medical technology, and Medicare policies. Significantly, the Federal Accounting Standards Board now requires the cost and funding of retiree benefits to be shown on each firm's annual financial statement and is considering disclosure of the unfunded obligations as a liability on corporate balance sheets. Finally, because of the limited and uneven work history of some elderly persons, no policy that operates through employers can reach the entire Medicare population. In this respect, the initial assumptions behind enactment of a public program to finance the health care of the elderly were correct.

The future of the partnership will undoubtedly be shaped by these considerations. In fairness to tomorrow's workers, tomorrow's elderly can probably count on having to pay for a larger share of their health care themselves. The issue is whether or not they and their employers will be encouraged by public subsidies to save now for that day. Although DEFRA limited the use of tax-preferred voluntary employee beneficiary associations (VEBAs) to fund the future health benefits of current workers (EBRI 1985),[5] several proposals make the shift from future, tax-supported Medicare benefits to current tax subsidies explicit. For example, the Health Care Savings Account Act of 1985 (HR 3505) would impose a higher Medicare deductible in retirement on employees who elect to participate in a tax-preferred, health individual retirement account (IRA).[6] Alternatively, rather than specifically involving health care, the issue can be seen as involving public policies to encourage retirement savings more generally (that would be sufficient to cover the cost of health insurance and health care, as well as other things).

Complicating matters is the long and uncertain planning horizon for both employers and employees. One of the biggest uncertainties is the future of Medicare itself. If there are indeed to be substantial cutbacks in Medicare, either through postponement of eligibility or changes in cost sharing, the announcement of this decision well in advance of its implementation would facilitate an efficient transfer of financing responsibility to employers and beneficiaries. In any event, in view of Medicare's uncertain future and the other uncertainties of inflation and changing medical practice, some employers are likely to move toward cash rather than in-kind retiree health benefits. Thus, instead of offering to pay whatever expenses Medicare does not cover, the employer would offer a specified cash amount to be used either to buy into the group plan or to pay medical expenses. Such an arrangement transfers the risk of inflation to retirees. However, because employers do not have the same flexibility as Medicare in terms of future adjustments, they may not be able to provide the same protection against such risks.

There will continue to be a substantial proportion of the Medicare population without access to employer-sponsored benefits, a fact with two important implications. First, a significant part of the cost of maintaining health benefits for an expanding elderly population cannot be financed through employers. Separate attention to elderly persons who purchase nongroup insurance or have no supplementary private insurance at all, who are disproportionately poor and disadvantaged anyway, will be a necessary part of any coherent policy. Second, if favorable tax treatment or other financial incentives are needed to encourage the involvement of employers, these inducements will discriminate against a large number of elderly persons who have no way to take advantage of them. As noted earlier, this bias is already inherent in the tax-free status of the health insurance premiums that employers pay for some retirees each year, in contrast to the premiums that other retirees pay directly to insurance companies out of their taxable income. Subsidies, if offered, should be structured in a more neutral fashion than the targeting of employers alone permits. But this line of reasoning brings one full circle. Rather than fund a universal program of implicit or explicit subsidies for private insurance or private retirement savings, the same tax dollars might be used more fairly and efficiently to fund Medicare directly.

Appendix 12.1: Data Sources and Definitions

The data used in this study were obtained from the 1983 SIPP and the 1977 NMCES. The following discussion briefly describes each data base, as well as the definitions of employment and insurance status derived from each.

1983 SIPP

SIPP, conducted by the Bureau of the Census, is a longitudinal household survey designed to provide detailed information on the economic circumstances of households and persons representing the noninstitutionalized population of the United States. Sampled households are interviewed every four months over a period of 2.5 years, with the reference period the four-month interval prior to the interview month. All persons fifteen years and older who are household members at the initial interview are included for the entire length of the survey. The data concerning these adults includes data about their children, so the survey covers the entire population. Within a given yearly panel, sample households are divided into four subsamples or rotation groups of approximately equal size, with one rotation group interviewed each month. One cycle of four interviews for an entire sample (i.e., one interview for each rotation group) is called a wave. Our estimates are derived from wave one of the SIPP panel, where June was the first reference month of the first reference group. Age, family income, insurance, and employment status in our estimates are defined as of the last reference month for each person, covering the last third of 1983.

During each interview, respondents to SIPP are asked about their labor force activity, the types and amounts of income received, and their participation in various public programs. With regard to the specific interests of this chapter, individuals are also asked about their labor force status and employment during each month of the reference period, whether they have ever retired from a job or business, and whether they were covered by private or public health insurance during the reference period. Details regarding private insurance include whether coverage is obtained through a current or former employer or union, whether a person is a primary insured or dependent on a health insurance plan, and the months in which the person was covered.

For purposes of our analysis, persons are considered retired if they reported ever retiring from a job and displayed no evidence of employment during the fourth month of the reference period (i.e., no job held during the month regardless of whether they were looking or on layoff). Persons were considered employed if they reported having a job during the month (regardless of whether they were looking or on layoff). Persons who had retired from a previous job but were currently working were also considered to be employed. It was not possible to determine whether employment-related insurance held by such persons was obtained through the current or previous (retirement) job. Once employment status was established, data on type of health insurance and primary insured/dependent status was used to establish employment and insurance classifications for persons sixty-two years of age and older.

1977 NMCES

The 1977 NMCES is a survey of the health insurance and medical care utilization and expenditures of 14,000 randomly selected households representative of the civilian noninstitutionalized population. The survey was undertaken to provide data for a major research effort in the NCHSR and was cosponsored by the National Center for Health Statistics.

Respondents to the survey were asked about their health insurance and expenditures for medical care in 1977 during five interviews conducted over an eighteen-month period from 1977 to early 1978. A variety of other sociodemographic and economic data were collected, including information on employment status and type of health insurance held by household members throughout the year.

Information regarding private health insurance from the household survey was verified and supplemented by the NMCES HIES. By surveying insurance companies, employers, unions, and other organizations named as the source of each household's coverage, HIES provided a detailed description of benefit provisions and premiums and the distribution of premiums among employers, employees, and other sources.

For purposes of our analysis, individuals sixty-two years of age and older were considered retired if they were without a job or out of the labor force at the last (round five) NMCES household interview. Individuals were considered employed if they held a job for pay during the week preceding the round five interview date. This distinction provides definitions of "retired" and "working" that are comparable to those developed using SIPP and yields estimates of labor force status for December 1977. These definitions have been combined with information on health insurance status during 1977 from both the household and HIES surveys to yield the employment and insurance classes presented in our analyses of NMCES data.

Notes

The views expressed are those of the authors. No official endorsement by the Department of Health and Human Services or NCHSR is intended or should be inferred. Programming assistance was provided by Kisun Han of Social and Scientific Systems, Inc., of Bethesda, Maryland. Mark Pauly's helpful comments led to improvements over an earlier version.

1. Somewhat ironically, there would be no change in the beneficiary's out-of-pocket expenses under either a carve-out or coordination of benefits, although the level of out-of-pocket expense maintained under the two arrangements differs substantially. Since carve-out benefits are reduced dollar-for-dollar by the Medicare benefit, any reduction in Medicare would be fully reflected in the plan benefit. By the same token, the plan benefits that are available to offset out-of-pocket costs under coordination of benefits are generally more than enough to offset the current amount of Medicare cost sharing. (Note in the example given, the employer's plan pays only about half the regular benefit.) Consequently, additional cost-sharing requirements would also be fully covered in most situations.

2. The incidence of retiree benefits on active workers versus employers is an open issue. In the long run, one can argue (although perhaps with some difficulty, since the future value of health benefits at retirement is quite difficult to predict) that workers implicitly pay for their own future health benefits through a reduction in current wages. However, the issue here is the short-run adjustment to a cutback in the Medicare benefits of workers who have already retired.

3. A much higher proportion of nonwhites are enrolled in Medicaid, but about 30 percent have no supplementary coverage at all, compared with about 20 percent of whites (Cafferata 1984).

4. The Bureau of Labor Statistics projects that female labor force participation will increase from 53.6 percent in 1984 to 60.3 percent in 1995. Male participation is projected to remain at just over 76 percent during this period (U.S. Bureau of the Census 1985).

5. Prior to DEFRA, tax law permitted employers to prefund retiree health benefits through Section 501(c)(9) trusts or VEBAs. DEFRA restricted the use of this funding mechanism by limiting the amount of qualified employer contributions to VEBAs by requiring actuarial assumptions to be based on current medical care costs and plan experience and by taxing investment earnings on reserves held in VEBAs. (See EBRI [1985] and U.S. Department of Labor [1986].)

6. See Bowen and Burke (1985) and the other proposals reviewed by EBRI (1986) as well.

References

Bowen, O. R., and T. R. Burke, "Cost Neutral Catastrophic Care Proposed for Medicare Recipients," *Federation of American Hospitals Review,* 42–45, November/December 1985.

Cafferata, G. L., Private Health Insurance Coverage of the Medicare Population, Data Preview 18, National Center for Health Services Research, National Health Care Expenditures Study, Rockville, MD: U.S. Department of Health and Human Services, Publication No. (PHS) 84-3362, September, 1984.

Chollet, D. J., *Employer-Provided Health Benefits: Coverage Provisions and Policy Issues,* Washington, DC: Employee Benefit Research Institute, 1984.

Davis, K., and D. Rowland, *Medicare Policy: New Directions for Health and Long-Term Care,* Baltimore, MD: Johns Hopkins University Press, 1986.

Employee Benefit Research Institute (EBRI), "Employer-Paid Retiree Health Insurance: History and Prospects for Growth," *EBRI Issue Brief* (Number 47), 1985.

———, "IRAs, 401(k)s and Employer Pensions—Must There Be Tradeoffs?" *EBRI Issue Brief* (Number 52), 1986.

Farley, P. J., *Private Health Insurance in the United States,* NHCES Data Preview 23, DHHS Publication No. (PHS) 86-3406, Rockville, MD: National Center for Health Services Research, 1986.

Health Insurance Association of America (HIAA), *Source Book of Health Insurance Data, 1984–1985,* Washington, DC: HIAA, 1985.

Kosterlitz, J., " 'Disaster' Stories May Spur Congress to Protect Health Benefits for Retirees," *National Journal,* 1743–1746, July 27, 1985.

Skolnik, A. M., "Twenty-Five Years of Employee-Benefit Plans," *Social Security Bulletin,* 3–21, September 1976.

Taylor, A., P. J. Farley, and C. M. Horgan, "Medigap Insurance: Friend or Foe in Reducing Medicare Deficits?" paper presented at the 1984 American Public Health Association Meetings, forthcoming in H. E. Frech III, ed., *Health Care in America: The Political Economy of Hospitals and Health Insurance,* San Francisco: Pacific Institute for Public Policy Research.

U.S. Bureau of the Census, *Statistical Abstract of the United States: 1986,* 106th ed., Washington, DC: U.S. Government Printing Office, 1985.

U.S. Bureau of Labor Statistics (BLS), *Employee Benefits in Medium and Large Firms, 1983,* Bulletin 2213, Washington, DC: U.S. Government Printing Office, August 1984.

———, *Employee Benefits in Medium and Large Firms, 1985,* Bulletin 2262, Washington, DC: U.S. Government Printing Office, July 1986.

U.S. Department of Labor, Office of Policy and Research, Pension and Welfare Benefits Administration, *Employer-sponsored Retiree Health Insurance,* unpublished staff paper, 1986.

U.S. Senate Special Committee on Aging, *Funding Post-Retirement Health Benefits,* unpublished staff report, 1985.

13. Increases in Beneficiary Burdens: Direct and Indirect Effects

❑ ❑ ❑

MARILYN MOON

Introduction

In recent years, many of the policy changes made under Medicare have focused on restrictions in reimbursements to providers. These changes have often been supported by the Congress and the administration as ways of increasing the efficiency of Medicare without harming individual beneficiaries. Yet such changes may have substantial effects on the out-of-pocket burdens of the elderly and disabled that are just now beginning to be recognized. Assessing these impacts is important both for evaluating the reimbursement changes themselves and in considering further changes that directly increase the out-of-pocket burdens on Medicare beneficiaries.

The Medicare program covered nearly $2,000 in benefits for the average enrollee in 1986. These benefits, however, paid for only about three-quarters of the costs of hospital stays and less than half the costs of physician services. The remaining expenses represent patients' liability under the Medicare program. The Health Care Financing Administration (HCFA) has estimated, for example, that patients' liability averaged $583 in 1985—or about 25 percent of the costs of Medicare-covered services.[1] These expenses arise directly from the Part B premium and Medicare cost-sharing provisions.

But limitations on coverage and other reimbursement changes may have indirect effects that are not captured by these standard out-of-pocket indicators, so the burdens may be even higher. For example, when beneficiaries substitute noncovered services, such as homemaker aides, for formerly covered hospital days, additional costs do not show up in out-of-pocket measures, such as those reported here.

This chapter examines the consequences of both direct and indirect impacts of policy changes since 1980 on the elderly and disabled under Medicare. At the outset, it is critical to understand who is covered and what Medicare enrollees must now pay. This chapter then examines how Medicare coverage has changed in recent years. To illustrate the potential impact on beneficiaries of reimbursement changes, a detailed discussion of Medicare's Prospective Payment System (PPS) for reimbursing hospitals is considered next. The likely distribution of increased burdens from this major reimbursement reform is then contrasted with the likely impacts of other more direct changes. The concluding section takes a broader perspective and argues that the financial impact on beneficiaries of reimbursement changes ought to be routinely considered in the decision-making process concerning future policy changes.

Medicare Coverage, Premiums, and Cost Sharing

Enrollees in the Medicare program are already required to share some of the costs of care for covered services—both through a premium for coverage under Part B (Supplementary Medical Insurance) and payment of a portion of the costs of services through deductibles and coinsurance.

Inpatient hospital care is provided to all enrollees through Medicare Part A (Hospital Insurance). Beyond the required deductible of $520 in 1987, the first 60 days of hospitalization for a spell of illness are covered in full. For each hospital day after that through day 90, a coinsurance payment of one-fourth of the deductible amount is charged. That is, in 1987, beneficiaries paid $130 per day for days 61–90. After 90 days of hospitalization, a beneficiary may draw upon a lifetime reserve of 60 days, with a required payment of one-half of the deductible amount for each such day. Once the lifetime reserve has been exhausted, the enrollee is liable for all hospital costs incurred until the next spell of illness begins—that is, until the patient has not been in a Medicare-covered institution for at least 60 days.

Currently, about one-fourth of all Medicare beneficiaries are hospitalized at least once in any given year. A smaller portion are assessed the deductible, however, because of the way that spells of illness are defined. Only a very small percentage of the enrollee population ever pays coinsurance—about 0.5 percent. And fewer still use their lifetime reserve days. Nonetheless, for those who are assessed coinsurance, the expenses can be very high. An individual with a

150-day stay (who is still eligible to use the lifetime reserve coverage) faced deductible and coinsurance costs of $20,020 in 1987 for inpatient hospital cost sharing alone. For longer stays or for individuals who have already exhausted their lifetime reserve, hospital costs would be even higher.

Stays in skilled nursing homes also are subject to coinsurance after 20 days of care. The coinsurance amount is tied to the hospital deductible and is set at $65 per day. Ironically, this amount is likely to be higher than Medicare reimburses institutions for providing an average skilled nursing facility (SNF) day. In 1984 the mean daily reimbursement was $54, an amount that had only risen by $5 over the 1981 amount. Thus, patients implicitly are limited to a 20-day covered SNF stay; beyond that point, they would in many cases pay more than the costs of the care they receive.[2] The average length of stay is about 28 days; in 1983 HCFA has estimated that coinsurance for a user of SNF services averaged $667.

Although the cost-sharing liabilities for a small group of individuals can be very great for Part A services, it is on the physician side of the equation where the largest average cost-sharing amounts arise. This high average amount reflects both a few very extensive users of care, and also the fact that most enrollees have physician or other ambulatory expenses in any given year. Under Part B, enrollees paid a premium—$17.90 per month in 1987—and the first $75 of covered charges incurred in a year. About 80 percent of all enrollees exceed the deductible each year. After paying that deductible amount, individuals are liable for at least 20 percent of the "reasonable" charges, as determined by Medicare for each service.

In addition, physicians may charge patients an additional amount above the reasonable fee. Although it is not known how many physicians actually collect these additional amounts, reported charges generally exceed allowed reasonable charges by about 25 percent. For patients who do pay these charges, liability for physician services would be about double the amount indicated by their 20 percent coinsurance. Before the physician fee freeze of 1984–85, about half of all bills were for physician services where assignment had been declined. The fee freeze—to be discussed below—has lessened the burdens for beneficiaries.

Medicare's Changing Coverage

Beginning with the Omnibus Budget Reconciliation Act (OBRA) of 1981, Medicare—like many other government programs—was subjected to a number of cost-saving legislative changes. And, in subsequent years, further changes have been made, cutting Medicare spending by approximately 15 percent in 1986, as compared with the spending level that would have occurred in the absence of the legislation. While not all of these changes have reduced benefits or increased costs to beneficiaries directly, some can have implicit impacts on use and cost of health care services. Consequently, two types of changes are described here: those that affect beneficiaries explicitly and those that pose implicit costs on Medicare enrollees.

Direct changes in beneficiary cost sharing

A number of legislative changes have altered the degree to which beneficiaries are required to pay additional shares of the costs of their Medicare-covered acute care. For example, in 1981, deductible amounts for both parts of Medicare were increased. The increase under Part B was from $60 to $75—a 25 percent one-time rise. For Part A, Hospital Insurance, the deductible rose by about 12 percent through a technical change in the formula. Although the hospital deductible increase was proportionally smaller than that for Part B, the dollar amounts were greater and, more importantly, this increase was permanently incorporated into the calculation of the deductible and coinsurance amounts. That adjustment thus increased the Part A deductible by about $53 in 1986. Coinsurance for Part A is tied to the deductible, so these charges also displayed similar proportional increases.

In addition, a number of other smaller changes also boosted the proportion of Medicare expenditures that beneficiaries must pay. For instance, hospital-based radiologist and pathologist charges used to be fully covered by Medicare. Now, these physician fees are subject to the normal 20 percent coinsurance that beneficiaries must pay. In another example, before 1981, some costs of physician services from the previous year could be carried over and applied to the current year's deductible. This is no longer allowed. While these limited changes were not very significant individually, they do generate substantial savings when added together.

The largest beneficiary cost to date from a direct change has resulted from the increased premium assessed for Part B services. When enacted in 1965, beneficiaries were required to pay one-half of the costs of Part B insurance coverage. But the rapid increase in the costs of the program outstripped the growth in Social Security benefits. The 1972 Social Security Amendments limited the rate of increase in premiums to the rate of increase in the consumer price index (which is used to adjust the rate of growth of Social Security). Consequently, Part B premiums came to represent a smaller and smaller share of the total costs of the program. Legislation in 1982 set the premium at one-fourth of the costs of the program for three years—and that requirement was later extended until the end of fiscal year 1987. The costs of this change to the beneficiaries also have long-term consequences since costs of the program have been rising rapidly in recent years. By 1987 the monthly premium would have risen to only $13.70 under the 1972 calculations but instead was set at $17.90.

Other changes in Medicare have expanded options or slightly reduced out-of-pocket burdens on the elderly. For example, the extension of Medicare coverage to include hospice benefits for the terminally ill expanded the range of choices open to the elderly, even though it was expected to achieve modest savings to the federal government over time. Similarly, as part of a move to establish a fee schedule for independent laboratory services, patient cost sharing has been eliminated.[3]

The combined impact of these changes has led to a reduction in Medicare benefits of about 4 percent but an 11 percent increase in enrollee liability for Medicare-covered services. Estimates from HCFA peg enrollee liability in 1985 at about $583 (including Part B premiums, Medicare cost sharing, and excess billing), while Medicare paid benefits (net of Part B premiums) of $1,778. The average shift in liability from Medicare to its enrollees totaled about $63 in 1985 (Table 13.1). To the extent that these changes have led to a reduction in the use of services, the reduction in federal costs might be greater still. The implications of reduced use of services on beneficiaries would be harder to assess, however, and no attempt to estimate either the size or the implications of such a change is attempted here.

On balance, direct changes in Medicare cost sharing increased what beneficiaries must pay for care. But, in general, these changes were of a lesser order of magnitude than were legislative initiatives aimed at altering reimbursement to the

TABLE 13.1
Direct Sources of Increased Enrollee Liability for Medicare Benefits, Fiscal Year 1985

	Per capita amounts (dollars)
Total enrollee liability	483[a]
Direct increase in liability from changes in	
Part B premiums	30
Part A deductibles and coinsurance	13
Part B deductible	13
Radiology/pathology	5
Miscellaneous	2
Total	63
Medicare's net contribution	1,778[b]

[a]Includes cost sharing, Part B premiums, and excess physician charges.
[b]Net of Part B premium contributions.
Source: Total liability and Medicare's contributions are from unpublished HCFA data; liability changes are author's estimates.

providers of such services. To the extent that these latter changes may affect beneficiaries, they have the potential for an even greater impact on the elderly and disabled.

Indirect costs imposed on beneficiaries

Reimbursement changes have dominated the cost-cutting efforts under Medicare. Although the OBRA changes of 1981 fell more heavily on beneficiaries, mainly through the increased deductible amounts, the Tax Equity and Fiscal Responsibility Act of 1982 (TEFRA) generated massive savings from the limits on hospitals that later became part of the constraints on reimbursements under the new PPS. Overall, savings from changes directed at providers have been of an order of magnitude about three times the level of changes that have fallen directly on beneficiaries. Although many of the reimbursement changes enacted to reduce Medicare's costs have been billed as affecting providers and not beneficiaries, the implicit consequences of some of the changes are to increase costs to beneficiaries as well.

The most important provider change in recent years has been the introduction of the new PPS for reimbursing hospitals that treat Medicare patients. Since this new payment system pays hospitals on the basis of the diagnosis, rather than on the costs actually incurred, hospitals have incentives to cut back on services offered and the length of the hospital stay for inpatients.

In many instances, these changes reflect a more efficient delivery of care, with no adverse consequences on beneficiaries. Prior to the introduction of PPS, the old cost-based reimbursement system was widely criticized as promoting excessive hospital stays for Medicare patients. For the elderly with chronic or complicating medical conditions, however, earlier discharges mean that other types of care must be substituted for at least part of the days that would otherwise have been spent in the hospital. If the substituted days of care are not covered by Medicare, the individual will incur additional costs for care (or do without) that will not be reflected by traditional measures of out-of-pocket spending. Thus, what appears at first glance to be a reimbursement change may actually constitute a decline in covered services and an implicit shifting of the costs of health care onto the beneficiaries.

More modest changes have been made in reimbursements to SNFs and home health agencies that may also limit beneficiaries' access to care. These two parts of the Part A program are currently very small, but the demands likely to be generated by PPS for follow-up care would suggest that use of SNFs and home health services would expand. But, dramatic growth has not occurred. Rather, reimbursement policies have discouraged participation by providers, so that even qualified beneficiaries may not be able to receive benefits. The Medicare patients would have to choose reduced care or privately purchase needed services.

For example, home health care reimbursement policies have been increasingly subjected to very stringent interpretations that seem to limit access to care (Leader 1986).

While the image of Medicare is usually one of increased usage over time, SNF utilization has fallen substantially since 1971. In 1984 there were 296 covered days of care for each 1,000 enrollees, a figure 18 percent below the 361 covered days of 1971. Over the same period, the percentage of covered charges actually reimbursed by Medicare fell from 77.7 percent in 1971 to 47.7 percent in 1984. Tough regulations on eligibility, coupled with these stringent reimbursement standards, likely explain a large portion in the decline in use of the SNF benefit.

The picture varies dramatically with physician and laboratory services. In these areas, federal activities to limit spending may have had complementary effects on beneficiaries' costs. The freeze on physician payments for fiscal year 1985 (and extended through May 1986) also restricted beneficiaries' cost sharing. Moreover, the freeze legislation provided for preferential treatment for physicians who agreed to accept Medicare's reasonable charge determination as the full payment for services. The result has been an increase in the number of physicians who do not charge patients additional fees for their services. HCFA has estimated that for the average enrollee, excess billing for physician claims fell by $16 in 1985, as compared with 1984. During the same period, however, per capita expenditures on physician services grew at a rate in excess of 10 percent, suggesting that some physicians may have billed for more complex procedures or may have seen patients more frequently in response to the freeze. Moreover, it is not known whether physicians will attempt to increase their charges at a more rapid rate in the future, or whether continued restrictions on reimbursements will result in problems of access to services.

Medicare has also moved to create a fee schedule for laboratory fees, requiring that providers accept assignment. Out-of-pocket costs for beneficiaries should also decline under such a system.

Developing specific estimates of the impacts of these changes on beneficiaries is difficult indeed. Yet such efforts need to be taken in an effort to evaluate fully the impact of these program changes and future legislative proposals. True efficiency effects of reduced costs of providing health care need to be separated from those that merely shift costs from one payment source to another.

Estimating the Beneficiary Burdens Imposed by PPS

The size and scale of the changes wrought by PPS make it a good candidate for illustrating the potential impact on beneficiaries from reimbursement changes. In the case of PPS, at least four types of potential beneficiary burden can be identified:

1. Increases in the Part A cost sharing as a result of the way that such liabilities are calculated.
2. Increases in burdens on patients and their families from earlier hospital discharges.
3. Increases in cost-sharing burdens from reducing the scope of services performed in the hospital setting.
4. Increases in burdens on patients when too little care is provided for inpatients.

Calculating Part A cost sharing

A primary way in which PPS may implicitly affect the elderly arises with the calculation of the hospital deductible and Part A coinsurance. Since PPS has induced shorter lengths of stay, the average cost per hospital day is rising faster than before, as more tests and procedures are delivered in a shorter period of time. Consequently, the average daily cost—which is used as the basis for calculating the deductible and coinsurance amounts—has risen much faster than the overall costs of the program. The deductible amount increased from $400 to $492 between 1985 and 1986—a 23 percent rise in just one year. And, although it was claimed that this would represent a one-time dramatic change, the 1987 deductible would have risen to $572, but the sixth OBRA (1986) froze the deductible at $520. Nonetheless, the 1986 increase remains part of the base for future years' calculations.

If the deductible rose at the same rate as per capita costs of hospital care over the period, the 1986 deductible would have been only $430. The $62 difference is larger than the estimated 1986 impact of the legislated deductible increase. And, all the coinsurance amounts tied to the Part A deductible would have been smaller as well. Across all Medicare beneficiaries, the burden would average $16—or almost $2 billion in total costs shifted to Medicare enrollees.

The effects of earlier discharges

As noted above, one of the most dramatic ways that PPS has changed hospital care has been through reduced lengths of hospital stays for Medicare patients. Indeed, the average length of stay for Medicare patients fell by more than 10 percent between 1983 and 1984, the first year in which PPS was in effect. The average inpatient hospital stay in fiscal year 1984 was 9.1 days—or more than eleven million hospital days less than if lengths of stay had remained unchanged from their 1983 levels. For 1985 the average fell further to 8.4 days—or an additional drop of about ten million days over 1984. While not all of this decline can be attributed to PPS, since there has been a long-term trend toward shorter hospital stays, the 1984 and 1985 declines were much greater than in the recent past.

Although on paper the Medicare program offers home health care and SNF services for those needing post-hospital care, these services are often not available. Moreover, early indications are that these two services, which together account for less than 3 percent of all Medicare spending, have not shown any unusual increases in expenditures in response to earlier hospital discharges. The increases in spending between 1983 and 1985 were at or below their recent average rates of change. In fact, covered days of care for SNFs declined by nearly 2 percent between 1983 and 1984.

Patients needing further care thus may not be able to count on Medicare. As a result, patients will have to purchase such care on their own, rely on other public programs such as Medicaid, turn to relatives and friends for informal care, or do without.

To get some idea of the order of magnitude of the potential problem, it is necessary to know how many of the elderly are likely to need follow-up care after a hospital stay and whether such individuals are as likely to be discharged earlier, as are their healthier counterparts. (Ideally, these individuals should be singled out for analysis of their use of services. It will be some time before such specific data are available, however. In the meantime, some orders of magnitude can be gauged from aggregate data.)

Studies of physical limitations of older Americans normally find that about one-fifth need assistance in meeting needs of daily living. These frail or disabled elderly persons are also more likely to be hospitalized than their healthier counterparts. As a group, elderly persons with needs for further care thus account for a greater than proportional share of all discharges. While some of these individuals will be discharged into a nursing home or other setting where they receive other services, Medicare will cover less than one in six of such individuals.

Were the earlier hospital discharges after 1983 concentrated among those with short stays or who left in relatively good health? If so, earlier discharges will have had a lesser effect on the need for follow-up care. The aggregate evidence suggests that reductions in length of stay have occurred across all types of discharges, lending little credence to the argument that needs for follow-up care will not increase.

Table 13.2 shows changes in lengths of stay for selected diagnosis-related groups (DRGs) between fiscal years 1981 and 1984. The first group represents DRGs that have been associated by Meiners and Coffey with the highest number of discharges to home health or nursing homes in Maryland in 1980 (Meiners and Coffey 1985). In some cases, the high proportions largely represent the overall size of the DRG in question, but in other instances the DRGs display disproportionate shares of long-term care patients (the latter group is identified in the table with a superscript "a"). For purposes of comparison, a second group of DRGs is also included—representing those top ten DRGs by discharge that are not associ-

TABLE 13.2
**Changes in Lengths of Stay and Average Stays in Days by Selected DRGs,
1981–84**

Code	Group description	FY1981	FY1984	Percent change
DRGs associated with follow-on care				
14	Specific cerebrovascular disorders, except transient ischemic attacks	15.1	12.6	−16.6[a]
201	Hip and femur procedures, except major joint, age > 69, and/or substantial comorbidity and complication (CC)	20.6	16.9	−18.0[a]
127	Heart failure and shock	10.5	8.9	−14.8
89	Simple pneumonia and pleurisy, age > 69, and/or CC[b]	11.1	9.6	−13.5[a]
320	Kidney and urinary tract infections, age > 69, and/or CC	9.1	8.2	−9.9[a]
209	Major joint procedures	18.8	15.8	−16.0[a]
182	Esophagitis, gastroenteritis, and miscellaneous digestive disorders, age ≥ 69, and/or CC	7.0	6.1	−12.9
296	Nutritional and miscellaneous metabolic disorders, age > 69, and/or CC	10.1	8.3	−17.8[a]
429	Organic disturbances and mental retardation	12.7	11.0	−13.4[a]
88	Chronic obstructive pulmonary disease	9.8	8.5	−13.3
132	Atherosclerosis, age > 69, and/or CC	9.1	7.0	−20.9
294	Diabetes, age > 35	9.8	8.3	−15.3
82	Respiratory neoplasms	11.6	9.9	−14.7
148	Major small and large bowel procedures, age > 69, and/or CC	19.7	17.8	−9.6
Other common DRGs				
96	Bronchitis and asthma > 69, and/or CC	8.4	7.3	−13.1
243	Medical back problems	9.7	8.0	−17.1
140	Angina pectoris	7.0	5.7	−18.6
	Total (all short-stay)	10.5	9.0	−14.3

[a]Those DRGs with disproportionate shares of nursing home or home health discharges.
[b]CC = critical care.
Source: Unpublished data from Prospective Payment Assessment Commission, Washington, DC, 1986.

ated with high use of follow-up care. There is no evidence to suggest that the frail and disabled elderly have been spared early discharges; long length-of-stay DRGs show comparable reductions to others.

Thus, of the twenty-one million fewer hospital days in 1985, as compared with 1983, perhaps 30 percent represented reductions in stays for individuals who were likely to require additional care after discharge. If so, the frail elderly probably had hospital stays between six and eight million days shorter in 1985 than if lengths of stay had remained unchanged. If these days had to be made up with privately financed formal or informal care, the potential burdens are very large. For example, costs of purchased care, or of lost wages to a family providing informal care, of $50 per day for the eight million needed days of care would sum to $400 million. The per capita impact of this conservative estimate would average about $12 across all enrollees in 1985.

The effects of unbundling

A third way that PPS has affected beneficiaries is through shifting services outside the hospital setting, for example, through use of more outpatient surgery and more tests done outside the hospital before or after an inpatient stay. Services outside the hospital are normally subject to high cost-sharing requirements, making this so-called unbundling of services a beneficiary issue, as well as a reimbursement concern.

While individuals of all ages are increasingly having surgery as outpatients, PPS has certainly increased the incentives for physicians to move to such settings. And, for some procedures, such as cataract surgery, physicians wishing to admit their patients to a hospital must seek special permission; otherwise, all of the procedures will be done on an outpatient basis. For the patient, this can often mean an increase in out-of-pocket costs—since 20 percent of outpatient charges (excluding surgery) must be paid by the beneficiary—and the need to find informal and unreimbursed ways of securing services during the recuperative period. A frail, older woman living alone may not be able to administer eye drops or change her own dressings after surgery, for example. Studies of cataract surgery have suggested that physician charges for such surgery are not less expensive in an outpatient setting. From the patient's perspective, there is little to be gained and much to be lost from such activity.

The effects of too little inpatient care

Finally, most important and perhaps most difficult to document, some enrollees will not receive needed care if hospitals become reluctant to accept some types of patients and physicians do not press for these admissions. While in the hospital, some patients may not receive tests or procedures that would be beneficial. Although these situations cannot be identified with certainty, the "burden of proof" has switched for care: in the past, errors were made on the side of delivering too much care, but now the incentives are to provide too little. PPS may be moving us to the brink of testing the notion of what is the marginal value of an additional unit of medical care.

These more intangible issues are given too little consideration in a chapter concentrating on cost shifting to beneficiaries. But they are particularly troubling because all Medicare beneficiaries are at risk when it is no longer a case of paying more to replace lost care but rather of not receiving such care at all. The possibility for harm is thus more widespread.

Potential Distributional Impacts of These Changes

Not all Medicare enrollees would be equally affected by the direct and indirect changes in Medicare discussed thus far. Needs and use of care vary dramatically across individuals, so it is also crucial to consider how additional financial burdens may be distributed. Many dimensions could be used to look at the burdens: income, sex, and age are but three variables that are likely to reflect considerable differences. For this analysis, age is used as the primary variable for examining differential burdens. The oldest of the old have both higher needs for medical care and greater use and fewer resources to devote to paying for such care. For example, incomes of families aged eighty and over were only two-thirds as high as for those aged sixty-five to sixty-seven in 1982 (Grad 1984).

Basic statistics on Medicare illustrate the enormous variation in use by age. Among the elderly, the likelihood of using any service rises with the age of the enrollee (Table 13.3). Skilled nursing care leads the list of Medicare services dominated by older beneficiaries. Persons aged eighty-five and above are more than eleven times more likely to have skilled nursing benefits paid for by Medicare. Indeed, all Part A services are particularly heavily used by the oldest beneficiaries.

Use of physician and outpatient services is much less correlated with age, however (HCFA 1985). Persons over age eighty-five are only 29 percent more likely to see a physician than is a younger beneficiary. This is a particularly dramatic statistic, given the much higher use of hospital care by the older beneficiaries, suggesting that ambulatory visits by older beneficiaries are actually lower than for younger beneficiaries.[4]

Dollars of expenditures on each of these service areas display a similar pattern. In each category, the oldest beneficiaries use more services than younger ones, but the differences are greatest for Part A services. Skilled nursing and

TABLE 13.3
Likelihood of Using Medicare Services by Age of Enrollee, 1981

Type of Medicare service	Ratio of persons served per 1,000 enrollees by age (65–69 as base)			
	70–74	75–79	80–84	85+
Skilled nursing facility	2.04	4.00	7.31	11.65
Home health care	1.64	2.51	3.62	4.60
Inpatient hospital	1.18	1.41	1.65	1.82
Physician services	1.08	1.16	1.22	1.29
Outpatient services	1.06	1.12	1.17	1.23

Source: Health Care Financing Administration, *Medicare and Medicaid Data Book, 1984*, Baltimore, MD: HCFA, June 1986.

TABLE 13.4
Per Capita Medicare Liability by Age, 1984

	Medicare liability (dollars) from:			
	Part A cost sharing	Part B cost sharing[a]	Part B premiums	Total
Age of enrollees				
65–69	78	211	172	461
70–74	92	226	172	490
75–79	104	234	172	570
80+	144	260	172	576
All enrollees	102	231	172	505
Ratio of liability of those 80+ to those 65–69	1.85	1.23	1.0	1.25

[a]Excludes excess billing from estimate.
Source: Author's simulations from 1978 Medicare History Sample.

home health benefits are most often used by those who have complications—including frailty associated with age—that lengthen periods of recovery from acute illnesses.

These age differences are borne out in the cost-sharing liability that individuals (or their insurance companies) must pay for covered Medicare services (Table 13.4).[5] Again, the greatest differences appear for Part A cost sharing. Such cost-sharing liabilities are, however, smaller on average than for Part B services; beneficiaries carry a greater share of the load for physician and outpatient services than for hospital care. Part B premiums also act to reduce the overall differential. Nonetheless, the oldest enrollees pay 25 percent more on average than their younger counterparts.

And the oldest old are more likely to experience very high cost-sharing burdens. In 1984, while persons over age eighty constituted less than 23 percent of over-sixty-five enrollees, they accounted for 31 percent of all the beneficiaries with reimbursed expenses of $5,000 or more (CBO 1983).

Thus, any change in cost-sharing or reimbursement policy that affects beneficiaries in one part of the program and not another will have differential effects by age. Only premium changes will be age neutral—affecting all beneficiaries. Changes in the physician deductible amount will also be relatively evenly distributed by age, as well as within each age group, since most Medicare beneficiaries (about 80 percent) have reimbursable Medicare physician expenses. Part A burdens are limited to those with hospital stays and the very small group of beneficiaries receiving skilled nursing care. Physician coinsurance will also fall more heavily on a small subgroup within each age category. (And, since heavy users of physician services are also very likely to have a hospital stay, they will suffer the double burden of having cost-sharing liability from both parts of the program.)

What about the specific burdens of the changes discussed above? About two-thirds of the direct changes described in Table 13.1 would be evenly spread across most enrollees. These include the changes in the Part B premium and the Part B deductible that raised average per capita burdens by $43 in that fiscal year and $45 in 1986—the year used for the distributional analysis in this section. The Part A deductible and coinsurance increases and the change in radiology and pathology services, which will be largely felt by those who are hospitalized, will be disproportionately shared by older beneficiaries.

In the case of the impact of PPS, we can only speculate on much of the impact. The two most straightforward changes discussed above were the higher Part A deductible and cost sharing that have resulted as a side effect of PPS and the likelihood of more individual responsibility for care following a hospital stay. The combined total of just these two changes total about 44 percent of all the direct changes in cost sharing described above. More sophisticated estimates of unbundling and foregone inpatient services would bring the total up considerably.

Reasonable predictions of the age-related burdens of the Part A deductible and cost-sharing changes from PPS would hit the oldest beneficiaries about twice as hard as younger elderly Medicare enrollees. As noted above, the deductible and coinsurance increases from PPS in 1986 were considerably greater than increases in the deductible legislated in 1981.

Several additional leaps of faith are needed for projecting the impact of unmet needs for more follow-up care after a hospital stay. As discussed above, it appears that the needs far outstrip the response by Medicare or even Medicaid. But some beneficiaries will be served. Are the oldest of the old more or less likely to gain access to Medicare-covered services? There is no hard evidence as yet to suggest how benefits may be "rationed" among eligible beneficiaries. But if regulations about the acute nature of Medicare's benefit are being more strictly observed, as anecdotal evidence suggests, the old old may be at a greater disadvantage.[6]

If unmet need parallels the age distribution for use of skilled nursing and home health services, then the impact of PPS will be very strongly skewed to greater burdens on the old. And, when combined with the deductible and coinsurance changes, the impact of these two parts of PPS look quite different than the impact of the direct policy changes estimated here (Table 13.5).[7] While largely illustrative, these findings underscore the danger of changes that create indirect effects on beneficiaries. They may be much less evenly distributed than are policies designed to increase beneficiary cost sharing. The legislative changes that gave birth to PPS were largely debated as provider changes seeking to alter Medicare's incentive structure. By paying little attention to the potential impacts on beneficiaries, the result was a highly skewed burden.

TABLE 13.5
Distribution of Per Capita Average Burdens
from Direct and Indirect Medicare Policy
Changes, FY 1986

	Increases in liability from:	
	Direct changes[a]	**PPS impact**[b]
Age of enrollees		
65–69	$63	$17
70–74	65	24
75–79	66	31
80+	72	46
All enrollees	$66	$29
Ratio of liability of those 80+ to those 65–69	1.15	2.71

[a]Includes same components as in Table 13.1, updated to 1986.
[b]Includes estimates of changes in Part A deductibles and coinsurance from PPS and purchases of own post-hospital care.
Source: Authors' estimates.

Policy Implications and Conclusions

The impact of PPS on Medicare enrollees raises broader policy questions than whether there are distributional effects from this particular policy change. More and more often, government policy is being set on the basis of attempts to "save costs" or "improve the efficiency" of various government programs. But, such policy is shortsighted if it takes into account only government costs when making those decisions.

At first blush, the changes sought by PPS would seem to be based on the economic goal of improving efficiency. That will indeed be the case if it leads to a system in which appropriate care is delivered in a less costly way—as measured by society's costs and not just the burden on the government. If "efficiencies" are instead achieved by merely shifting burdens onto beneficiaries, government costs will indeed fall but costs to society may not.

The "cost savings" to the government from PPS can be readily documented. Average hospital lengths of stay are decreasing dramatically, and costs for the care received by beneficiaries have risen at a much slower pace than before. But, can we conclude from this that Medicare has become a more efficient health care system than before? The answer correctly is no, until we have established that society as a whole has achieved savings, without reductions in needed care.

The additional costs to beneficiaries from various reimbursement changes might not equal 100 percent of the savings to the federal government, and some real efficiencies may be obtained through these changes. Along with such legitimate reductions in costs, however, will be cases in which individuals must extend considerably their recuperation at home or in another setting and must pay for services out-of-pocket. Services may be purchased from private suppliers, or relatives may take time off from work to aid the returning patient. In these cases, costs have not been "saved"; rather, they have merely been shifted from the federal government to individuals.

The next level of analysis must then be to consider the effects of such cost shifting in the decision-making process to determine whether the resulting impact is acceptable or even desirable. The type of analysis described in this chapter would contribute to an informed debate over such reimbursement changes. In that debate, a number of factors ought to be addressed.

First, are burdens too high? The current levels of cost sharing through Medicare are already higher than for average private, employer-based cost-sharing provisions, for example. And, if indirect changes also increase burdens, future debate over cost sharing increases the need to recognize the total burden on beneficiaries, regardless of source.

Second, reimbursement changes may affect how well cost sharing works for the elderly. PPS, for example, may have implicitly made much of Part A cost sharing obsolete by strongly curtailing incentives to stay longer in the hospital. At a minimum, the structure of that cost sharing now makes little sense; the calculation of the deductible is based on the concept of per diem costs that are no longer valid.

Finally, when indirect means are used to raise the costs on beneficiaries, the impacts may be more complex than from simple cost-sharing changes. Reimbursement changes may implicitly reduce the coverage offered to enrollees and thus pose the choice between less care or greater out-of-pocket burdens. But as in the case of PPS, for example, coverage for some inpatient services may be reduced in such a way as to eliminate or severely inhibit beneficiary choice, regardless of ability to pay.

Notes

Theresa Varner provided valuable assistance in collecting some of the data reported in this chapter.

1. The figures presented here are from unpublished HCFA data.

2. Covered charges for such services, however, are much higher. Individuals purchasing care directly might have to pay charges greater than the current coinsurance. Again, the sources for these figures are from unpublished HCFA data. Another reason for seeking Medicare coverage is that Medigap policies often will pay the coinsurance portion of an SNF stay but normally will not pay for any services not formally covered by Medicare.

3. A discussion of these and other legislated changes in Medicare can be found in a report by the Committee on Ways and Means (1986).

4. Disabled beneficiaries are less likely to use services overall than are their elderly counterparts. Part A service use is greater than for the elderly, however, while Part B services are less likely to be used. But even in the case of Part B, per enrollee expenditures are higher for the disabled. Like the elderly, the probability of using services tends to increase with age.

5. These estimates do not include cost-sharing liability for excess billing by physicians who do not accept assignment or for services not covered by Medicare. Liability for disabled beneficiaries (excluding end-stage renal disease [ESRD] patients) are estimated to have averaged $520. These estimates represent authors' simulations from the Medicare History Sample derived for a Congressional Budget Office study (CBO 1983). The age breakdowns have not previously been published.

6. For example, intermittency requirements under home health regulations make it more difficult for the very frail to qualify. Anecdotal stories on skilled nursing care point to less coverage for problems, such as recovery from a broken hip, that may also be more closely associated with the very old.

7. One of the major omitted impacts of PPS—the shift to more outpatient services—would seem at first consideration to fall more heavily on the young, who have traditionally used more of such care. But the imposition of PPS seems also to have shifted use of outpatient services, so that we might expect a fairly substantial burden of this change to fall on the old old as well. For any overall reductions in the quality of inpatient care, the distribution of burdens might parallel that for changes in the Part A deductible.

References

Beebe, K., W. Callahan and A. Mariano, "Medicare Short-Stay Hospital Length of Stay, Fiscal Years 1981–85." *Health Care Financing Review,* 7:119–125, Spring, 1986.

Gornick, M., J. Greenberg, P. Eggers, and A. Dobson, "Twenty Years of Medicare and Medicaid: Covered Populations, Use of Benefits, and Program Expenditures." *Health Care Financing Review,* Annual Supplement, 13–59, 1985.

Health Care Financing Administration, *Medicare and Medicaid Data Book, 1984.* Washington, DC: U.S. Government Printing Office, June 1986.

Leader, S. (1986), "Home Health Benefits Under Medicare." American Association of Retired Persons, Public Policy Institute, Washington, DC (mimeographed).

Meiners, M., and R. Coffey, "Hospital DRGs and the Need for Long-Term Care Services: An Empirical Analysis." *Health Services Research,* 20:359–384; August 1985.

Moon, M., "The Effects of Medicare Cost-Sharing on Beneficiaries." Paper presented at the American Public Health Association Meeting, November, 1983.

Ruggles, P. and M. Moon, "The Impact of Recent Legislative Changes in Benefit Programs for the Elderly." *The Gerontologist,* 25:153–160, April 1985.

U.S. Congress, U.S. House of Representatives Subcommittee on Ways and Means, *Background Material and Data on Programs Within the Jurisdiction of the Committee on Ways and Means, 1986 Edition,* March 3, 1986.

U.S. Congress, Congressional Budget Office, *Changing the Structure of Medicare Benefits: Issues and Options,* Washington, DC, March, 1983.

Waldo, D. R. and H. C. Lazenby, "Demographic Characteristics and Health Care Use and Expenditures by the Aged in the United States: 1977–1984." *Health Care Financing Review,* 6(1):1–29, Fall 1984.

Wilensky, G. and M. Berk, "The Poor, Sick, Uninsured, and the Role of Medicaid," in *Hospitals and the Uninsured Poor,* New York: United Hospital Fund, 1985.

V

Medicare and Appropriate Medical Care

14. Relation of Surgical Volume to Outcomes and Charges: Pilot Study of Total Hip Replacement Using Northern California Medicare Data

□ □
□

JINNET FOWLES, JOHN P. BUNKER,
MARJORIE ODA, DAVID J. SCHURMAN, AND
MARGARET LOFTUS

Introduction

Following the introduction of total hip replacement in the United States in the late 1960s, this important new surgical procedure was disseminated rapidly throughout the country. Thus, half of the nearly 1,500 acute care hospitals reporting to the Commission on Professional and Hospital Activities (CPHA) in Ann Arbor performed at least one total hip replacement in 1974 or 1975 (Luft, Bunker, and Enthoven, 1979). Teaching hospitals and large medical clinics, particularly those that specialize in this technology, have collected and published their results from the outset, but the national experience with total hip replacement, based on outcome data from all hospitals, is not known. While there is no single source of data for all medical and surgical procedures in this country, claims data for care provided to Medicare beneficiaries do offer the opportunity to examine the experience in patients over the age of sixty-five and for a limited number of disabled at younger ages. In the study reported herein, we demonstrate the use of Medicare claims data to monitor mortality, complications, and professional charges for the Medicare beneficiaries of Northern California, following total hip replacement.

In a period in which the Medicare program is increasingly concerned about quality of care, as well as cost, this study demonstrates a quality control mechanism that can be implemented either independent of or as part of broader reforms.

Methods

In collaboration with Blue Shield of California, the Part B intermediary for Medicare in Northern California, we identified a total of 1,324 operative procedures billed and coded as primary or revisions of total hip replacements (California Relative Value Study Nomenclature codes 27130 and 27135) in 1980.[1] Access to the data was approved, given a guarantee of anonymity for patients, providers, and hospitals. These cases were then followed through their claims history until November 1982, providing a follow-up history of twenty-two to thirty-two months. Abstracting forms and procedures for identifying and coding the initial and follow-up encounters for these cases were developed. A total of six abstractors, who were already experienced Blue Shield medical claims review personnel, were trained to use the forms in two two-hour training sessions. Ten percent of each coder's work was randomly selected for validation, following the initial training period. Phase I abstracting (the initial operations) required 457 hours. Three abstractors trained and worked on the second phase. Phase II abstracting (review of subsequent medical claims histories) required 640 hours.

All of the cases had provider codes associated with them. However, these provider codes represented groups for 42.7 percent of the cases; individual surgeons were not represented as billing entities. Since part of the analysis depended on an accurate measure of the individual surgeon's surgical volume, we attempted to ascertain the specific surgeon performing the operation. Subsequently, the initial claims data were re-reviewed by a consulting orthopedic surgeon, and from the operative reports or the original claims the identity of the individual surgeon was determined. We were able to identify the individual surgeon in 94.7 percent of the cases. Identification of the individual institutions and surgeons remained confidential through the use of blind codes.

A second problem of data ambiguity existed in identification of the side (left or right) of the initial operation. The 1969 California Relative Value Study Nomenclature coding, as used for Medicare billing, does not indicate the side on which the procedure was performed. Again, all available data were screened by our consulting orthopedic surgeon. The side of the original operation was determined in 81.9 percent of the cases.

Deaths are reported to Medicare carriers by the Social Security Administration and appear on the beneficiary research documents. Although there may be a lag time in this procedure of up to six months, our final analysis of the follow-up period took place one year later (e.g., we identified and analyzed data from November 1982 in November 1983). Mortality was defined in this study as death occurring within ninety days of operation.

Major and minor complications were recorded from the claims data by reviewing all subsequent hospitalizations. Major complications included all operations requiring hospitalization and revision: exchange of prosthesis, removal, and deep infection. Minor complications included hospitalization for dislocation and minor revision surgery.

In tabulating major complications, we summed exchange of prosthesis, removals, and deep infections. However, multiple major complications in one case counted as a single case only. As a result, the total number of exchanges, removals, and deep infections exceeds the total number of cases with any major complication.

Hospitalizations that may have occurred outside the Northern California region were not captured in this analysis. However, any hospitalization in the region was captured, whether or not the rehospitalization took place at the same hospital as the initial operation.

The relationship between the mortality rate and the number of operations performed by the surgeon was examined by grouping the cases by outcome (survival or not) and thus comparing the surgical volume for the surgeons associated with the outcome in the two groups. The significance was calculated using the two-tail Student t-test. Complication rates were examined in the same way, as was the relationship between survival and hospital volume, and complication rate and hospital volume.

In order to determine the relative contributions of surgeon volume and hospital volume to mortality rate (and also complication rate), the binary outcome (survival or not) was regressed on surgeon volume and hospital volume and several other control variables (patient age, patient sex, teaching or nonteaching hospital, and urbanness).

Results

The initial sample represents all 1,324 operations performed in 1980, coded as total hip joint replacement or revision. The age and sex distributions shown in Table 14.1 indicate that 89.6 percent of the operations were performed in patients sixty-five years of age or older, and almost two-thirds were female patients. Of these 1,324 cases, 91.7 percent were billed as primary procedures, while 8.3 percent were billed as revisions of total hip replacements. Operative reports (available for 64.1 percent of the cases) indicated that 83 percent of this subsample were confirmed as primary total hip joint replacements, 11.8 percent were revisions of total hips, 4.9 percent were hemiarthroplasties, and 0.3 percent were other operations.

The distribution of diagnoses as given on the claim is indicated in Table 14.1. This distribution is similar to that reported nationally (Sutherland et al. 1982; Stauffer 1982; Vakili et al. 1981), with the exception that academic medical centers generally have a larger proportion of patients suffering from rheumatoid arthritis.

Results from analysis of the initial procedures demonstrate how widely total hip replacement surgery has diffused into the medical community. Fig. 14.1 shows that 399 providers[2] (individual surgeons or surgical groups) performed the 1,324 operations, averaging 3.32 Medicare total hip replacements each in 1980. However, 144 providers (36.1 percent) performed a single Medicare total hip replacement, and 95.7 percent did ten or fewer such operations during the year. The distribution of hospital operative rates shows a similar pattern. There are 261 acute care hospitals in Northern California, and among these one or more total hip replacements were carried out in 148, as shown in Fig. 14.2. These 148 hospitals accounted for 1,210 operations, averaging 8.2 Medicare total hip replacements. There were 114 operations (8.6 percent) for which the hospital could not be determined. A single Medicare total hip replacement was performed in 45

TABLE 14.1
Description of Sample

	N	Percent
Sex (N = 1,324)		
Male	480	36.3
Female	844	63.7
Age (N = 1,314)		
21–54	53	4.0
55–64	83	6.3
65–74	605	46.0
75–84	466	35.5
84+	107	8.1
Operation per claim (N = 1,324)		
Total hip replacement	1,214	91.7
Revision of total hip replacement		
(as initial procedure)	110	8.3
Preoperative diagnoses (N = 932)		
Osteoarthritis	548	58.8
Prosthesis complication	131	14.1
Fracture of femur	103	11.1
Avascular necrosis	71	7.6
Rheumatoid arthritis	43	4.6
Other	36	3.9

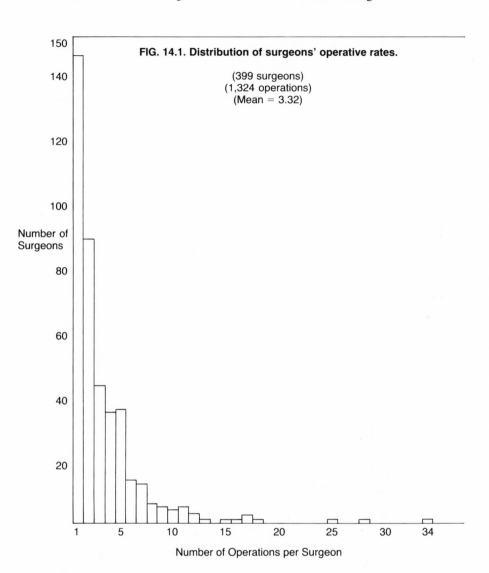

FIG. 14.1. Distribution of surgeons' operative rates.

(399 surgeons)
(1,324 operations)
(Mean = 3.32)

hospitals (30 percent), and there were ten or fewer Medicare operations in 71 percent of the hospitals.

Seventy-eight patients, constituting 8 percent of the operations, died in the
twenty-two- through thirty-two-month period of observation. Twenty-eight (2.1
percent) died within ninety days of surgery, and sixty (4.6 percent) died within
one year, as shown in Table 14.2. Thirty-nine hip replacements (3.8 percent of
those for which the original side was known) required subsequent exchange of

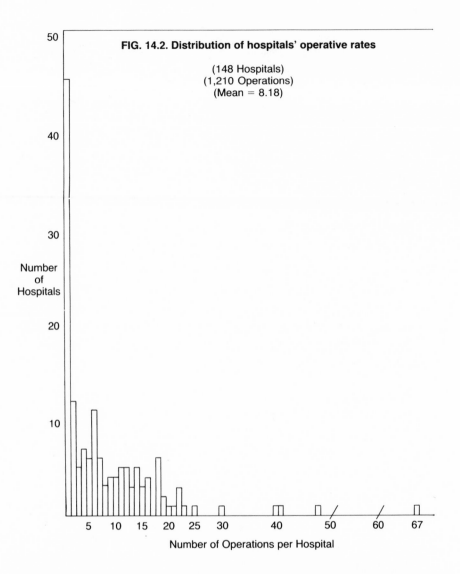

FIG. 14.2. Distribution of hospitals' operative rates

(148 Hospitals)
(1,210 Operations)
(Mean = 8.18)

prosthesis, seven required removal for deep infection, and five were removed for unspecified reasons. Dislocation requiring hospitalization was reported in thirty-nine patients.

The relationship of outcomes to surgical volume

Table 14.3 illustrates the unadjusted relationship of both the surgeon's surgical volume and the hospital's surgical volume to complications and death. There is a highly significant inverse relationship between the surgeon's operative volume and postoperative mortality. The several categories of complication are also in-

TABLE 14.2
Frequencies of Complications in the Follow-Up Period

	N	Percent
Postoperative death within 90 days	28	2.1
Postoperative death within 1 year	60	4.6
One or more major complications requiring revision	48	4.6
Exchange of prosthesis	39	3.8
Removal of prosthesis	5	0.5
Deep infection requiring hospitalization	7	0.7
One or more minor complications requiring hospitalization	44	4.2
Dislocation	39	3.8
Minor revision surgery	9	0.9

TABLE 14.3
Relationship of Surgeon Surgical Volume and Hospital Surgical Volume to Outcome (ANOVA)

Outcome		Mean surgeon volume		Mean hospital volume
Postoperative death within 90 days				
Yes	($N = 25$)	3.72[b]	($N = 22$)	13.82[a]
No	($N = 1{,}250$)	7.40	($N = 1{,}139$)	19.77
Major complication (exchange of prosthesis, removal, or deep infection)				
Yes	($N = 48$)	5.17[a]	($N = 46$)	14.17[a]
No	($N = 989$)	6.94	($N = 933$)	18.71
Exchange of prosthesis				
Yes	($N = 39$)	5.54	($N = 37$)	18.63
No	($N = 998$)	6.91	($N = 942$)	15.35
Removal of prosthesis				
Yes	($N = 5$)	3.20	($N = 5$)	18.55
No	($N = 1{,}032$)	6.88	($N = 974$)	9.2
Deep infection requiring hospitalization				
Yes	($N = 7$)	3.14	($N = 7$)	9.14
No	($N = 1{,}030$	6.88	($N = 972$)	18.57
Dislocation				
Yes	($N = 39$)	6.41	($N = 38$)	20.87
No	($N = 998$)	6.88	($N = 941$)	18.41
Minor revision				
Yes	($N = 9$)	6.67	($N = 9$)	15.67
No	($N = 1{,}028$)	6.86	($N = 970$)	18.53

Note: Significance test values were computed using two sample t-tests to compare mean volumes for the operations classified as shown in the first column.
[a] $p \leq .10$
[b] $p \leq .001$

TABLE 14.4
Comparison of High-Volume and Low-Volume Surgeons in High-Volume and Low-Volume Hospitals (ANOVA)

Outcome	High-volume physicians (>6) in high-volume hospitals (>25) (N = 156)	Low-volume physicians (≤6) in high-volume hospitals (>25) (N = 66)	Low-volume physicians (≤6) in low-volume hospitals (≤25) (N = 740)
Postoperative death (within 90 days)	0.0	0.0	0.0218[a]
Major complication	0.0215	0.0455	0.0604
Exchange of prosthesis	0.0215	0.0455	0.0461
Removal of prosthesis	0.0	0.0	0.0079
Deep infection	0.0	0.0	0.011
Charges	$2,688.08	$2,825.68	$2,999.48[b]

[a]$p \leq .05$
[b]$p \leq .001$

versely related to surgeon volume, but taken separately they are not statistically significant. When the major complications (exchange of prosthesis, removal, or deep infection) are considered together, the differences between surgeon volumes is significant at the 7 percent level. There is no similar association with minor complications.

The same inverse relationship is seen for postoperative death and for major complications versus the hospital's surgical volume, although, again, neither reaches the 5 percent level of significance ($p = .08$ for death, .06 for complication). We used only those major complications in the analysis for which we could identify the side of the complication as corresponding to the side of the initial surgery. In following this process, we may have underestimated the number of complications because the side of the original operation or reoperation could not be identified in every case. Taking the total number of major complications (same side or side unknown), as representing the maximum number of complications possible, the relationship to the physician's surgical volume is stronger ($p = .0288$).

Correspondingly, considering the total number of major complications (same side or side unknown) as the maximum, the relationship to the hospital's surgical volume is highly significant ($p = .0081$).

The physician's surgical volume and the hospital's surgical volume are themselves related ($R = 0.64$). Therefore, the question arises as to which measure of surgical volume—physician or hospital—is more strongly related to poor outcomes. One approach is to examine the performance of low-volume surgeons in low-volume hospitals, low-volume surgeons in high-volume hospitals, and high-volume surgeons in high-volume hospitals. The results of this analysis indicate that low-volume surgeons in low-volume hospitals have poorer mortality rates than low-volume surgeons in high-volume hospitals ($p = .05$). This trend is maintained for complications but does not reach statistical significance.

Another approach to examining this question is the use of a linear regression model, in which both volume measures are entered. This method also allows us to control for additional patient and hospital characteristics. Using this model to analyze death rates and also major complications, we entered the physician's surgical volume and the hospital's surgical volume, along with control variables for the type of patient (age and sex) and the type of hospital (teaching or nonteaching and relative urbanness).

The resulting analysis shown in Table 14.5 suggests that the surgeon's volume is much more strongly related to death than is hospital volume, and that each contributes very nearly equally to the association of volume with major complications. The number of deaths on which this analysis is based is scanty, however, and none of the effects reaches the 5 percent level of significance. When two measures are as highly correlated as these, there may be some danger of unstable results due to multicolinearity. However, the regression results appeared stable in several alternative test versions.

Billed physician charges ranged from \$1,100 to \$5,720; the median charge was \$2,860. Charges were inversely related to both the surgeon's volume and the hospital's surgical volume: low-volume surgeons charged significantly more than high-volume surgeons. These results are shown in Tables 14.6 and 14.7.

TABLE 14.5
Estimated Conditional Effects of Physician Surgical Volume and Hospital Surgical Volume on Death and Major Complications (standardized beta coefficients)

	Physician volume	Hospital volume	Patient age	Patient sex	Teaching hospital	Urban-ness
Death within 90 days[a]	−0.066	−0.009	−0.055	−0.035	−0.039	−0.018
Major complications[b]	−0.032	−0.036	−0.060	−0.050	−0.006	−0.018

[a]Physician volume significant at 0.116, age significant at 0.090.
[b]Age significant at 0.063.

TABLE 14.6
Relationship of Surgical Volume to Charges (ANOVA)

Charges (dollars)	Mean surgeon volume		Mean hospital volume
1,000–2,500 ($N = 227$)	10.98[a]	($N = 212$)	25.43[a]
2,501–3,000 ($N = 653$)	7.90	($N = 608$)	20.33
3,001–3,250 ($N = 189$)	3.86	($N = 153$)	13.35
Over 3,250 ($N = 204$)	4.72	($N = 186$)	16.15

[a]$p < .00005$

TABLE 14.7
**Estimated Conditional Effects of Physician Surgical Volume and Hospital
Surgical Volume on Physician Charges (standardized beta coefficients)**

	Physician volume	Hospital volume	Patient age	Patient sex	Teaching hospital	Urban-ness
Physician charges	−0.177[a]	−0.042	−0.080[a]	−0.035	0.009	−0.170[a]

[a]$p < .001$

Discussion

The results presented demonstrate the potential feasibility of the use of routinely collected claims data to monitor the outcomes of a surgical procedure. Wennberg has previously reported the use of Medicare claims data to monitor mortality following lens extraction (1980) and following prostatectomy (1982). A similar result has also been demonstrated in Canada (Roos et al. 1985), where claims data are available for the entire population under their National Health Service.

The method is not without error, however, as reflected in the nearly 10 percent error rate in classification of operation by claims data, when compared with the original operative report. Primary procedures were overestimated by claims data, and revisions were underestimated.

An additional serious problem in the use of claims data that emerged is that procedure codes currently in use do not distinguish between right and left side. It is, therefore, not possible—using routinely computerized claims data alone—to determine whether a second hip operation is a primary procedure on the opposite side or a reoperation on the same side. Similar uncertainty can be expected for other procedures involving bilateral organs or limbs. By abstracting both the claims and the operative report, we were able to identify the side of the operation in 82 percent of the cases.

The results reported above have immediate and important clinical implications. From previous reports, it appears that the rate per year at which total hip components are revised because of complications or failure is constant from one year to the next for the first ten years (Sutherland et al. 1982). Many well-known surgeons or single institutions have reported excellent revision rates over long periods, including the Hospital for Special Surgery, with 1.8 percent for 10 years (Ranawat et al. 1984), the University of Iowa, with 1.5 percent for 10 years (Johnston and Crowninshield 1983), and Dr. John Charnley, initiator and developer of the operation, with 2.0 percent for 11.5 years. Rates for other institutions tend to be somewhat higher and include 7 percent cumulative revisions in ten years at the Mayo Clinic, (Stauffer 1982), 10.4 percent at Stanford University (Tapadiya et al. 1984), and 23.2 percent at the Cleveland Clinic (Sutherland et al. 1982). These rates are probably reasonably accurate, but in no situation were life table statistics used and thus failure rates may have been exaggerated or minimized, according to individual rules of follow-up reporting. In the current study involving a region rather than a single hospital or surgeon, the revision rate was at least 4.9 percent (removal, exchange of prosthesis, and deep infection) for twenty-seven months, which projected for ten years would be approximately 26 percent. Thus, it would appear that the revision rate for this popular procedure is much greater when the denominator includes all hospitals and practicing surgeons in a large area, compared with the reportings of selected tertiary care institutions. These data are even more striking in view of the fact that the analysis of Northern California revision rates is for 1980, and most published studies concern operations performed a decade earlier, when total hip replacement methods were relatively primitive by comparison.

The observation of increased mortality following total hip replacement, when carried out infrequently in a given hospital or by an individual surgeon, is consistent with the previous report of an inverse relationship between surgical volume and mortality for this and other procedures (Luft et al. 1979; Flood et al. 1984). (An exception for total hip replacement has been reported by Riley and Lubitz [1985]. However, their analysis is based on Medicare Part A data, which has less precise diagnostic data.) These previous reports have limited their analyses to the hospital relationship only, however, and the present study suggests that the low-volume surgeon may have a stronger relationship than the low-volume hospital. In addition, the data suggest an inverse relationship between major complications and surgical volume. Of particular note is the apparent large number of surgeons and hospitals that carry out very small numbers of Medicare total hip replacements, many as few as one per year. Even adjusting for those hip operations not covered by Medicare (we assume that the Medicare claims data reflect approximately half of the total hip replacements performed), the large majority of hospitals carried out many fewer procedures than previous reports indicate to be associated with a low mortality.[3]

Two explanations have been offered for the superior results of hospitals and surgeons with greater volumes: (1) the greater skill that accompanies practice or experience or, alternatively, (2) that patients are referred preferentially to hospitals and surgeons with better results (Luft 1980). Presumably, both mechanisms are active, although their relative strengths are unknown. Additionally, procedures as complicated as joint replacement surgery require a variety of complex and expensive equipment, a team of trained technicians, and a need for an almost open-ended assortment of different-sized prostheses that might be required for unexpected or unusual cases. The greater the hospital volume, the more likely it is that the necessary equipment (appropriate prostheses) and teamwork will be in place and functioning properly.

The increasing death rate associated with decreasing frequency on the part of the surgeon might also be explained by the fact that the "seldom" surgeon has less expertise in choosing appropriate patients and also more difficulty in carrying out the procedure. The postoperative regimen is overseen by the surgeon, and the less experienced surgeon is less likely to be aware of critical points in the postoperative management.

The striking inverse relationship between volume of procedures and surgeon charges bears special comment. Poor results, whether caused by inexperience or not, certainly do not justify increased reimbursement. Presumably, the increased fee charged by the seldom surgeon is a reflection of the perceived difficulty of the procedure to this surgeon. Paradoxically, the increased complication rate lends veracity to the perception.

Such routinely collected volume data do not allow us to identify specific poor performers, either hospitals or surgeons (Moses 1986; Luft and Hunt 1986). This identification is not feasible because of the limited number of patients seen and the low occurrence of adverse outcomes. Nonetheless, the relationship can be repeatedly demonstrated across large numbers of low-volume hospitals and surgeons.

From the original claims data used for this study, it would have been impossible to track the performance of individual physicians. Billing numbers are assigned in the Medicare system to billing entities, not to individuals. When an individual practices with more than one group, he or she has more than one billing number. Furthermore, an entire group of physicians may have only one billing code. Thus, billing codes alone may either overestimate or underestimate an individual's surgical experience. Routine monitoring of claims data, in the hopes of tracking individual performance, is not a useful exercise with the current data base. However, there are other providers of medical care who do routinely employ unique provider identifiers. In these settings, one might realistically require the quality-assurance programs already in place to carry out such monitoring. It is interesting to note that the Joint Commission on the Accreditation of Hospitals, in its new outcome-oriented quality-assurance program, has opted not to include the monitoring of these volume-outcome measures. Even more disappointing is its decision not to examine physician-specific outcomes (*American Medical News* 1986).

Another approach for the application of such findings is directed toward the consumers of health care, both purchasers and patients. The knowledge of the correlation of surgical experience and medical outcomes needs to become part of the informed consumer's decision-making process. Regardless of whether low volume causes poor performance or only signals poor performance, volume should affect one's choice of surgeon. Such information should be used as employers make decisions about contracting with health care systems. This knowledge should also be incorporated as individuals make decisions regarding their own medical care choices.

Conclusions

Routinely collected Medicare claims data are a valuable source of information by which to monitor the outcomes of hospital care. This information is of considerable potential value to third-party payers, to the government, to Medicare-established medical peer review organizations (PROs), and to the public. Third-party payers of medical claims are in a strategic position to survey the quality of medical care. For example, when patients are readmitted to hospitals for treatment of complications resulting from previous hospitalization and treatment, the claims submitted for reimbursement provide a unique record of the major events. An important potential use by medical insurers is to identify providers (both hospitals and physicians) with demonstrated superior outcomes, and to offer to their subscribers policies with economic incentives to patronize those "preferred providers." Thus, Blue Shield of California is currently implementing selective coverage for major organ transplantation, percutaneous transluminal angioplasty, and a number of new medical technologies to institutions with superior clinical results, as well as negotiated (e.g., lower) charges (*American Medical News* 1986). On the basis of our results, total hip replacement would appear to be an important candidate for selective coverage.

Claims data are also potentially valuable as a source of epidemiological information on the quality of hospital care provided to the population as a whole. Unfortunately, except for patients over the age of sixty-five and for some disabled, medical insurance coverage in the United States is a mix of multiple third-party payers, virtually precluding any comprehensive use of their total experience for epidemiological purposes. Even if it were possible to link the very large number of insurers and third-party administrators into a single information system, there would remain the problem of multiple coverage, with a single episode of care often covered and reimbursed by two or more agencies (Luft 1981). Despite these limitations, much can be learned from Medicare claims data, particularly concerning those conditions primarily affecting the elderly, as demonstrated for total hip replacement in the present study. Roos and colleagues urge that algorithms based on claims data also be developed for "medical admissions . . . common in the elderly" such as heart failure, chronic obstructive lung disease, and pneumonia (Roos et al. 1985).

Claims data will be of great potential value to the Health Care Financing Administration in monitoring the patterns of hospitalization and possible abuses under the Medicare Prospective Payment System (PPS) based on diagnosis-related groups (DRGs). Readmissions for complications of surgery at present are reimbursed as separate and legitimate medical events. A hospital (or surgeon, if DRGs are extended to reimbursement of physicians), is thus fiscally rewarded for its (or his or her) mistakes (Anderson and Steinberg 1984). If the goal of prospective payment is to provide incentives for cost-effective medical care—including fewer costly complications—the reimbursement per episode-of-care formula should logically include all complications, including readmissions. To do so would, of course, be one further step toward full prepayment or capitation, a direction in which DRGs are generally acknowledged as already taking us.

We have noted before (Bunker and Fowles 1985) that in espousing claims data as a basis for medical audit, it is important to recognize their inherent limitations and errors. In the present investigation of the use of claims data to identify complications of total hip replacement, we found an approximate 10 percent discrepancy between claims data and procedure, as recorded on the operative report. In using claims data as a technique for medical audit, one is faced, therefore, with a trade-off between accuracy that might be obtained by reference to the medical record itself and the efficiency and low cost of a fully automated audit using claims data. In recommending the latter, we emphasize that the goal of such automated audits should be a limited one—to measure overall performance of institutions and to identify problem areas for further study. The computer-based audit cannot be expected to provide information on the basis of which one can pass judgment on the quality of care provided by individual physicians to individual patients or as the basis for disciplinary actions against physicians or institutions.

The responsible and appropriate use of claims data, as a source of information on the quantity and quality of medical care, will become increasingly important. The government is now committed to the release of information documenting the quality of care of individual hospitals, and claims data are an obvious primary source. Employers as purchasers of medical services are already demanding access to claims data, in an effort to determine how and where their health care dollars are being spent, for what illnesses, and to what effect. It is essential, therefore, that the widespread availability of these data be coupled with their thoughtful and informed correlation with individual medical records, and that physicians and other health professionals actively participate in their interpretation.

Notes

The statistical advice of Byron W. Brown is gratefully acknowledged. We are indebted to the California Blue Shield Medicare staff and to Ralph Schaffarzick, Medical Director of Blue Shield of

California, for their extended cooperation. This study was funded in part by a grant (HS 04853) from The National Center for Health Services Research and Technology Assessment.

1. The Health Care Financing Administration divides California for administrative purposes into two groups of counties, with approximately equal Medicare claims. To achieve this division, several counties (e.g., Ventura, San Bernardino, Kern) in Southern California have arbitrarily been assigned to Northern California.

2. Since we were able to identify the surgeon in only 94.7 percent of cases, the number of "providers" may not be exactly the same as the number of surgeons. In 1980 there were 794 surgeons certified by the American Board of Orthopedic Surgery in practice in this Northern California region. Of the individual surgeons we could identify in this study, 92.4 percent were board certified. Therefore, it can be assumed that approximately half of the board-certified orthopedic surgeons performed one or more total hip replacements during the year.

3. Various estimates for the rate of Medicare total hip replacements to all total hip replacements have been derived from separate data sources, using age sixty-five and older as a proxy for the Medicare population. (In fact, in our study 10.2 percent of the Medicare total hip joint replacements were performed in patients under sixty-five.) In Manitoba, with universal health coverage, 51 percent of total hip replacements are done in patients sixty-five and older. At Stanford University Hospital (a tertiary care facility), 45 percent are performed on patients sixty-five and older. At the University of California, San Francisco, the rate is 42 percent; and in a national study of chronic disease, 57 percent of total hip replacements were performed on people sixty-five and older.

References

Anderson, G. F., and E. P. Steinberg, "Hospital Readmissions in the Medicare Population," *New England Journal of Medicine,* 311:1349–1353, 1984.

Bunker, J. P., and J. Fowles, "Medical Audit by Claims Data," *American Journal of Public Health,* 75(11)1261–1262, 1985.

Farber, B. F., D. L. Kaiser, and R. P. Wenzel, "Relation between Surgical Volume and Incidence of Postoperative Wound Infection," *New England Journal of Medicine,* 305:200–203, 1981.

Flood, A. B., W. R. Scott, and W. Ewy, "Does Practice Make Perfect?" Parts I and II, *Medical Care,* 22(2):98–124, 1984.

"JCAH to Review Clinical Outcomes," *American Medical News,* September 19, 1986.

Johnston, R. C., and R. D. Crowninshield, "Roentgenologic Results of Total Hip Arthroplasty: A Ten-Year Follow-Up Study." *Clinical Orthopaedics and Related Research,* 181:92–98, 1983.

Klett, S. V., and L. Lopez, "Transplant Center's Approval Stirs Quality, Access Issues," *Business and Health,* 52–53, June 1986.

Luft, H. S., "The Relation Between Surgical Volume and Mortality: An Explanation of Causal Factors and Alternative Models," *Medical Care,* 18(9):940–959, 1980.

———, "Diverging Trends in Hospitalization: Fact or Artifact?" *Medical Care,* 19(10): 979–994, 1981.

Luft, H. S., J. P. Bunker, and A. C. Enthoven, "Should Operations Be Regionalized? The Empirical Relation Between Surgical Volume and Mortality," *New England Journal of Medicine,* 301:1364–1369, 1979.

Luft, H. S., and S. S. Hunt, "Evaluating Individual Hospital Quality Through Outcome Statistics," *Journal of the American Medical Association,* 255:2780–2784, 1986.

Maerki, S. C., H. S. Luft, and S. S. Hunt, "Selecting Categories of Patients for Regionalization: Implications of the Relationship Between Volume and Outcomes," *Medical Care,* 24:148–158, 1986.

Moses, L. E., "The Evaluation of Hospital Death Rates," *Journal of the American Medical Association,* 255:2801, 1986.

National Center for Health Statistics, Division of Health Care Statistics, *Detailed Diagnoses and Surgical Procedures for Patients Discharged from Short-Stay Hospitals, United States, 1979,* Washington, DC: U.S. Government Printing Office, January 1982.

Ranawat, C. S., R. E. Atkinson, E. A. Salvati, and P. D. Wilson, "Conventional Total Hip Arthroplasty for Degenerative Joint Disease in Patients Between the Ages of Forty and Sixty Years," *The Journal of Bone and Joint Surgery,* 66-A:745–751, 1984.

Riley, G., and J. Lubitz, "Outcomes of Surgery among the Medicare Aged: Surgical Volume and Mortality," *Health Care Financing Review,* 7:37–47, 1985.

Riley, G., J. Lubitz, and M. Newton, "Outcomes of Surgery Among the Medicare Aged: Mortality After Surgery," *Health Care Financing Review,* 6:103–115, 1985.

Roos, L. L., S. M. Cageorge, E. Austen, and K. N. Lohr, "Using Computers To Identify Complications after Surgery," *American Journal of Public Health,* 75(11):1288–1295, 1985.

Stauffer, R. N., "Ten-Year Follow-Up Study of Total Hip Replacement With Particular Reference to Roentgenographic Loosening of the Components," *The Journal of Bone and Joint Surgery,* 64A:983–990, 1982.

Sutherland, C. J., A. H. Wilde, L. S. Borden, and K. E. Marks, "A Ten-Year Follow-Up of One Hundred Consecutive Muller Curved-Stem Total Hip-Replacement Arthroplasties," *The Journal of Bone and Joint Surgery,* 64-A:970–982, 1982.

Tapadiya, D., R. H. Walker, and D. J. Schurman, "Prediction of Outcomes of Total Hip Arthroplasty Based on Initial Postoperative Radiographic Analysis: Matched, Paired Comparisons of Failed Versus Successful Femoral Components," *Clinical Orthopaedics and Related Research,* 186:5–15, 1984.

"Transplant Criteria Published By Blues," *American Medical News,* July 12, 1985.

Vakili, F., P. Aglietti, and G. C. Brown, "A Ten-Year Follow-Up Study of Our First One Hundred Consecutive Charnley Total Hip Replacements," *The Journal of Bone and Joint Surgery,* 63A(5):753–767, 1981.

Wennberg, J. E., and A. Gittelsohn, "Variations in Medical Care Among Small Areas," *Scientific American,* 246:120–129, 1982.

Wennberg, J. E., R. Jaffe, and L. Sola, "Some Uses of Claims Data for the Analysis of Surgical Practices," in *New Challenges for Vital and Health Records,* DHHS Publication No. (PHS) 81-1214, December 1980.

15. Health Promotion and Prevention: A Medicare Issue

❏ ❏ ❏

SHELDON ROVIN AND ZOE BONIFACE

Introduction

Over the last twenty-odd years, the concept of prevention has gained popular support in American society. Magazines such as *Prevention* and *Today's Health* sell in the millions of copies. Many businesses and industries sponsor health promotion programs for their employees. New industries from health foods to running shoes have sprung up to meet consumer demand. Restaurants have adopted no-smoking sections and low-calorie or salt-free entrees. Millions of Americans apparently are willing to spend billions of dollars for prevention.

The popular image of prevention to date has been rather youth oriented. But the rising costs of Medicare, the increasing proportion of elderly within the general population, and expanding ambitions for high quality of life in old age have engendered increasing attention to prevention for the elderly.

Medicare generally does not pay for prevention. The only preventive services covered by Medicare are (1) pneumococcal vaccinations and (2) a limited amount of respite care if a Medicare recipient has chosen the hospice care option (U.S. DHHS 1986). It specifically disallows many goods and services that could be called preventive.

1. Standard medical prevention activities—routine physical examinations, tests directly related to those exams, most immunizations, and eye, hearing, and dental examinations.
2. Some products and services which compensate for loss of functional ability and may slow further deterioration, such as supportive devices for the feet.

3. Some services which could delay institutionalization—homemaker ser-
    vices, full-time nursing care in the home, services performed by immediate
    relatives or members of one's own household; and meals delivered to one's
    home (U.S. DHHS 1986).

Should Medicare begin to emphasize, or at least allow, coverage for preventive care? The Medicare guidelines do not even address some of the behavior
modifications (e.g., diet to slow osteoporosis). Should there be a Medicare-based
preventive policy? Dealing with these questions requires us to confront at least
four crucial issues:

1. What are we trying to prevent?
2. What parameters define the boundaries of prevention—that is, what goals
    or activities may or may not be called "preventive"?
3. What possible forms of prevention are in fact clinically effective?
4. How should we evaluate the outcome of investment in prevention? (In lay
    terms, is it cost effective?)

In our chapter, we introduce these issues, concluding with suggestions for
how Medicare may play a part in their resolution.

Goals

Conventional wisdom suggests that prevention is a good idea, a logical strategy
for managing many if not most health care problems. In contrast, research tends
to suggest that many preventive medical services are not cost effective (Russell 1986). So the issue comes down to asking, What exactly do we wish to prevent? Conceivably, Medicare coverage of preventive services could further goals
such as:

- [ ] Lengthened life
- [ ] Postponed onset of disease
- [ ] Increased quality of life
- [ ] Delayed onset of institutionalization and decreased aggregate use of nurs-
      ing homes
- [ ] Increased capacity for independent living
- [ ] Decreased dependence upon one's children
- [ ] Increased control over one's own health and life
- [ ] Reduction of total Medicare costs

At face value, none of these goals is especially controversial, but as a group
they may be incompatible. Strategies that bring progress toward one may reverse
progress toward another. For example, increasing Medicare benefits in order to

delay the onset of disease or institutionalization could increase Medicare's costs. Some measures to lengthen life may reduce quality of life, for example, extending life chemotherapeutically. Sooner or later we must determine, specify, and prioritize the trade-offs among our goals for prevention.

Parameters

Assuming we can agree upon our goals for prevention, we must define the range of acceptable means. A wide variety of activities can be called "prevention." This variation must be understood, in order to avoid making inappropriate generalizations or placing unintended restrictions upon the range of options considered. As illustration, we discuss societal versus individual and active versus passive preventive measures.

Societal measures of prevention address the ways communal life may increase or decrease the risks to our health (Castillo-Salgado 1984). Initial preventive measures against acute infectious disease—quarantine and sanitation—recognized that the danger to society could be minimized by controlling the spread of contagion (Terris 1981). Little could be done to reduce the risk for a given individual until the development of vaccines. Even then, public health officials promoted vaccines among a suspicious populace (to the point of mandating vaccination before entry into public schools) because an increasing percentage of vaccinated population reduced the spread of disease across an entire community (Russell 1986).

Societal measures often are controversial at their inception because they require community investment and/or sanction, are perceived to restrict individual freedom, and commonly threaten some vested interest (Castillo-Salgado 1984). Fluoridation is a good example. Furthermore, the range of changes that can be described as "preventive" has no clear limits. The fifty-five-mile speed limit has reduced the number of fatal car accidents. Traffic signs prevent accidents from occurring. The shutdown of nuclear power plants removes the health hazards of a nuclear meltdown. Even distributing needles to intravenous drug users is being tested as a preventive measure to curb the spread of the acquired immune deficiency syndrome (AIDS). Examples of preventive societal measures that would directly affect the elderly include cleaning streets and sidewalks to prevent falls and broken hips and placing greater restrictions on the renewal of the impaired person's driver's license to prevent accidents. But not all potential societal forms of prevention may be perceived as issues of public health, and not all are worth their social or financial cost.

In contrast, the individual approach to prevention recognizes that the way an individual lives can affect his or her chances of disease or injury. If an individual adopts healthy behaviors or eschews unhealthy ones, he or she will reap the benefit (Berkanovic 1976; Castillo-Salgado 1984; Fielding 1979). Society also may benefit from a lower aggregate rate of morbidity if enough individuals participate and if the cost of care is covered by insurance and from the control of unhealthy behavior that affects more than the individual (e.g., smoking that harms others as passive smoke). However, often it is considered inappropriate, infeasible, or inefficient for society to coerce individuals into altering their behavior. Instead, they must be persuaded to choose the benefits of healthful behaviors (Brennan 1981).

The individual approach has gained prominence as chronic disease emerged as the major cause of death. Chronic diseases are perceived to stem in large part from the health habits of individual life-style; thus, their prevention emphasizes the alteration of individual behavior (Berkanovic 1976; Castillo-Salgado 1984). Nevertheless, societal measures against chronic disease are no less important. Occupational and environment hazards such as dust, toxic chemicals, and air pollution contribute to the development of chronic disease (Castillo-Salgado 1984). Also, individual choice does not occur in a societal vacuum. Individual health behaviors can be encouraged or discouraged by the laws or norms of the community where we live or work (Berkanovic 1976).

Another consideration is active versus passive modes of prevention. Active measures require individuals to commit substantial personal effort toward prevention. Smoking cessation, weight loss, fitness, and redesign of one's home to reduce the risk of falls all demand one's time, money, and sometimes painful behavior change. Passive measures, such as immunization or fluoridation, require only minimal personal effort in order to be effective. Although active measures often focus upon the individual and passive measures focus upon the entire society, there are exceptions. Immunization, for example, directly reduces the risk of the individual but requires no more effort than an occasional or one-time visit to the physician. Societal measures demand tax support, political compromise, and restriction of individual freedom, all of which can entail large individual sacrifice (Warner 1979).

Since the boundaries of prevention are broad, how we define them may restrict our choices. For example, the medical model stresses treatment of disease. It also stresses a physician-patient relationship that gives to the physician, tacitly or overtly, the role of in loco parentis. But physicians generally are not specially trained in technical matters, such as toxic waste disposal or how to deal with environmental pollutants. Nor are they trained very well in the concept of prevention as a health care discipline (Silver 1978). Their traditional schooling may ill-equip them to facilitate the negotiations and political efforts required for enactment of societal prevention measures. Defining the boundaries of prevention requires both technical expertise and societal consent.

Clinical Effectiveness

Given the wide range of possible prevention activities, a comprehensive assessment of their clinical effectiveness is necessary to identify those to be incorporated into a sound policy design. However, to date there is no truly comprehensive review of the literature. At least three studies have attempted a comprehensive approach. In 1985 the Ciba Foundation sponsored a symposium entitled "The Value of Preventive Medicine" (Evered and Whelan 1985). Participants addressed topics ranging from genetic screening to control of tobacco-related disease to issues of experimental design and cost-effectiveness. Perhaps due to its medical basis, the symposium did not address societal forms of prevention. The American Medical Association's Council on Scientific Affairs reported in 1983 its reassessment of the periodic health examination (American Medical Association 1983). This work was based in part upon the previous work of a Canadian task force. The council concluded that the standard yearly exam consisting of a uniform list of procedures should be replaced by a list and schedule of exam procedures tailored to the individual patient's age, medical history, and known risk factors. The Foundation for Health Services Research in 1983 developed a research agenda for health promotion and disease prevention for children and the elderly. This work defined the following four classes of prevention targets for the elderly:

1. *Problems that can be addressed in traditional prevention terms* (i.e., primary, secondary, or tertiary prevention).
2. *Behaviors likely to produce beneficial or adverse effects on health status.* These health behaviors are risk factors rather than diseases or impairments, . . . [for example], . . . smoking, diet modification, weight control, social participation, and stress reduction.
3. *Problems requiring attention from caregivers* (i.e., problems such as hearing impairments or alcoholism which cause a loss of functional ability but which may be detected and treated by physicians or other caregivers).
4. *Iatrogenic problems* (which result from the caregiving system (e.g., drug reactions and functional disability deriving from "overprotective" environments or inappropriate placement into a nursing home) (Kane, Kane, and Arnold 1985).

This work described the evidence regarding various risk factors as thorough or deficient, but it did not systematically present or test the validity of the assumptions upon which prevention strategies are based. The summary included some societal aspects of prevention, but it did not attempt to define boundaries for societal prevention measures.

Several researchers have suggested lists of health habits or risk factors to be targeted for modification. Lester Breslow and others (Belloc and Breslow 1972; Breslow and Enstrom 1980) have identified seven personal health practices that correlate with subsequent better physical health: never smoking cigarettes, regular physical activity, moderate or no use of alcohol, seven to eight hours of sleep per day on a regular basis, maintenance of proper weight, eating breakfast, and not eating between meals. Jonathan Fielding (1979) has suggested six similar targets for health promotion programs; his recommendations have influenced the design of health promotion programs in business. Neither of these two researchers particularly address the elderly; however, the Lifetime Health Monitoring Program proposed by Breslow and Somers (1977) prescribes health goals and professional services for each age group. Their recommendations for the Medicare-aged group include both specific goals and professional services (see Appendix 15.1).

Rather than trying to develop our own comprehensive review of the clinical effectiveness of prevention, we shall attempt to describe the complexity of proving clinical effectiveness. According to Russell, most studies of effectiveness suffer from design or standardization problems. In her recent book, *Is Prevention Better than Cure?* (1986), she separately discussed three categories of intervention—vaccination, screening, and life-style modification—because she found they differ somewhat in the logical steps necessary to prove clinical effectiveness or cost-effectiveness.

Immunization programs are a popular preventive strategy and are often dramatic in their results. Even so, debate occurs with each new vaccine over whom to vaccinate (everyone or high-risk groups) and how to evaluate the costs and benefits of a given vaccine (discussed later). One issue that is relevant when considering immunization programs for the elderly, if prevention is being touted in terms of potential cost savings, is the cost of future medical care for those whose lives are saved because they received a vaccination. It is well known that the beneficiaries that consume the largest proportion of Medicare expenditures are the old old (i.e., those over seventy-five years). Consequently, interventions such as vaccinations have the potential of costing Medicare more over the long term than it saves through avoiding hospitalization for a particular illness because of the chronic illness that often characterizes the last years of the very old. Here is a clear case where cost-benefit or cost-effectiveness outcomes depend on the assumptions underlying the evaluation.

Screening by itself, as Russell (1986) points out, has no health benefit since it only identifies people who may benefit from treatment. To evaluate the benefits of screening, one must weigh the costs of screening *and* treatment against the benefits associated with absence of the disease. The cost-benefit or cost-effectiveness ratio can be dramatically altered, depending on the frequency of screening that is deemed necessary, the risks associated with screening, the treatment that is chosen, the compliance with the treatment, the side effects of the treatment, and the likelihood that treatment will result in cure or remission.

The value of life-style modification is harder to prove or disprove than that of vaccination or screening. Many life-style modifications work indirectly upon a given disease, targeting a risk factor that is associated with but not conclusively proved to cause the disease. For example, control of hypertension might decrease one's risk for death from heart disease. Moreover, life-style modification is harder to achieve, enforce, and measure. It requires frequent, even daily, intervention and, therefore, much more commitment and effort on the part of the individual. Participation either must be voluntary or must be relatively easily enforced because the professional sector has less control over administration of the intervention (Russell 1986) and because measurement must rely on the individual's self-reports of his or her behavior.

An additional assumption concerning life-style, particularly appropriate in regard to the elderly, is that decrease of a risk factor or unhealthy life-style will reduce one's risk for disease. For example, at least one study has found that smoking cessation correlates with a lesser risk for disease (Rosenberg et al. 1985). However, if the unhealthy life-style or risk factor has persisted for some time, it may already have caused damage that cannot be undone. Most commonly recommended life-style modifications have not yet achieved this degree of proof of clinical effectiveness.

A final questionable assumption, applicable to all forms of prevention activities, is that proof of clinical effectiveness among the general adult population can be generalized to apply to the elderly. This assumption generally has not been proved because to date little clinical evaluation of prevention measures has focused upon the elderly. Kane, Kane, and Arnold (1985) state that many prevention measures are conceived as occurring in earlier adulthood, with the goal of mitigating the diseases and conditions of old age. It is difficult to know when during the lifespan these interventions are most useful.

Evaluation of the Investment in Prevention

Cost-effectiveness analysis and cost-benefit analysis both must verify similar hierarchies of assumptions. Most important, both presume that the prevention activities in question possess some degree of clinical effectiveness: an activity that is not clinically effective is a waste of money. Some guidelines in the design

of tests for clinical effectiveness, cost-effectiveness, or a favorable ratio of benefits to costs are common to all forms of social science research. For example, one
should not assume the cause and effect between two correlated events, such as
presence of disease and risk factor (Russell 1986). A controlled experimental
design is essential for measuring the individual effects of multiple factors.

In addition, several guidelines more specifically apply to evaluation of prevention. Diseases, risk factors, and preventive activities are aggregate in nature: a
single disease may be associated with several risk factors; a single risk factor may
correlate with several diseases and may be modified through several strategies.
Therefore, an experimental design must anticipate and separately measure these
components (Russell 1986). There may be no defined or natural dividing line
between normal and abnormal levels of disease states or risk factors. For example, designation of normal versus high blood pressure is somewhat arbitrary
(Russell 1986). Moreover, the intervention should not be worse than the disease
or risk factor it is intended to combat. For example, the suggestion that hysterectomies be performed prophylactically to preclude ovarian and uterine cancer,
unwanted pregnancies, and painful menstruation was found unreasonable (Goodman and Goodman 1986).

Russell (1986) suggests a further guideline for tests of cost-effectiveness or
determination of cost-benefit ratios. Cost-effectiveness explicitly compares alternative strategies to achieve a given outcome. Often, the alternatives differ greatly
in clinical nature and, therefore, require divergent designs to test clinical effectiveness (e.g., vaccine administration vs. treatment of the disease). Nevertheless, comparison of the alternatives' relative cost-effectiveness requires that both
be measured using equivalent parameters. The level of a single such parameter
can determine whether or not an alternative is judged cost effective. Therefore, if
the results of individual cost-effectiveness studies are to be compared, each
should use the same measure of outcome. Cost-benefit studies should use the
same financial parameters: discount rate, amount of medical care costs per added
year of life, and so on (Russell 1986).

Banta and Luce (1983) recently surveyed 240 journal articles loosely categorized as cost-benefit or cost-effectiveness analyses of various prevention measures. They concluded that the majority of these articles were flawed by serious
conceptual or analytical errors. Some errors were due to the inherent difficulties
of applying cost analysis to prevention, such as the inability to precisely predict
the nature and magnitude of future streams of preventive cost and benefits. Other
common errors resulted from neglect of an inexpert application of cost-analytic
principles, such as failure to discount future discounts and costs or failure to
measure cost of a program as the cost of one's next best alternative (i.e., opportunity cost). Banta and Luce suggest that researchers can produce higher-quality

cost analyses through adherence to the general principles of cost analysis methodology recently developed by/for the U.S. Congress Office of Technology Assessment.

Numerous authors have discussed the relative merits of cost-effectiveness analysis versus cost-benefit analysis. Both methods may be suitable for the evaluation of prevention for the elderly. However, the "human capital" approach, which determines the financial value of a life saved in terms of earnings (or other productivity) saved, may be particularly inappropriate in regard to the elderly, who may retire by age sixty-five.

Recommendations

Very little evaluation of prevention measures has been performed in relation to the elderly. Their clinical effectiveness and cost-effectiveness largely has not yet been proved or disproved. How does this affect development of a Medicare policy on preventive services? A recent Hastings Center Report (Goodman and Goodman 1986) criticized policymakers who "jump the gun," advocating preventive measures before they have been proved to work. Yet policymakers in any field caution us that proof is never perfect. And, the timetable of politics cannot delay a policy solution until all the evidence is in; we simply must do the best with what we know. Advocates of this position note that Snow shut down the Broad Street pump and stopped a London cholera epidemic before he could explain why cholera cases correlated with families who used that particular pump. Quarantine and sanitation reduced the spread of infectious disease before the germ theory of disease was developed. Each side of this issue is right; we must find an acceptable balance for the given situation.

Pilot programs are a useful compromise. They can examine administrative innovations on a small scale, eliminating obvious failures, and identify ideas with greatest chance for success. When, as in the case of prevention, the knowledge base needed for policy and administrative innovation is far from complete, innovatively designed pilot programs can both enlarge the general knowledge base and answer immediate questions.

A literature search showed that, to date, numerous programs have been developed to test the delivery of preventive services to the elderly. Unfortunately, most of these programs merely test the feasibility of the delivery process (e.g., ability to attract eligible elderly to use the service) or measure only short-term outcomes, such as subjects' acquisition of knowledge of prevention or the lowering of blood cholesterol levels. The true outcomes of interest—documented decrease of morbidity (e.g., heart attacks) or mortality due to the preventive intervention and attendant cost effects—are not reported. Measurement of these outcomes of interest requires that pilot programs follow up on the health status of their subjects for at least several years (and the longer the better). Lack of reporting of the outcomes of interest may reflect either the relative youth of the programs (i.e., the idea of prevention for the elderly is relatively new, and pilot programs, to date, may not have existed long enough to measure the health effects of interest) or a tendency not to support pilot studies over the period of time necessary for long-term health effects to become manifest.

We feel that Medicare, through well-designed pilot programs, is particularly equipped to take a leading role in the definition and evaluation of prevention for the elderly. Since Medicare is the major payer for the entire population of U.S. citizens over sixty-five, existing data collection procedures could be used, with perhaps some modification to collect long-term morbidity and mortality measures for participants in pilot programs, comparing them with any number of natural control groups. Medicare has already initiated some pilot programs to consider how coverage for prevention services should be designed. At this writing, three such programs have already begun: one dealing with the prevention of falls and two concerned with screening and health education (HCFA, Office of Research and Demonstrations 1986). Details of these current and planned research programs are included in Appendix 15.2. In April 1986 Congress authorized five additional programs to be started in the coming year (PL 99-272).

In October 1986 the Health Care Financing Administration (HCFA) announced an agenda for future research, which included further investigation of prevention services for both Medicare and Medicaid populations. HCFA stressed its interest in the cost effects of coverage for prevention (*Federal Register* 1986).

While we applaud Medicare's cautious yet activist use of pilot programs, Medicare's current activities will not answer questions regarding cost-benefit. When their plans are compared with the conceptual framework we have described, it appears that the design of programs to date has occurred backwards: a focus upon cost-effectiveness has eclipsed attention to clinical effectiveness. Specifying minimum reimbursement for a polyglot package of services delegates the responsibility for selecting particular services to be included, but it also does not effectively allow observation of the effects of individual services. Whether the particular package should prove clinically or cost effective (or ineffective), the aggregate results preclude us from maximizing our contribution to the knowledge base or incrementally improving the composition of the original package. Furthermore, since the research agenda, so far, includes only a small range of traditional means, it appears that means were specified before goals were identified.

We suggest that Medicare draw from a clear conceptual framework when designing future initiatives in prevention. It first should identify and prioritize its goals. Such a beginning point could expand the range of means considered, illuminating nontraditional means such as, for example, discounting premiums for nonsmokers. Since cost-effectiveness presumes clinical effectiveness, and since we wish to identify the most cost-effective means from a set of alternatives, expansion of the range of means considered could help us avoid premature approval of a particular strategy. It could protect us from abandoning prevention entirely, if the few means considered proved unsatisfactory.

In particular, Medicare can help us fill the gap regarding how a particular means of prevention may differ in clinical effectiveness or cost-effectiveness, when applied to an *elderly* rather than to an average adult population. Individual programs should be designed to separate and compare the effects of various means. The design could differentiate the various levels of a hierarchy of means. For example, lowering of serum cholesterol is a possible means to avert a heart attack; alteration of one's diet is a possible means to lower serum cholesterol; health education is a possible means to achieve alteration of diet. A class led by a nurse practitioner is a possible means of health education. Another example, brought to the public's attention by its occurrence in President Reagan, is cancer of the colon. The issue is whether colonoscopy, an uncomfortable procedure and one whose clinical effectiveness is yet to be determined as a preventive measure, should be a routine screening procedure for the group most at risk—the elderly. Other suggested pilot programs could include peer support groups to assist independent living and day care and home care as a potential means for delaying institutionalization. The evaluation of prevention is a long-term endeavor. Medicare should not have to wait for others to generate the information and experience needed to institute a national policy on coverage for prevention. Well-designed pilot programs can simultaneously answer our immediate and our more fundamental questions about prevention.

Appendix 15.1: Recommended Health Goals and Preventive Services for the Elderly (Breslow and Somers 1977, p. 604)

The elderly (sixty to seventy-four years)
Health goals

1. To prolong the period of optimum physical/mental/social activity.
2. To minimize handicapping and discomfort from onset of chronic conditions.
3. To prepare in advance for retirement.

Professional services

1. Professional visits with the healthy adult at sixty years of age and every two years thereafter, including the same tests for chronic conditions as in older

middle age, and professional counseling regarding changing life-style related to retirement, nutritional requirements, absence of children, possible loss of spouse, and probable reduction in income as well as reduced physical resources.

2. Annual dental prophylaxis.
3. Periodic podiatry treatments as needed.

Old age (seventy-five years and over)
Health goals

1. To prolong period of effective activity and ability to live independently and to avoid institutionalization so far as possible.
2. To minimize inactivity and discomfort from chronic conditions.
3. When illness is terminal, to assure as little physical and mental distress as possible and to provide emotional support to patient and family

Professional services

1. Professional visit at least once a year including complete physical examination, medical and behavioral history, and professional counseling regarding changing nutritional requirements, limitations on activity and mobility, and living arrangements.
2. Annual immunization against influenza (unless the person is allergic to vaccine).
3. Periodic dental and podiatry treatments as needed.
4. For low-income and other persons not sick enough to be institutionalized but not well enough to cope entirely alone, counseling regarding sheltered housing, health visitors, home help, day care, and professional services.
5. Professional visit at least once a year including complete physical examination, medical and behavioral history, and professional counseling, recreational centers, meals-on-wheels, and other measures designed to help them remain in their own homes and as nearly independent as possible.
6. Professional assistance with family relations and preparations for death, if needed.

Appendix 15.2: Medicare's Current and Planned Research in Prevention for the Elderly

Existing pilot programs

Recently, Medicare initiated some pilot programs to study prevention among the elderly. At present, the following three sites have initiated programs.

The Kaiser Foundation Research Institute, Portland, Oregon, is conducting a two-year randomized clinical trial (2,400 total participants) to prevent falls in the elderly. The experimental group will receive self-management education, as well as minor home renovations and safety equipment. The project began recruitment of participants in September 1985. It is cosponsored by the HCFA, The National Institute on Aging, the Robert Wood Foundation, and Kaiser Foundation Hospitals, Inc.

The University of North Carolina—Department of Social and Administrative Medicine, Chapel Hill, North Carolina, has begun a six-year randomized clinical trial for a package of preventive services. Eligible services include a menu of annual screening exams provided by a physician and a health education/promotion program conducted biannually by a community health nurse. Reimbursement is limited to $100 per year per person. Approximately 1,500 total participants (solicited by their regular physicians) will be tracked to monitor health outcomes, such as death and hospitalization.

Blue Cross of Massachusetts, Boston, Massachusetts, has begun a six-year randomized clinical trial similar to the University of North Carolina's program. The program will provide similar annual screenings and biannual health education/promotion; however, both types of services will be provided by a geriatric nurse practitioner. In addition, experimental group participants identified as high-risk individuals will be seen every three months and also will receive medication monitoring. Medicare beneficiaries of a given geographical area will be invited by the HCFA to participate. Of approximately 10,000 eligible individuals, 3,000 are expected to enter the experimental program; of these, 600 may be identified as high-risk individuals. Health outcome data will be drawn from death certificates, payer records, and a telephone survey (U.S. DHHS, Office of Research and Demonstration 1986).

Future pilot programs

The Comprehensive Omnibus Budget Reconciliation Act of 1985 (PL 99-272, April 7, 1986) has authorized a four-year Medicare demonstration (pilot) program for preventive services. Five sites—schools of public health or departments of preventive medicine—should offer the following services:

☐ Health screenings
☐ Health-risk appraisals
☐ Immunization

In addition, counseling on the following should be offered:

☐ Diet and nutrition
☐ Reduction of stress
☐ Exercise and exercise programs
☐ Sleep regulation
☐ Injury prevention
☐ Prevention of alcohol and drug abuse

☐ Prevention of mental health disorders
☐ Self-care, including use of medication
☐ Reduction or cessation of smoking

Proposals for this program will be solicited in January 1987 (Michael Spodnick, personal communication). Beyond this mandated project, the HCFA plans continuing study of preventive services, for both Medicare and Medicaid populations (*Federal Register* 1986).

References

American Medical Association, Council on Scientific Affairs, "Council Report: Medical Evaluations of Healthy Persons," *Journal of the American Medical Association*, 249:1626–1633, March 25, 1983.

Banta, H. D., and B. R. Luce, "Assessing the Cost-Effectiveness of Prevention," *Journal of Community Health*, 9(2):145–165, 1983.

Belloc, N. B., and L. Breslow, "Relationship of Physical Health Status and Health Practices," *Preventitive Medicine*, 1:409–421, 1972.

Berkanovic, E., "Behavioral Science and Prevention," *Preventitive Medicine*, 5:92–105, 1976.

Brennan, A. J. J., "Health Promotion in Business: Caveats for Success," *Journal of Occupational Medicine*, 23:639–642, September 1981.

Breslow, L., and J. E. Enstrom, "Persistence of Health Habits and Their Relationship to Mortality," *Preventitive Medicine*, 9:469–483, 1980.

Breslow, L., and A. R. Somers, "The Lifetime Health Monitoring Program: A Practical Approach to Preventive Medicine," *New England Journal of Medicine*, 296:601–608, March 17, 1977.

Castillo-Salgado, C., "Assessing Recent Developments and Opportunities in the Promotion of Health in the American Workplace," *Social Science and Medicine*, 19:349–358, 1984.

Evered, D., and J. Whelan, eds., "The Value of Preventive Medicine," *Proceedings of Ciba Foundation Symposium 110*, London: Pitman, 1985.

Federal Register, "Medicare and Medicaid Programs: Health Care Financing Research and Demonstration Cooperative Agreements and Grants; Amendment," 51: 36795–36990, October 16, 1986.

Fielding, J. E., "Preventive Medicine and the Bottom Line," *Journal of Occupational Medicine*, 21:79–88, February 1979.

Goodman, L. E., and M. J. Goodman, "Prevention—How Misuse of a Concept Undercuts Its Worth," *Hastings Center Report*, 16:26–38, April 1986.

Kane, R. L., R. A. Kane, and S. B. Arnold, "Prevention and the Elderly: Risk Factors," *Health Services Research*, 19:945–1006, February 1985.

Rosenberg, L., D. W. Kaufman, S. P. Helmrich, and S. Shapiro, "The Risk of Myocardial Infarction After Quitting Smoking in Men Under 55 Years of Age," *New England Journal of Medicine*, 313:1511–1514, December 12, 1985.

Russell, L. B., *Is Prevention Better than Cure?* Washington, DC: The Brookings Institution, 1986.

Silver, G. A., *Child Health: America's Future,* Germantown, MD: Aspen Systems Corp., 1978.

Spodnick, M., Health Care Financing Administration, Office of Research and Demonstrations, Office of Operations Support. Baltimore, MD: Personal Communication, November 1986.

Terris, M. "The primacy of prevention." *Preventitive Medicine,* 10:689–99, 1981.

U.S. Comprehensive Omnibus Budget Reconciliation Act of 1985, Pub. L. No. 99-272, 9314, 100 Stat 82, 194-96 (April 7, 1986).

U.S. Department of Health and Human Services, Health Care Financing Administration. 1986. *Your Medicare Handbook.* Publication No. HCFA-10050, ICN-461250.

U.S. Office of Research and Demonstrations, *Health Care Financing Status Report: Research and Demonstrations in Health Care Financing.* Publication No. HCFA-03219, 245, 247–248, 1986.

Warner, K. E., "The economic implications of preventive healthcare." *Social Science and Medicine,* 13C:227–237, 1979.

16. Post-Acute Care: Packages, Bows, and Strings

ROBERT L. KANE

Introduction

The introduction of the new Medicare Prospective Payment System (PPS) has had a number of important effects on the program. Among these is the renewed interest in post-hospital care. Under the current funding scheme, there are attractions for various post-acute care (PAC) efforts; these often seem tied up with pretty bows. The counterstrategy is to repackage hospital care and PAC into a single bundled service or to go even farther toward a capitated approach; each of these proposals has a number of strings attached.

Medicare might have chosen Lewis Carroll for its patron saint. As Somers (1972) has noted, the arrangements for the elderly under this program often look as though they had been designed in Wonderland. Indeed, the discussions about the program sometimes take on the same flavor. Considerations of one or another element remind one of Humpty Dumpty's principle that things mean exactly what he wants them to mean. As we set about to tinker with the program by adding a bit here and there, we are at great peril of creating confusion unless we take great pains to be specific. However, the message of this chapter is simply that the field does not permit the necessary level of specificity. We are, and will likely remain, in a state where we can better address what we want to accomplish than to specify precisely how we wish to get there. This dilemma has not kept a number of professional constituencies from offering very dogmatic statements about just what should be included in a legitimate service package. The result has produced a rather encumbered system, reminiscent of the White Knight. When Alice asked him why he traveled with so much paraphernalia—like a beehive, a mousetrap, and a candlestick—he explained that he never knew when he might want to raise bees, trap mice, or light a candle.

The framers of Medicare had intended to produce an insurance program that would provide elderly persons with generally the same benefits as those they could not easily buy in the private market. In 1965 that meant coverage of hospital care. With commendable foresight, these framers recognized that hospitals were expensive places, and that a creative insurance program should provide incentives to reduce hospital use. Although they avoided addressing the primary incentive by offering a payment system other than cost reimbursement, they did provide some options for care. They anticipated that a substantial portion of post-hospital recuperation could occur in settings less sophisticated and hence less expensive. They envisioned such institutional care in something called an extended care facility, the name implying an extension of the work begun in the hospital. They also made provisions for recuperation at home under the doubly covered home health care benefit. Both of these benefits were initially intended as extensions of hospital care and not to become entities on their own. Careful stipulations were built into the eligibility criteria to assure this.

Post-Acute Care Under Medicare

Three types of PAC can be recognized. Each offers some specific attributes that argue for separate consideration, but all share enough common characteristics to make a general discussion feasible and questions about their interchangeability important. One form of such care is terminal care. This is generally identified by a determination of impending death; the expectations of such care are essentially palliative, with an emphasis on maximizing the patient's comfort. Such care seems to stand in sharp contrast to rehabilitative care, where the expectation is improvement in function. Still a third form of PAC lies somewhere between these poles. It might be thought of as recuperative or convalescent care. As with rehabilitation, the expectation is for improvement, but the clinical course has already been established by the acute care, and thus the actual mix of services may more closely resemble terminal care. To some degree, each of these forms of PAC in turn blend into long-term care. Although Medicare regulations have been developed to attempt to distinguish carefully between PAC and long-term care (Medicare takes great pains to disallow "custodial" care), the separation is more difficult in practice.

These post-acute provisions have changed slightly in the ensuing twenty years. The extended care facility became the skilled nursing facility (SNF), a term certainly no more accurate. Home care benefits were made more generous, on the one hand, by removing the limitations on numbers of visits but more restricted by more careful attention to strict enforcement of the eligibility criteria. Among those using these benefits to deliver care, there emerged a culture of praiseworthy outlaw behavior in the tradition of Robin Hood, in which the principled care-giver acted nobly in his or her client's behalf to find ways around the rules to allow the client to remain covered (and his or her agency to get paid) (Mundinger 1983).

The Tax Equity and Fiscal Responsibility Act (TEFRA) of 1982 added another component to the montage of aftercare; namely, hospice care. Hospice care is pursued as an alternative to expensive hospitalizations. Hospice care can be delivered in several forms; basically, it is customarily divided into hospital-based units (including some free-standing programs) and home care, but it can also be viewed in terms of organized programs and adapted programs; the latter are usually equivalent services provided without an official designation.

The patient must elect the hospice benefit and sign a waiver to other types of care. Five percent of total direct patient care hours are to be furnished by volunteers and documentation maintained of the cost savings achieved with the use of volunteers. Four levels of hospice care have been established for payment purposes: (1) routine home care, (2) continuous home care, (3) inpatient respite care, and (4) general inpatient care. The number of inpatient days used by all beneficiaries of the hospice may not exceed 20 percent of the total number of days of hospice coverage.

Because the Medicare payment rates for hospice care are often lower than those for regular home health care visits, many agencies have opted to provide a hospicelike service without official designation. Patients cared for in this manner can be paid for under Medicare without a special hospice waiver.

A fourth component of the PAC picture had existed as a quiet (almost silent) player until the change in hospital payment. Rehabilitation had not received very much attention until it was exempted from prospective payment. Prior to that, rehabilitation was treated very much like any other hospital service, although it had certain differences, as recognized under the Professional Standards Review Organization (PSRO) program utilization review activities. For example, lengths of stay that would be considered excessive for acute hospital stays were acceptable for rehabilitative care.

With the introduction of prospective payment for Medicare in 1983, the situation changed rather dramatically. Under this new system, the hospitals faced strong incentives to discharge patients as quickly as possible and potential financial incentives to retain the care of these same patients under other auspices, if such care could generate additional revenue, especially if such care could generate generous revenue. Thus, with the introduction of PPS, interest in PAC grew appreciably. It is important to note, however, that PAC was not a product of PPS. Indeed, PAC had existed as long as acute care, but few had noticed it. Some hospitals had developed home health care programs, and some had even begun exploring creative ways of diversifying their activities into long-term care and even housing. Now PAC represents both a means of relieving pressures on the acute care hospital and an opportunity for hospital diversification.

The PPS program exempted rehabilitative care along with psychiatric, pediatric, and chronic hospital care because the nature of such care did not fit the diagnostically based groupings that lay at the heart of the payment system. Rehabilitative care was thus allowed to continue as a separate service if the units providing such care met certain criteria. These included some tests of orthodoxy (e.g., directed by a rehabilitation specialist, certain amounts of rehabilitative therapies provided to each patient daily) and a general limitation on the kinds of problems treated (a requirement that at least 75 percent of admissions be for care of ten specified conditions). Such cautions seem in order to prevent misuse. However, on careful examination the problems treated, especially the problems treated among the elderly—the group one might expect Medicare to be most concerned about—look very similar to the kinds of problems treated in other post-acute settings, like home health care and nursing homes.

Defining and Evaluating Post-Acute Care

We have now begun to confront the first dilemma of PAC. Are things that look alike necessarily alike? Early administrators of the PPS era at the Health Care Financing Administration (HCFA) cast occasional troubled glances at the issue of rehabilitative care and asked periodically why the seemingly same patients treated in a nursing home cost so much less than those receiving rehabilitation in a certified unit. The puzzlement was all the greater when the nursing homes (SNFs) billed for rehabilitative services, like physical therapy and occupational therapy. The first response from the rehabilitation community was fairly predictable. These SNFs were denounced as pretenders; their care was not considered true rehabilitation.

A careful review of the literature on rehabilitation raises new questions. There is little hard evidence that rehabilitation rehabilitated anyone. Despite the enthusiastic descriptions of improvements in rehabilitative technology and case series, there are few carefully done studies that compare rehabilitation patients to controls. Moreover, the best studies are ambiguous or discouraging in their results (Johnston and Keith 1983). Many patients do indeed improve, but much of the improvement seems to be spontaneous and does not occur with impressively greater frequency among those receiving formal rehabilitative care. As with many other parts of medical care, it seems that the earlier one begins treatment, the better the results; but the same problems of bias and artifact haunt these studies as those in cancer detection. The controlled trials do not substantiate the enthusiasm of the field.

The problem is further complicated by the lack of a consistent definition of the goals of rehabilitation. Is the purpose to improve the functional capacity of the patient, or is it to assure that the patient actually functions at a higher level? This distinction is not merely semantic. The first alternative charges rehabilitation with the responsibility of working with the patient to assist him or her in regaining function. The test of such activity would be the patient's performance under controlled conditions. The latter charge looks at the ultimate outcome. It asks, in essence, what is the real value of all this unless the patient is able to return to his or her natural environment as a more functional person? Rehabilitation is thereby charged with assuring that the environment can indeed support the patient. Many might argue that this represents a rather tall order.

PAC is surely a different entity from acute care—but how different? On the one hand, it is a continuation of the work begun in the hospital. On the other, it is the beginning of long-term care. In acute care, the emphasis is on diagnosis and intervention. By the stage of PAC, the mystery is usually solved; the goals are recuperation and restoration. Rehabilitation was exempted from PPS because the simple four-part marker system of diagnosis-related groups (DRGs) did not seem likely to work. Indeed it did not. In an analysis of some 8,000 rehabilitation records, the Rand study found that DRG-like items could explain only about 12 percent of the variance in total charges, whereas a regression equation that addressed functional status could explain almost 35 percent (Hosek et al. 1986). Nonetheless, there was considerable variation in costs across rehabilitative facilities, even when these factors were controlled. Free-standing facilities cost more than units within hospitals, and there was up to 65 percent variation in cost across the various regions.

A special variant on the PAC theme is the case of the geriatric evaluation unit. Some observers have argued that Medicare's present prospective payment arrangement discriminates against geriatrics. Although most elderly patients do not need special attention, geriatrics addresses the 20 percent or so who do. The DRG system recognizes only a primary diagnosis and the presence of other problems; it fails to recognize the classic geriatric paradigm, in which one must contend with an older patient with chronic disability created by the interaction of multiple simultaneous problems. However, the situation may not be as bleak as some geriatricians protest. Jencks and Kay (1987) suggest that older, sicker Medicare patients did not really cost more prior to DRGs. Nonetheless, the current Medicare funding has created a troublesome paradox, in which a program designed for the elderly fails to recognize the geriatric patient and, in fact, discourages the hospital from treating such a patient.

There is now good evidence to show that careful geriatric assessment can make a dramatic difference in the course of these patients (Rubenstein et al. 1984). When assessments are carefully targeted, there is the potential for substantial benefits in terms of reduced mortality and increased functioning. There is now a growing body of literature to support the claims of cost-effectiveness from such an approach (Rubenstein 1987).

The geriatric evaluation unit in essence represents a merger between good medical care and good case management. It is seen as part of, rather than a substitute for, ongoing community care. It is, however, something not easily funded under the current reimbursement regulations.

The World Health Organization (1980) carefully distinguishes among disease, impairment, disability, and handicap. This progression may be attacked at any point. By the time of rehabilitation, the sequelae of the disease (i.e., the disability) may be more significant in determining treatment costs and prognosis than the diagnosis. However, we are also told that rehabilitation begins in the acute stages of an illness. Under such a scheme, the process is more continuous. The earlier the patient is identified, the more difficult the prognosis, and hence potentially the more difficult it is to determine the most appropriate mode of care.

Research on Post-Acute Care

At this point, we lack even the most basic data about PAC. We cannot say who goes where, let alone why or what difference it makes. Not surprisingly, part of the variation in the choice of post-acute resources is directly attributable to the availability of care. Some parts of the country have special chronic care facilities, others have well-developed home care programs. But simply noting such variation or relating it to available resources is unsatisfactory. That one service is substituted for another is not the same as one being equivalent to another.

More work is needed on defining the attributes of patients sent to various resources when several alternatives are simultaneously available. We can begin by asking how the patients using different services differ. The more pressing question is whether they are subsequently different as a result of the services they receive. If there is no evidence of differential impact, the argument for buying the cheapest service makes more sense. Indeed, some services begin by promising a better outcome and end up simply being less expensive.

The experience with hospice care is quite instructive in this regard. In a number of studies on hospice effects, the major concern has been cost. Lubitz and Prihoda (1984) provide a financial justification for hospice care in their analysis of health care services use and Medicare expenditures in the last two years of life. Using a 1978 cohort, they estimate that the 5.9 percent of beneficiaries who died accounted for 27.9 percent of expenditures for these two years. Moreover,

46 percent of the costs of the last year of life are spent in the last sixty days. Of course, a hospice's ability to save these dollars is greatly compromised if the bulk of the cost is already accrued before the patient is deemed appropriate for hospice care.

A study in Ohio using Medicare Part A and Blue Cross hospital insurance claims matched terminal cancer patients served by a home care hospice with those treated conventionally. The hospice patients used 50 percent less hospital care and ten times as much home care. There were associated cost savings (Brooks and Smyth-Staruch 1984).

In looking at the issue of evaluating hospice care, it seems most appropriate to focus on the question of effectiveness. Although the pressures for policy-relevant information call for *cost*-effectiveness data, it is important first to establish whether the new therapy is indeed effective. If the efficacy can be established, then one can go on to ask questions about how one can maintain the performance level, while reducing the cost. Experience with hospice care has shown that much of the cost question is going to be established by external events at any rate. Certainly, once hospices became covered as a Medicare benefit, the question quickly became how much care could one provide for the price being paid.

Two major evaluations of hospice care have been reported. The University of California, Los Angeles (UCLA) study is a randomized controlled trial of a VA hospital-based hospice program. The National Hospice Study used a quasi-experimental design to compare hospital-based and home care hospice with conventional care in forty sites across the country; twenty-six of these were funded under special Medicare demonstration waivers. These two major evaluations of hospice care created substantial controversy when the results were made public. They basically reported that hospice care was not generally better than conventional care, but it was no worse. Where there were differences, they tended to be around the levels of satisfaction, expressed by patients or their families; differences did not occur around pain control, effect, or symptoms (Greer et al. 1986; Kane et al. 1984, 1986; Kane, Bernstein, Wales, and Rothenberg 1985; Kane, Klein, Bernstein, Rothenberg, and Wales 1985). The National Hospice Study found that the cost of home-based hospice care was cheaper than conventional care (Birnbaum and Kidder 1984). The UCLA study, which employed largely a hospital-based model of hospice care, found no difference in the cost of care (Kane et al. 1984).

Hospice care has a unique attribute in the spectrum of PAC; it is usually time limited. Although some error in prognosis is possible, and indeed occurs in as many as a quarter of the cases (Kane et al. 1984), for the most part hospice care is terminal care.

For other types of PAC, the questions of cost may be better posed over a

longer time horizon. Although PAC is primarily viewed as a less expensive substitute for hospital care, the full cost implications may not emerge until one looks
at the full episode. In the case of rehabilitation, for example, the variation in cost
differences between free-standing and hospital units was less than those for the
components (i.e., average length of stay and cost per day). Some washout occurred. Similarly, when comparing the cost of care provided at home or in an
SNF, the true cost differences should recognize the possibility of additional costs
resulting from iatrogenic consequences or inadequate attention.

The basic principle underlying rehabilitation is one of investment. Spending
resources to improve function should pay savings dividends later on. The critical
issue in assessing the true benefit and cost savings of a rehabilitation program
thus depends on the time frame for the analysis. Under the conditions of many
demonstration programs, the time available to measure the potential savings from
such an investment strategy is inadequate. The basic paradigm used to evaluate
such a demonstration recognizes that there will be an initial increase in expenditures of effort and money in the experimental group in the early phases of the
project. At some point, the lines for expenditures among the experimental and
the control groups will cross. The longer one has to observe such programs, the
greater the opportunity to see subsequent savings from the intervention. When
the follow-up study is foreshortened, the possibility of demonstrating this savings is essentially precluded. In this sense, the demonstration project may be a
very bad predictor, certainly an underestimator, of the potential benefits of an
ongoing operational program. The economist may be quick to argue the need to
discount the value of delayed benefits, but the period of observation is rarely so
long as to make that concern a pressing issue.

Policy Implications

As we look toward the future, three funding options are available beyond the continuation of the current fragmented special handling of PAC. The first of these
options would be to expand the concept of prospective payment to cover one or
more PAC options. Hospice payment is presently based on this method. The earlier noted Rand/MCW study on rehabilitation was designed to test the feasibility
of such an approach for that type of care. In general, such an approach is indeed
feasible if one can obtain data not currently collected systematically, particularly
information on the functional status of the client, or to assume, as in the case of a
hospice, that all patients are essentially alike at some point in their disease.

The second option would be some effort to combine the payment for PAC with
the current PPS for acute care. This approach is usually referred to as "bundling." The general configuration of such an approach allows for probability cal-

culations as the proportion of people in each group who would need PAC and the estimation of the average cost for such care. This would then be apportioned over all such cases as a general add-on payment to the acute care payment. The implications are multiple. Resources might be more evenly distributed between acute care and PAC. Decisions about acute care might consider more closely the PAC consequences. Providers would not necessarily have any strong incentive to pursue the most effective course of care if a cheaper option were available. There is always a danger that where the providers of PAC are also the providers of acute care, they might select out the most desirable cases for their own organization and send the rest out to their competitors.

The final option would be to move directly toward some broad capitation system, such as that currently being tested with expanded coverage under the TEFRA regulations for Medicare health maintenance organizations (HMOs). For both the capitation and bundling approaches, one needs much better information on how to identify which groups of clients need what kinds of service. Without such information, we are not in a position to act as a prudent buyer to generate appropriate requirements for a benefit package. An important research agenda now is to look closely at what kinds of patients are most likely to benefit from what kinds of interventions in PAC. Here, we have reason to suspect that functional status will be an important predictor, but certainly diagnostic groupings in one form or another should also have an important bearing on the prognosis of the clients and the likelihood of benefit from various different forms of interventions. A great deal of work must ensue before we will be in a position where we can feasibly consider an empirically driven capitation approach. The alternative is to jump into capitation and hope somehow to counter the ill effects of both selective marketing and selective servicing by retrospective regulation. In light of our past history with such efforts, one would not be optimistic about such a strategy.

References

Birnbaum, H. G., and D. Kidder, "What Does Hospice Cost?" *American Journal of Public Health,* 74:689–697, 1984.

Brooks, C. H., and K. Smyth-Staruch, "Hospice Home Care Cost Savings to Third Party Insurers," *Medical Care,* 8:691–703, 1984.

Greer, D. S., V. Mor, J. N. Morris, S. Sherwood, D. Kidder, and H. Birnbaum, "An Alternative in Terminal Care: Results of the National Hospice Study," *Journal of Chronic Diseases,* 39:9–26, 1986.

Hosek, S., et al., *Charges and Outcomes for Rehabilitative Care: Implications for the Prospective Payment System,* Rand, R-3424-HCFA, Santa Monica: Rand Corp. 1986.

Jencks, S. F., and T. Kay, "Do Frail, Disabled, Poor, and Very Old Medicare Beneficiaries Have Higher Hospital Charges?" *Journal of the American Medical Association,* 257:198–202, 1987.

Johnston, M. V., and R. A. Keith, "Cost Benefits of Medical Rehabilitation: Review and Critique," *Archives of Physical Medicine and Rehabilitation,* 64:147–154, 1983.

Kane, R. L., L. Bernstein, J. Wales, and R. Rothenberg, "Hospice Effectiveness in Controlling Pain," *Journal of the American Medical Association,* 253:2683–2686, 1985.

Kane, R. L., S. J. Klein, L. Bernstein, and R. Rothenberg, "The Role of Hospice in Reducing the Impact of Bereavement," *Journal of Chronic Diseases,* 39:735–742, 1986.

Kane, R. L., S. J. Klein, L. Bernstein, R. Rothenberg, and J. Wales, "Hospice Role in Alleviating the Emotional Stress of Terminal Patients and Their Families," *Medical Care,* 23:189–197, 1985.

Kane, R. L., J. Wales, L. Bernstein, et al.,"A Randomized Controlled Trial of Hospice Care," *Lancet,* 1:890–894, 1984.

Lubitz, J., and R. Prihoda, "The Use and Costs of Medicare Services in the Last Two Years of Life," *Health Care Financing Review,* 3:117–131, 1984.

Mundinger, M. O., *Home Care Controversy: Too Little, Too Late, Too Costly,* Rockville, MD: Aspen Systems Corporation, 1983.

Rubenstein, L. Z., L. J. Campbell, and R. L. Kane, eds., *Clinics in Geriatric Medicine: Geriatric Assessment,* vol. 3, no. 1, Philadelphia: W. B. Saunders, February 1987.

Rubenstein, L. Z., K. R., Josephson, G. D. Wieland, P. A. English, J. A. Sayre, and R. L. Kane, "Effectiveness of a Geriatric Evaluation Unit: A Randomized Clinical Trial," *New England Journal of Medicine,* 311:1664–1670, 1984.

Somers, A. R., "Who's in Charge Here?—or Alice Searches for a King in Mediland," *New England Journal of Medicine,* 287:849–855, 1972.

World Health Organization, *International Classification of Impairments, Disabilities, and Handicaps,* Geneva, Switzerland: World Health Organization, 1980.

Index

Access to care, 92, 219; HMOs and, 240, 246–48, 265; PPS and, 235; under capitation, 277–278. *See also* Quality of care
Accreditation Association For Ambulatory Health Care (AAAHC), 293
Activities of daily living (ADL), 157–58, 329; of HMO enrollees, 252–56
Acute care: benefits, 16–21; resources, 247. *See also* Post-acute care
Adjusted average per capita cost (AAPCC), 29, 243–44; health status adjustments, 259
Adjusted community rate (ACR), 243
Adverse risks, 290
Adverse selection, 78, 160, 161, 171, 174, 253, 257; and capitated payment, 279; in HMOs, 260; under vouchers, 35–38. *See also* Biased selection
Aid to Families with Dependent Children (AFDC), 74
Ambulatory care, 276–77
American Association of Retired Persons (AARP), 42
American Hospital Association (AHA), 16–19, 233; Annual Survey of Hospitals, 236
American Medical Association (AMA), 17, 22, 233; Council on Scientific Affairs, 361; Socioeconomic Monitoring System (SMS), 236
American Medical Care Review Association, 265
American Public Health Association, 175
Ancillary services, 216, 217, 224–25
Assignment of benefits, 18, 19, 124–25; under capitation, 280; under DEFRA, 142
Average length of stay (ALOS): hospital, 141, 215–17, 218, 225, 233, 328; nursing home, 130, 323

Baucus amendment, 12, 144, 192; effects of, 190, 191, 198, 199, 203; requirements, 135, 143, 185, 187
Beneficiaries, Medicare, 57–60, 65; access to care, 219, 235, 246–48, 265, 277–78; employed, 305; HMO disenrollment, 254–56; HMO enrollment, 243, 247–49, 250, 252–56, 265, 278; hospitalization rate, 120, 254–55, 322; knowledge about coverage, 14–15, 41, 161–62, 169–70, 171, 176; lack of other coverage, 140, 308–09; liability, 11–15, 17, 19, 20, 117–46, 321, 334–36; medical preferences, 33, 35, 40–42; Medigap coverage, 60–61, 144–45, 162, 181–203; out-of-pocket costs, 5–9, 11–15, 17–19, 39, 56–59, 65–67, 68–69, 117–46, 183, 306–07, 321–36; PPS and, 324–31, 334–36; and quality of care, 293; requirements for benefits, 5–6, 14, 182, 308; risk of deductible expense, 121; risk under HI, 120–23; risk under SMI, 125–29, 131; taxation, 92–93; and vouchers, 31–32, 33, 38, 161
Benefits, Medicare: average amount of, 321; current structure of, 3–15, 56–60, 75–77; means-test for, 62; period, 17; problems of, 11–15, 33; proposed reforms, 15–21; retiree, 304–08; under capitation, 278
Biased selection, 256–60, 279, 295. *See also* Adverse selection; Favorable selection
Bishop, Christine E., 175
Blacks. *See* Minorities
Bloomrosen, Meryl F., 211
Blue Cross and Blue Shield Association, 76, 77, 94; Medigap insurance, 182, 192–203
Blue Cross/Blue Shield United of Wisconsin, 250
Blue Cross of Massachusetts, 250, 369
Blue Shield of California, 342, 353
Body systems count, 218
Boniface, Zoe, 357
Bovbjerg, Randall R., 25
Bowen, Otis R., 15
Bowen-Burke proposal, 16–20
Breslow, Lester, 362, 367